Mastering Problem-Based Learning in Health Profession Programs

Santiago Lorenzo · Bei Zhang
Editors

Mastering Problem-Based Learning in Health Profession Programs

Principles, Procedures, and Best Practices

Springer

Editors
Santiago Lorenzo
Lake Erie College of Osteopathic Medicine
Bradenton, FL, USA

Bei Zhang
College of Medicine
University of Vermont
Burlington, VT, USA

ISBN 978-3-032-05404-3 ISBN 978-3-032-05405-0 (eBook)
https://doi.org/10.1007/978-3-032-05405-0

This Springer imprint is published by the registered company Springer Nature Switzerland AG
The registered company address is: Gewerbestrasse 11, 6330 Cham, Switzerland

Preface

Problem-Based Learning (PBL) has become one of the most transformative approaches in health professions education. At its core, PBL encourages students to take ownership of their learning by working collaboratively to solve complex, real-world problems. This approach not only fosters critical thinking and clinical reasoning but also cultivates the habits of teamwork, self-directed inquiry, and lifelong learning that are essential to the practice of medicine and other health professions.

Mastering Problem-Based Learning in Health Profession Programs was conceived with a dual purpose. Foremost, it is intended for program directors, administrators, and curriculum designers who wish to adopt a PBL curriculum and build it from the ground up. For these readers, the book provides guidance on planning, implementation, faculty development, and the institutional structures required to support a thriving PBL program. Equally, it serves as a comprehensive guide for faculty who facilitate PBL, offering practical strategies, frameworks, and insights to strengthen their teaching practice and enhance student learning.

The chapters are designed to be both practical and reflective. They examine the historical foundations of PBL, present frameworks for effective facilitation, and address the nuances of assessment, feedback, and faculty development. Examples and case studies illustrate how PBL can be adapted across disciplines and cultures, while highlighting innovations that enhance its effectiveness in an ever-evolving educational landscape.

This book is the result of collaboration among educators, researchers, and practitioners who share a deep commitment to preparing future health professionals to meet the demands of patient care with competence, compassion, and integrity. We hope it serves as a resource for those who are new to PBL as well as for experienced educators seeking to refine their practice.

Ultimately, *Mastering Problem-Based Learning in Health Profession Programs* reflects our belief that learning is most powerful when it is active, collaborative, and grounded in authentic problems. We invite readers to engage with the ideas presented here, to experiment with them in their own classrooms and curricula, and to contribute to the ongoing evolution of PBL in health professions education.

Bradenton, USA Santiago Lorenzo
Burlington, USA Bei Zhang

Acknowledgements

Professional Acknowledgements

This book evolved from the many years of exemplary practice in Problem-Based Learning (PBL) at the Lake Erie College of Osteopathic Medicine (LECOM) in Bradenton, Florida. The continued success of the program is a result of an unwavering institutional commitment to active, student-centered learning, which is wholeheartedly embraced by both the administration and the faculty. The book is inspired by their dedication to implementing PBL with care, creativity, and consistency, and it reflects the collective effort of educators who believe deeply in the power of active and self-directed learning.

We wish to extend our special thanks to Sarah Tjioe, Ph.D., Mark Coty, Ph.D., Ross Longley, Ph.D., and Paul Danahy, M.D., who were instrumental in establishing and organizing PBL at LECOM in its earliest years. Their vision, leadership, and mentorship provided the foundation upon which the program has flourished. Their thoughtful input during the development of this book was invaluable, and their example continues to shape the way we think about PBL and its role in health professions education.

We are also grateful for the invaluable support provided throughout the publication process by Evelien Bakker, Prasad Gurunadham, Saheli Roy Choudhury, Corina van der Giessen, and Ann Ruth at Springer. Their guidance, patience, and expertise ensured that the book moved from an idea to a finished work that we are proud to share.

Finally, we extend our sincere thanks to all the chapter authors—Mark A. Best, M.D., MBA, MPH, M.S. (Med Ed), Sarmad Ghazi, MBChB, Shaan Kunwar, D.O., Todd A. Nolan, Ph.D., Teresa M. Hunter-Pettersen, M.D., M.P.A., M.S., Voicu S. Ciobanu, M.D., Varna Taranikanti, M.B.B.S., M.D., Ph.D., Srineil Vuthaluru, M.B.B.S., Mark Coty, Ph.D., and Serene Shaham, MBChB. Their thoughtful reflections on teaching practice and their willingness to share insights from their experience have enriched this book immeasurably and will serve as an ongoing source of inspiration for fellow educators.

Personal Acknowledgements (Editor Lorenzo)

I extend my deepest and most heartfelt gratitude to my wife, Birgit, and to my children, Isabella and Matteo. Your unwavering love, patience, and support have been the true foundation of everything I have been able to accomplish, including this book.

Birgit, you have been my constant source of strength. Your encouragement and quiet confidence in me, even in the moments when I doubted myself, fueled my determination to keep moving forward. You have carried so many unseen burdens with grace so that I could dedicate the long hours needed for this work. I am endlessly grateful for your partnership, your wisdom, and your belief in me.

Isabella and Matteo, your understanding during the many evenings and weekends I spent writing instead of being fully present with you has touched me deeply. The joy you bring into my life and the pride I feel as I watch you grow remind me daily of what truly matters. It is for you, and because of you, that I strive to be better not only as a professional but as a person.

I would also like to honor the memory of my father, Gerardo, who passed away earlier this year. His example of hard work, integrity, and perseverance has guided me throughout my life. The values he instilled in me—discipline, humility, and a deep sense of purpose—shaped who I am and made it possible for me to pursue this work with dedication. Though he is no longer here, I carry his lessons with me every day, and this book is, in many ways, a tribute to the foundation he laid.

This book could not have been completed without the love and support of my family. You are my inspiration, my grounding, and the cornerstone of my success. From the bottom of my heart, thank you for walking this journey with me.

With love and gratitude,
Santiago Lorenzo, Ph.D., M.S., M.S. (Med Ed), B.S.

Personal Acknowledgements (Editor Zhang)

To Chunqi, Tao, John and William, you are the wind under my wings.

Bei Zhang, MD, PhD, MLS (ASCP)CM

Contents

Chapter 1
Building a Pre-clinical Curriculum of Problem-Based Learning

Santiago Lorenzo

1.1 Understanding the PBL Curriculum

The Problem-Based Learning (PBL) was first introduced by McMaster University School of Medicine in 1969 (Neufeld & Barrows, 1974) and has been adopted by many schools worldwide, usually with some variation to meet the school's specific needs. For a successful PBL program to develop, it is crucial for faculty and administration to understand the tenets and purpose of PBL and to believe in the process.

1.1.1 Principles and Purpose of the PBL Curriculum

The overarching purpose of a PBL curriculum is for health professional students to learn and master the basic medical or health sciences using clinical cases as the framework (Schmidt, 1983). It is characterized by the application of problems for knowledge acquisition and practical skills that can be applied to any health professional program (Alrahlah, 2016; Walton & Matthews, 1989). Students use clinical cases to identify knowledge gaps and understand basic medical or health sciences, which promotes critical thinking as well as clinical reasoning skills. Contrary to traditional didactic pedagogy, the PBL approach puts the students in the driver's seat by making them responsible for their own learning. The PBL approach is distinguished by its student-centered nature; it fosters active learning by encouraging students to engage in discussions centered around pre-prepared problems. This participatory framework empowers students to take ownership of their learning, facilitating personal growth and development throughout the process (Holen et al., 2015; Tsai

S. Lorenzo (✉)
Lake Erie College of Osteopathic Medicine, Bradenton, FL, USA
e-mail: slorenzo@lecom.edu

S. Lorenzo and B. Zhang (eds.), *Mastering Problem-Based Learning in Health Profession Programs*, https://doi.org/10.1007/978-3-032-05405-0_1

et al., 2018). The students themselves are the ones who read and learn from textbook chapters (and other potential learning resources, such as journal articles, educational videos, and various internet sources), identify essential concepts, and extract key takeaways from each topic. The primary objective of the PBL approach is to foster the integration of acquired knowledge and skills, rather than merely imparting information. By presenting students with real-world problems to solve, PBL encourages learners to draw upon their existing knowledge base and apply it in novel contexts. This process not only deepens understanding of the subject matter but also enhances the ability to think critically, solve complex problems, and make connections among various concepts of different subjects (Bodagh et al., 2017). Empowering students to assume ownership of their learning, ultimately, PBL aims to equip students with the skills necessary for lifelong learning and professional success (Gao et al., 2020).

The main objective of the PBL approach to learning is to foster the educational and personal development of health professions students who will:

- Take personal responsibility for learning, both during and following formal education and training programs.
- Command a relevant knowledge base characterized by depth, breadth, and flexibility.
- Master the skills in critical evaluation and acquisition of new knowledge.
- Develop proficiency in clinical reasoning.
- Excel at finding and evaluating resource material and formulating diagnostic hypotheses.
- Possess good interpersonal skills.
- Enhance readiness for clinical clerkships.

1.1.2 Pedagogy of the PBL Curriculum

The mechanism of achieving the objectives above (educational and personal development) is an approach that will:

- Shift the emphasis of the program from teaching to learning, by requiring students to be active, independent, self-directed learners and problem solvers, rather than passive recipients of information.
- Emphasize the development of attitudes and skills, which stress the understanding of the new information in a clinical context, rather than the memorization of facts.
- Limit the amount of information that students are expected to memorize.
- Provide a small group environment, within which students can work cooperatively to solve common problems analytically, with faculty who are facilitators of the discussion rather than teachers.

In the PBL curriculum, clinical cases serve as a platform for learning and applying the basic medical, clinical, and health sciences. The objective of PBL is not to diagnose the case but to identify learning issues, which act as topics for further study (Dalrymple et al., 2007; Dolmans et al., 1993). Students work independently on their learning issues before the next group meeting, at which time the new information is discussed and refined in the context of the clinical case. If necessary, more learning issues are then identified and studied. With this approach, the memorization of isolated facts, taken out of context, is de-emphasized. Instead, the skills that help students develop into self-directed, independent learners are emphasized. Along with learning the basic medical, clinical, and health sciences, the "process" of learning is stressed (Schmidt, 1983).

Students are organized into small groups comprising approximately eight to ten peers. Each group is assigned a faculty member whose role is to facilitate discussions within the group. Unlike traditional didactic teaching where the instructor is viewed as the primary source of knowledge, in PBL, the faculty member serves as a facilitator rather than an authority figure. Faculty facilitators in PBL are not necessarily expected to possess expertise in all topics discussed. Instead, they guide the discussion, encourage critical thinking, and provide support as needed. By adopting this approach, students are encouraged to take responsibility for their own learning and collaborate with peers to deepen their understanding of the subject matter. This shift from teacher-centered to student-centered learning empowers students to actively engage with the content and develop problem-solving skills essential for their future careers in healthcare. The small group setting also fosters the development of a sense of community among students, who learn to work together in a problem-solving and collaborative capacity. They learn both trust and responsibility as active members of the group. They become adept at both receiving and providing constructive criticism, comfortable with having their viewpoints questioned without taking it personally, and asking others without fear of offending. The small group process also provides valuable practice in sharpening students' clinical reasoning skills.

1.1.3 Potential of the PBL Curriculum

One critical feature that could place the PBL approach to teaching/learning above any other pedagogical approaches in healthcare professional programs is that students integrate all basic medical/health sciences during every case throughout the pre-clerkship years (Zaveri et al., 2019). This approach makes a tremendous difference in the student's preparation for their pre-clerkship, clinical rotations, and post-graduate studies, as they constantly must integrate healthcare sciences and clinical reasoning across different disciplines. In traditional subject-based didactic learning, for example, students take a physiology course for one semester and after that, they do not get many opportunities to integrate and apply the physiology learned previously. On the other hand, the students in a PBL curriculum learn physiology (and every other basic medical/health science subject) over 2 years (or however long the PBL curriculum is at a particular institution). This approach allows students to revisit and reinforce complex concepts and mechanisms multiple times. Ultimately, spaced repetitive exposure to basic medical/health science concepts, coupled with the continual process of making connections and understanding how these concepts interrelate across various disciplines, greatly enriches students' learning experiences. By immersing themselves in the foundational principles of health sciences over an extended period, students develop a comprehensive understanding of the underlying mechanisms and principles that govern the human body.

Furthermore, the PBL approach holds promise in diminishing the necessity for extensive "board review" before student licensing board examinations, particularly when PBL learning is evaluated using the same testing format as the licensing board examinations. By aligning the assessment methods with the format of the licensing board exams, students are continuously exposed to scenarios and questions that mirror those they will encounter during their licensure assessments. This approach not only fosters a deeper understanding of the material but also cultivates the critical thinking and problem-solving skills essential for success in such examinations.

Emphasizing the importance of the PBL model, it's crucial to recognize its foundation in self-directed learning within a collaborative team setting. In PBL sessions, students are tasked with actively contributing to group discussions, fostering teamwork and collective problem-solving. Moreover, students are encouraged to take ownership of their learning journey, relying on each other to grasp complex concepts in basic medical or health science. This dual emphasis on independent learning and interpersonal skills underscores the significance of the PBL approach in preparing students for the challenges they will encounter in their academic and professional pursuits.

The adoption of the PBL pre-clerkship approach has revolutionized the traditional dynamics between teaching and learning (Fig. 1.1). Unlike the conventional model where students passively listen and take notes (mainly via PowerPoint lectures), PBL encourages active student participation and engagement (Jones, 2006). By presenting students with authentic, real-world problems to solve, PBL prompts them to take ownership of their learning process and exercise subjective initiative. This shift empowers students to delve deeper into the subject matter, explore diverse perspectives, and develop critical thinking and problem-solving skills. Ultimately, the PBL approach fosters a more dynamic and interactive learning environment, where students play a central role in constructing their knowledge and solidifying understanding.

1.2 The PBL Case

The PBL case discussed in the PBL session is organized along the lines of the progressive disclosure model (Barrows, 2000). The outline below is typical for the PBL discussion in medical school, but can be modified to represent clinical reasoning in other healthcare professional education. The case is processed via structured small-group discussions with an organized agenda.

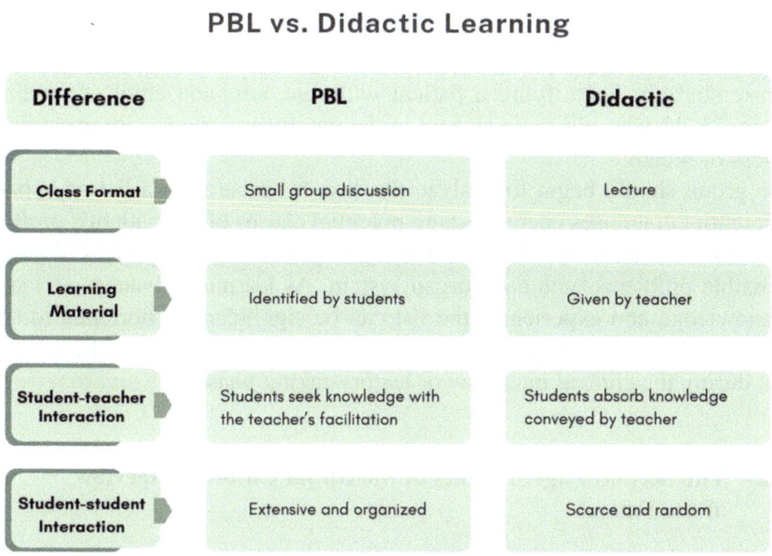

Fig. 1.1 Major differences between PBL and didactic learning, highlighting the differences between the two approaches in terms of class format, learning materials, student-teacher interaction, and student-student interaction

1.2.1 The Outline of the PBL Case

In healthcare professional education, the PBL cases are based on actual or fictional, real-like patient conditions. The information concerning the patient will be distributed over several pages, presented one at a time, in a logical sequence based on approximately the same order in which it would be available to the practitioner. Thus, the first page will usually contain only the information that would be available to the practitioner at the onset of a visit: the patient's age and gender, and the chief complaint(s) that prompted the patient to seek medical attention. After a brief discussion, the group will decide what additional information is required to understand the patient's problem(s). The data provided on subsequent pages will include such information as responses to predictable questions concerning patient history, other possible symptoms, physical exam, results of selected laboratory tests, and, ultimately, a diagnosis and course of treatment. In summary, the student will, as in an actual clinical situation: (1) initially be given only the name, age, and gender of the patient, along with the chief complaint, (2) be expected to follow this with an appropriate history and physical exam, plus requests for appropriate laboratory tests and diagnostic procedures, and (3) be given additional information over time, allowing for generating hypothesis/hypotheses and ordering testing at every step.

1.2.1.1 The First Page: Chief Complaint

- Name, sex, and chief complaint

The case starts by identifying a patient with age, sex, and chief complaint. For example, "A 43-year-old male arrived at the emergency room with chest pain and shortness of breath."

The group should begin to analyze the case by generating a list of hypotheses or differential diagnoses encompassing potential causes of the patient's problem(s). Initially, this list can be very long, consisting of possible organ systems involved and the possible problems with each organ system. As learning advances and students gain knowledge and experience, the list can be significantly shortened to specific diseases. Students should then compile a list of information to be gathered from the patient during the clinical interview or history-taking phase.

1.2.1.2 The Second Page: Results of the Initial Clinical Interview of the Patient

- History of present illness
- Medical history
- Medications/allergies
- Social and family histories
- Review of systems

This page can be processed via role-playing, that is, the facilitator can take on the role of the patient and one student may assume the role of the physician. The patient history page provides students with practice interviewing a patient and understanding the role of the patient. This page provides critical information needed to support or rule out existing hypotheses and for the formulation of new hypotheses.

1.2.1.3 The Third Page: Results of Physical Examination

- Vital signs
- Results of general and all appropriate systemic exams

The next step should be the physical exam. Students should give some thought to the clinical signs that the physician should look for, based on the history. Students should request all routine vital signs and list the specific elements of the physical exam that they would like to see evaluated. Results will be disclosed using terms that might appear in the official record. This page provides more data to support or eliminate existing hypotheses or may require the addition of new hypotheses. Like in real-life clinical practice, much of the information needed for diagnosis is found in the clinical case history and physical examination, yet students are not expected to reach the diagnosis right after the physical exam.

1.2.1.4 Additional Pages: Additional Patient Information Must Be Requested by the Students

- Laboratory and diagnostic test results, e.g., CBC, urine analysis, imaging, ECG, and specific organ function tests.
- Any other relevant facts and findings

At this point, the students should begin to engage in the generation of more focused hypotheses. Students should also consider ideas for learning issues, and begin to identify tests and procedures, the results of which will help clarify the patient's problem. Properly chosen laboratory tests or clinical procedures will help rule in or out the hypotheses/diagnoses being considered for the patient.

Please note, the first three pages of a case are standard:

1. Chief complaint
2. Patient history/interview
3. Physical exam

The remaining pages must be requested by the students, based on the data needed to support the hypotheses/differential diagnoses being considered for that patient.

1.2.2 The Agenda of the PBL Session

Below is a description of how a typical case in PBL progresses. Note this is for illustrative purposes only. A specific PBL case usually spans over 2–3 PBL sessions, so not all these steps are present in one single PBL session.

1. Chief complaint page
   (a) Brainstorm differential diagnosis.
2. History page (Dr/Patient interview). The facilitator acts as the patient, and one student from the group is the "Doctor" who takes the history. Every student in the group is required to take notes
   (a) Brainstorm more differential diagnoses.
   (b) Discuss all pertinent basic medical/health science mechanisms responsible for the signs and symptoms presented in the patient.
3. Physical exam page
   (a) Encourage the group to go through each section of the physical exam in order.
   (b) Update the differential diagnosis list and continue to explore the basic medical/health science mechanisms responsible for the findings presented on this page.

4. Clinical diagnostic tests
   (a) Before revealing each test, ask the students to predict what they might see and why.
   (b) At the end of each test, have a student summarize "What does this mean?"
5. Diagnosis page
6. Treatment page
   (a) Have students find treatment options before providing this to them.
7. Outcome page
8. Final questions about the case that may need to be reviewed.
9. Wrap-up. Before ending each PBL session, all students provide their thoughts on how the session went, how they performed individually and as a group, and what they can do to improve for the next session.

As the case progresses, the culmination often involves reaching a definitive diagnosis. Through thorough examination, discussion, and application of acquired knowledge, students work collaboratively to identify the underlying health issue or condition presented in the case. This diagnostic conclusion represents a significant milestone in the PBL journey, showcasing students' ability to synthesize information, apply critical thinking skills, and arrive at informed decisions based on evidence and reasoning. After making a diagnosis, the students need to consider the treatment and management of the patient and, if appropriate, information related to any follow-up of the patient.

Following the completion of each case, students are responsible for submitting their list of examination topics in the following way:

- At every meeting, the board scribe writes all the learning issues from the clinical case that was just completed.
- When the case is finished, examination topics are chosen from the learning issues list. Exam topics are specific chapters from the approved PBL-required basic medical/health science textbooks list. For example, *Physiology Ch. 38: Pulmonary Ventilation.* Detailed descriptions of learning issues and examination topics can be found in Chap. 6.
- The facilitator is present during the deliberation of topics chosen for examination but is not involved in the decision.
- Exam topics are **NOT** allowed to be submitted outside of group sessions.
- The topics are submitted electronically **BEFORE** they are allowed to begin the next case.

1.3 PBL Strategies and Process

1.3.1 The Clinical Reasoning Process

The clinical reasoning process is how clinicians diagnose patients and is the basic means by which students in PBL progress through case studies (Dolmans et al., 1993). In clinical practice, the clinical reasoning process is crucial as the health-care provider must understand the patient's clinical background to provide optimal care. The clinical reasoning process could be considered the scientific method of the physician, implying a remarkable similarity between scientific research and clinical diagnostics. Both involve the formulation of hypotheses to be tested, followed by the application of tests designed to eliminate all hypotheses except the correct one.

Initially, students may find the clinical reasoning process challenging as it involves eliminating potential diagnoses that were originally proposed by them. This may feel psychologically unpleasant at first as inexperienced PBL students might be hesitant to rule out certain diagnoses to prove themselves wrong. There might be a concern about appearing less competent to their peers by suggesting ideas that later turn out to be incorrect, as there is often an emphasis on providing correct answers in our education system. Overcoming this challenge requires accepting that ruling out potential diagnoses is a crucial part of the learning process. Students should recognize that eliminating possibilities, even their own suggested diagnoses, brings them closer to discovering the correct diagnosis.

The clinical reasoning process can be learned by addressing the following questions step-by-step (Fig. 1.2):

1. Given the available information, such as the patient's name, age, gender, and chief complaint, the initial question is: What could be the possible cause of the patient's condition? At this stage, the diagnostic grid (presented later) serves as the appropriate starting point.
2. After listing hypotheses based on broad differentials covering all possible organ systems, the next question is: What additional information, whether from history, physical examination, tests, etc., is needed to eliminate or confirm each of the hypotheses proposed?
3. Upon obtaining new information, especially from the history-taking process, another question emerges: Can we now dismiss any of the hypotheses initially listed? Conversely, could this new information reveal previously overlooked hypotheses as the case unfolds?

As mentioned earlier, experienced healthcare providers often possess sufficient information to accurately diagnose a patient by the end of the history-taking process, a skill that may not yet be well-developed in PBL students. Nonetheless, it's crucial to encourage considering broad differentials to prevent misdiagnosis. After completing step 3, the process loops back to step 1, continuing with each phase of the case until its conclusion. Subsequently, the second round of new information typically arises from the results of the physical examination, followed by any necessary laboratory

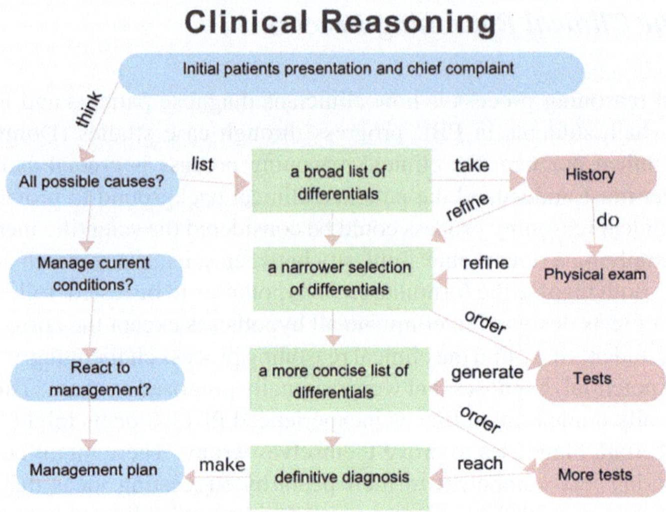

Fig. 1.2 Clinical reasoning process of PBL mimics clinical practice in real life, which is a systemic approach involving stepwise patient assessment, diagnosis, and management

tests and diagnostic procedures as determined by the group. Rather than employing a "shotgun" approach with numerous tests, the focus should be on judiciously selecting tests that address specific questions related to the proposed hypotheses.

Tests should be selected based on the following considerations:

1. Will this test contribute to the rejection (help rule out) of one or more of the hypotheses? It is also appropriate to consider how the test might support (help rule in) any of the hypotheses.
2. What are the expected results if the hypothesis being tested is correct or incorrect? This consideration helps guide the interpretation of test results about the hypotheses under consideration.

Another question that often arises when considering a test is whether that test is appropriate from a perspective of clinical practice. Questions addressing whether the test is cost-effective should be phrased along the lines of: "Is this test really necessary? Will the results of the test affect either the diagnosis or clinical management of the patient?" If the answer to this two-part question is "no," then the students need to question the necessity of the test to be ordered.

The construction of PBL cases is designed to facilitate the clinical reasoning process that mirrors the approach employed by healthcare practitioners when assessing and treating patients clinically. The process outlined here applies to students across various healthcare professions.

1.3.2 *Small Group Discussion and Independent Study of PBL*

At the core of problem-based learning lies small group discussions, typically consisting of 8–10 students alongside a facilitator. These discussions kick off with introductions from both students and the facilitator. Each student briefly shares their background with the group to establish the levels of existing expertise. The initial session commences with the distribution of the first page of the case, usually outlining the chief complaint, to be deliberated upon. See Chap. 2 for more details about the design and development of PBL cases.

The PBL case study process can be divided into three phases (Fig. 1.3). In the *first phase*, one student reads the case while another serves as a "board scribe" and records information on a whiteboard. The whiteboard could be divided into separate areas that are labeled, "facts; ideas/questions/hypotheses; learning issues/references." Facts are listed as they are read, and the students then discuss the facts and decide what is important and what is irrelevant. Students then probe for scientific explanations and correlate information relating to the clinical picture presented. The existing knowledge of the group members serves as the basis of further discussion at that time. Students must challenge any information presented for accuracy and understanding. Progress at this stage requires that group members have appropriate resources available so that topics can be investigated. While a considerable portion of investigation can occur outside the PBL discussion session, students are encouraged to utilize their PBL textbooks and any other credible resources available to delve into the topics being discussed during the session. Students' reading habits vary, with some preferring printed textbooks while others opt for electronic versions. There could be a PBL book cart available to the group during the discussion session. This cart contains one printed copy of each required PBL textbook, plus any supplementary textbooks. As general ideas emerge, they are recorded on the whiteboard, while questions are also documented by the designated board scribe. Over time, hypotheses begin to take shape. Each hypothesis may lead to the identification of one or more learning issues, which are areas where there is either insufficient knowledge to comprehend the clinical scenario or inadequate understanding to test the hypothesis effectively. At the end of the session, the group collectively decides which learning issues warrant further exploration and determines the appropriate resources to address the identified learning issues and deepen their understanding of the case.

Throughout this process, students must remain mindful not to fixate solely on reaching a diagnosis but rather to stay focused on the primary goal of PBL, which is learning and comprehending the basic science of the human body. In essence, students aim to elucidate the observed phenomena from the case by exploring the

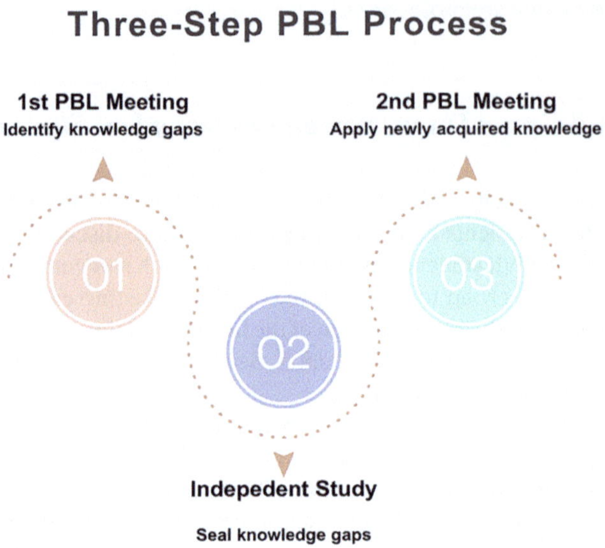

Fig. 1.3 The process of PBL features a combination of collaborative and individual learning, with small group meetings and independent study occurring alternately

underlying processes, encompassing physical, biological, and psychosocial mechanisms (Schmidt, 1983). Maintaining a holistic approach is crucial for the learning process, necessitating the examination of the "whole picture" etc. After each session, the group participates in a final activity known as "wrap-up," during which students assess their adherence to these principles and offer suggestions to enhance the group's performance going forward. This reflective practice fosters continuous improvement and ensures the consistent fulfillment of PBL's learning objectives.

During the *second phase*, the students engage in "independent study" outside the PBL session, addressing the learning issues adopted during the group session. Appropriate resources for acquiring this knowledge include textbooks, journals, microscope slides, radiographs tomographic scans, and audio-visual materials. The term "independent study" is meant in the broadest sense to refer to any activity outside the small group meeting. Students are allowed and encouraged to work in teams or small groups.

During the *third phase*, the students meet to discuss their newly acquired knowledge and use it to evaluate their hypotheses. In place of the new information, they approach the case again, listing new ideas, and formulating new hypotheses and learning issues, followed by another group self-evaluation, another period of independent study, and another PBL meeting. This process may be repeated several times during a single case, as additional learning issues are added until the group is satisfied that it has gained sufficient knowledge of basic scientific concepts to understand the basic mechanisms underlying the clinical picture presented in the case. At that time, a final self-evaluation occurs, and the group evaluates its activities and summarizes what it has learned. Every member of the group has responsibilities that are important if the process is to succeed (see more details on group dynamics in Chap. 5). Communication among members of different tutorial groups is likewise encouraged once the case has been completed by all groups.

The amount of information provided during a single PBL discussion session may vary with the progress of the group. Each group should identify its learning issues and select from its list as many learning issues as can be reasonably addressed in the allotted time before the next meeting. Occasionally, larger learning issues may be identified that can be carried over several class meetings. A case will require more than one session to complete.

1.3.3 Learning Basic Medical and Health Sciences in PBL

The primary learning resources that should be used by students to master basic medical and health sciences in PBL are the PBL-required textbooks. Faculty members who write questions for the PBL examinations are asked to mimic those encountered on the national licensing board examinations and use the PBL textbooks as their resource. Therefore, exams in PBL are constructed from questions written by content experts using the required PBL textbooks. The facilitator must encourage PBL students to read and learn from the required basic medical and health science textbooks.

Numerous resources can potentially aid with the learning of basic medical and health sciences in PBL such as flashcards (Anki, Quizlet, etc.), videos (YouTube, Sketchy, Pathoma, etc.), and review questions. Every student is unique and therefore has a specific learning preference. These resources could be used to complement and potentiate the learning that occurs via the reading of basic medical and health science textbooks. Students in PBL may be tempted to primarily use or only use these alternative resources for studying for all sorts of reasons. The PBL facilitator must ensure that students do not go down this path as learning through shortcuts is too often heavily reliant on memorization of isolated facts, resulting in superficial understanding. The process of reading and learning from classical textbooks ensures students have a broader and deeper understanding of the basic medical and health science concepts and mechanisms that are discussed during the PBL session.

1.4 Role of the Participants

1.4.1 Facilitator

The PBL session is quite structured, and the "structure" is maintained by the facilitator, who guides the group through progressive disclosure of the case content. The facilitator must observe the group dynamics and actively listen to the discussions so appropriate questioning can take place if needed. More specifically, the ***facilitator*** is responsible for providing the case information at the appropriate times during the discussion. He or she also assures that each member of the group participates by prompting, if necessary, the timid members, and monitors how accurately the group is addressing the desired learning objectives. The facilitator monitors the direction of the group and redirects them if they digress too far. The students are given the latitude to pursue alternative or tangential concepts and to decide for themselves that a particular learning issue is not germane to understanding the patient's problems.

During the PBL session, the facilitator should discourage students from relying on review books and instead encourage them to consult classic textbooks or other reliable resources. Facilitators should avoid directly answering student questions; instead, they should respond with guiding questions that prompt students to think critically about how to approach the question or which resources to use. Hostile attitudes should not be tolerated, and the facilitator should promote an atmosphere of respect for everyone. While it's acceptable for students to disagree and challenge each other, it must be done constructively and respectfully. At the end of the PBL session, the facilitator must ensure there is enough time for an adequate "wrap-up," where each group member shares their reflections on how the session went. This part of a PBL session is crucial, as it allows each student and facilitator to reflect on the session they just finished. They often have good comments to share with the group and help them have better subsequent PBL sessions. The facilitator should also share his or her thoughts or feedback on the session, which students also appreciate as they take the facilitator's constructive comments to improve their own PBL group dynamics.

In general terms, successful PBL facilitators are characterized as being "student-centered", particularly with well-seasoned PBL students, such as those students in the second year of the PBL curriculum. Their philosophy is not to intervene in group discussions unless they need to. The facilitator has the option to sit at the table with the group or sit away from the table. Indeed, students tend to feel more comfortable during PBL sessions when the facilitator is not at the table. Facilitators should consistently encourage the discussion of basic concepts and mechanisms during the PBL group discussions, as well as during any student presentation that may take place at the beginning of each session. Details of how to facilitate PBL sessions can be found in Chap. 5 (Fig. 1.4).

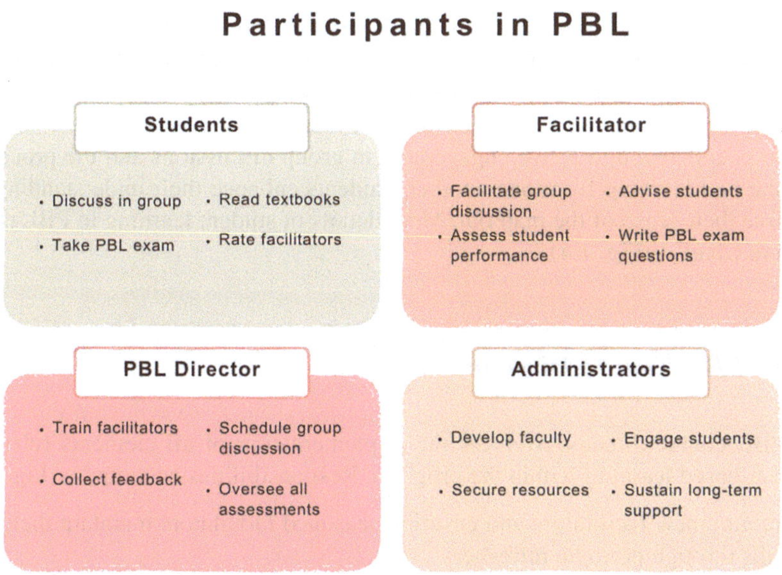

Fig. 1.4 All participants have distinct roles in PBL, with students, facilitators, the PBL director and administrators each having different responsibilities

1.4.2 Student

Students bear the responsibility of actively participating in group discussions during PBL sessions. This entails being open to giving and receiving constructive criticism, acknowledging areas of knowledge deficiency, and diligently completing independent study assignments to contribute meaningfully to the group's collaborative learning process. Additionally, students are assigned specific roles during PBL sessions, such as reader, board scribe, and presenter, as outlined in Chap. 5.

Students learn in the PBL curriculum primarily by reading required textbooks. To encourage textbook reading, all exam questions are written based on the assigned textbooks. Some students may also use electronic resources such as e-books and YouTube videos to supplement the assigned readings. In PBL, the reliance on lectures, PowerPoint presentations, or bullet-pointed notes with "high-yield facts" to know is discouraged. Instead, students take full responsibility for their learning by engaging with classic textbooks and determining the important concepts and mechanisms within each section. To achieve this, students must thoroughly read the entire section, allowing them to grasp the "big picture" before extracting the most relevant information. After completing the necessary readings, students are encouraged to convene in small groups, typically consisting of two or three members. These small group discussions outside the PBL session provide more opportunities for students to vocalize their understanding, tackle challenging concepts, and pose questions to one another. This collaborative approach often reveals gaps in understanding, as students may realize they do not comprehend a topic as thoroughly as they initially thought when unable to answer a peer's question. Furthermore, these study sessions serve to reinforce comprehension as students attempt to explain mechanisms and concepts to their peers. Through active engagement in group discussions and the process of teaching and learning from one another, students enhance their understanding and reinforce their grasp of the material. More details of student learning in PBL can be found in Chap. 4 (Fig. 1.4).

1.4.3 PBL Course Director

The PBL course director oversees the implementation of all elements related to problem-based learning within the program. Responsibilities encompass (Fig. 1.4):

1. Training new facilitators and ensuring seasoned facilitators maintain their PBL skills through periodic refreshers
2. Scheduling and preparing informational materials such as case schedules
3. Facilitating regular meetings to disseminate information and fostering a platform for facilitator feedback
4. Overseeing PBL sessions, including periodically attending sessions to evaluate the progress of new facilitators and review the skills of seasoned facilitators, and acting as a backup facilitator for all groups in the event of unexpected absences
5. Managing and overseeing assessments at all levels, including PBL examinations, student performance evaluations, facilitator evaluations, and course evaluations
6. Compiling, reviewing, and implementing any necessary changes to ensure continuous improvement of the PBL course.

Amid the lengthy to-do list, scheduling is one of the major responsibilities of the PBL course director, who works closely with the designated administrator (e.g. Assistant Dean of Pre-clerkship Education) or faculty group responsible for curriculum scheduling, such as the curriculum committee, and the PBL facilitators. This collaboration ensures the smooth operation of the PBL program. The director assists in preparing schedules and determines PBL group and facilitator assignments for each semester. This coordination helps in ensuring that the PBL course aligns effectively with the broader curriculum and educational objectives.

The PBL course director manages PBL cases and has responsibility for the organizational preparation, review, modification, scheduling, posting, and monitoring of all cases in PBL daily. The PBL course director works closely with a PBL case review committee, whose members assist in the review and modification of new and existing PBL cases (see details in Chap. 2). The PBL course director is responsible for putting all case materials and modifications into a web-based design format, which is distributed electronically to all PBL groups during the PBL sessions. The electronic posting of all PBL cases follows the PBL case schedule and is done by the PBL course director. Preparation and modification of facilitator guides for each case are also the responsibility of the PBL course director (see details in Chap. 2) Before the beginning and during each PBL session, the PBL director is available to assist facilitators with hardware or software problems within their group session or any minor network problems and seek assistance from computer services when necessary and when they are available.

The PBL course director is the primary point of contact for all student inquiries related to PBL. The director prepares information on test results, study tips, and reading and test-taking strategies. This information is presented to students during scheduled talks held three to four times throughout the semester. The PBL course director should maintain an open-door policy, being available to students for advisement through appointments or drop-in visits. From time to time, the PBL director meets with PBL groups experiencing difficulties to facilitate group solutions to any problems. The director dedicates significant time to identifying and providing academic counseling to students who are at risk of failing PBL. Additionally, the PBL course director serves as an ad-hoc member of the Student Promotions and Graduation Committee, representing failing students in relevant proceedings.

1.5 Assessment of PBL

PBL undergoes assessment through formative, summative, or a combination of both approaches. Students, facilitators, and learning material, along with their interactions, all need to be assessed regularly.

Formative assessments, detailed in Chap. 7, are geared towards learning purposes. They serve as feedback mechanisms crucial for developing expertise in learning and facilitating PBL. An example of formative assessment within PBL occurs during the wrap-up session after each PBL session. Here, students and facilitators provide feedback on what went well and areas for improvement. Regular formative assessment/feedback, involving self, peer, and group evaluations, is recommended after each PBL session. These evaluations can address group dynamics, student contributions, communication skills, and professional behavior.

Relying solely on PBL sessions for assessing knowledge has limitations. Hence, additional methods are necessary. Summative assessments, such as written PBL examinations (explained in Chap. 6), evaluate student learning at the culmination of an instructional unit, like a block of PBL cases. They compare student performance against predefined standards or benchmarks. Summative assessments should align with the program's objectives and expected learning outcomes and competencies. Each school has its own processes and forms for conducting formative and summative assessments within the PBL framework, and those tools themselves need to be assessed for validity.

A robust PBL program relies heavily on the effectiveness of its facilitators, making comprehensive training and evaluation essential for the program's success (see details in Chap. 3). As outlined earlier in this chapter, the PBL Director plays a pivotal role by periodically attending sessions to assess the progress of new facilitators and review the skills of seasoned ones. This hands-on evaluation ensures that facilitators are equipped to effectively guide students through the PBL process. Furthermore, student feedback is invaluable in evaluating the PBL program's efficacy. Through the Student Evaluation Form (SEF), students provide insights into their PBL experience, including feedback on the course itself and the performance of their facilitators. This feedback loop allows for ongoing refinement and improvement of the program.

Additionally, continuous assessment of learning materials is essential. The careful selection of textbooks and online resources significantly influences student learning outcomes (Robinson et al., 2014). Regular evaluation ensures that these materials remain relevant, up-to-date, and aligned with the program's objectives. Equally critical is the assessment of PBL cases. These cases must be periodically reviewed for accuracy, relevance, and alignment with the learning objectives of the health profession program. Updates to treatment options and advancements in medical knowledge necessitate ongoing scrutiny of PBL cases to ensure they remain effective tools for student learning (see details in Chap. 2). By maintaining a commitment to continuous improvement, PBL programs can provide students with a dynamic and impactful learning experience.

1.6 Challenges Implementing a PBL Curriculum and Potential Solutions

Implementing a PBL curriculum presents several challenges, including resistance to change, ensuring facilitator competency, maintaining student engagement, developing fair assessment methods, securing resources, and sustaining long-term support (Abdul-Ghaffar et al., 1999; Park, 2012). Faculty, students, and administrators may resist transitioning from traditional lecture-based teaching to PBL. Ensuring that facilitators are well-trained and competent in guiding PBL sessions is crucial for the curriculum's success. Furthermore, maintaining student engagement and motivation can be challenging, especially if students are accustomed to passive learning, such as traditional lectures. Also, developing fair and reliable assessment methods to measure student learning outcomes in PBL can be complex, as will be described in Chap. 6. Implementing a PBL curriculum may require additional resources, including faculty time, technology, and administrative support. Finally, maintaining momentum and support for PBL over the long term can be challenging, particularly if there is turnover in leadership or faculty (Fig. 1.5).

To address these challenges, institutions should provide comprehensive training and professional development opportunities for faculty to familiarize them with the PBL philosophy, methodology, and procedures, and address any concerns. Engaging in open dialogue with stakeholders to discuss the benefits of PBL and address misconceptions is essential. Offering robust training programs for facilitators that cover PBL principles, facilitation techniques, group dynamics, and assessment strategies,

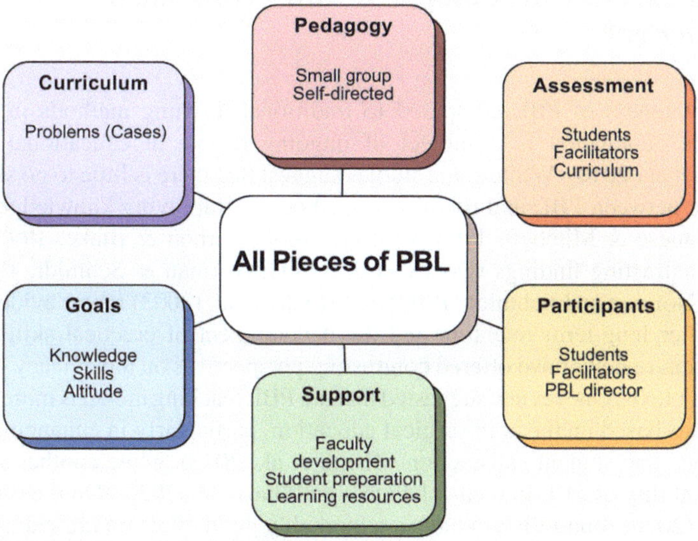

Fig. 1.5 PBL is a puzzle of multiple pieces, requiring collaborative efforts among students, faculty and administration

as well as implementing a mentorship or peer observation program, can support new and seasoned facilitators. Designing PBL cases that are relevant, authentic, and intellectually stimulating, incorporating active learning strategies, and providing opportunities for self-directed learning can keep students engaged. Using a variety of assessment tools to assess different aspects of student learning, aligning assessment criteria with learning objectives, and providing clear feedback can improve evaluation processes. Securing adequate funding and institutional support, strategically allocating resources, and seeking external partnerships and grants can address resource needs. Finally, fostering a culture of continuous improvement and innovation, developing mechanisms for ongoing faculty development and support, creating opportunities for collaboration and knowledge sharing among faculty members, and documenting and disseminating best practices can ensure sustainability and long-term success. By proactively addressing these challenges and implementing appropriate solutions, institutions can successfully implement and sustain a PBL curriculum that enhances student learning and prepares graduates for real-world challenges in their respective fields.

1.7 Efficacy of PBL Compared with "Traditional" Curricula

The effectiveness of PBL compared to traditional teaching methods in terms of knowledge acquisition is a subject of ongoing debate in educational research (Hartling et al., 2010). While some studies suggest that there is little to no significant difference between PBL and traditional methods in improving knowledge acquisition (Albanese & Mitchell, 1993; Colliver, 2000; Vernon & Blake, 1993), others present contrasting findings (Dochy et al., 2003; Norman & Schmidt, 1992). For instance, Norman and Schmidt (1992) and Dochy et al. (2003) report evidence indicating better long-term retention and the development of practical skills through PBL. Recent reviews have offered contrasting perspectives on the efficacy of PBL in specific contexts. One review suggested that the PBL teaching model is more effective than lecture-based methods in surgical education, particularly in enhancing clinical competence and student satisfaction (Zheng et al., 2023), while another supported the applicability of PBL in medical education (Gao et al., 2020). On the other hand, Solomon (2020) found PBL to have a remarkably good effect on immediate knowledge retention, but it was not statistically different from the traditional lecture method in nursing students (Solomon, 2020). In contrast, a meta-analysis offers a comprehensive examination of various studies and suggests several potential advantages of PBL (Koh et al., 2008). According to their findings, PBL may lead to improved competencies in communication skills, a deeper appreciation for legal, ethical, and cultural aspects of care, enhanced self-directed learning abilities, and better coping mechanisms for dealing with uncertainty. A recent review has concluded that students in a PBL curriculum score the same, if not better, than non-PBL students, on licensing board examinations (Forbes et al., 2023). Moreover, PBL students demonstrated better clinical competence and interpersonal skills when on rotations than their non-PBL peers (Forbes et al., 2023). However, it's crucial to acknowledge that drawing definitive conclusions from these studies is often hindered by a lack of methodological rigor or consistency, which may affect the reliability and generalizability of the results. This inconsistency underscores the complexity of assessing the efficacy of different teaching methodologies.

Beyond purely academic outcomes, studies indicate that students generally find PBL to be more enjoyable and engaging compared to traditional methods (Dolmans et al., 2016; Schmidt et al., 2007). Additionally, PBL has been shown to promote enhanced self-directed learning, empowering students to take ownership of their educational journey and fostering a deeper understanding of the material (Barrows & Tamblyn, 1980; Hmelo-Silver, 2004).

Overall, while the evidence regarding the impact of PBL on knowledge acquisition may be mixed, there are indications that it offers unique benefits in fostering certain skills and attitudes crucial for success in health profession fields. Further research with robust methodologies is necessary to provide clearer insights into the effectiveness of PBL compared to traditional teaching approaches.

References

Abdul-Ghaffar, T. A., Lukowiak, K., & Nayar, U. (1999). Challenges of teaching physiology in a PBL school. *The American Journal of Physiology, 277*(6 Pt 2), S140–S147. https://doi.org/10.1152/advances.1999.277.6.S140

Albanese, M. A., & Mitchell, S. (1993). Problem-based learning: A review of literature on its outcomes and implementation issues. *Academic Medicine: Journal of the Association of American Medical Colleges, 68*(1), 1. https://doi.org/10.1097/00001888-199301000-00012

Alrahlah, A. (2016). How effective the problem-based learning (PBL) in dental education. A critical review. *The Saudi Dental Journal, 28*(4), 155–161. https://doi.org/10.1016/j.sdentj.2016.08.003

Barrows, H. S. (2000). *Problem-based learning applied to medical education* (Revised ed.). Southern Illinois University, School of Medicine.

Barrows, H. S., & Tamblyn, R. M. (1980). *Problem-based learning: An approach to medical education.* Springer Publishing Company.

Bodagh, N., Bloomfield, J., Birch, P., & Ricketts, W. (2017). Problem-based learning: A review. *British Journal of Hospital Medicine (London, England: 2005), 78*(11), C167–C170. https://doi.org/10.12968/hmed.2017.78.11.C167

Colliver, J. A. (2000). Effectiveness of problem-based learning curricula: Research and theory. *Academic Medicine: Journal of the Association of American Medical Colleges, 75*(3), 259–266. https://doi.org/10.1097/00001888-200003000-00017

Dalrymple, K. R., Wuenschell, C., Rosenblum, A., Paine, M., Crowe, D., von Bergmann, H. C., Wong, S., Bradford, M. S., & Shuler, C. F. (2007). PBL core skills faculty development workshop 1: An experiential exercise with the PBL process. *Journal of Dental Education, 71*(2), 249–259.

Dochy, F., Segers, M., Van den Bossche, P., & Gijbels, D. (2003). Effects of problem-based learning: A meta-analysis. *Learning and Instruction, 13*(5), 533–568. https://doi.org/10.1016/S0959-4752(02)00025-7

Dolmans, D. H., Gijselaers, W. H., Schmidt, H. G., & van der Meer, S. B. (1993). Problem effectiveness in a course using problem-based learning. *Academic Medicine: Journal of the Association of American Medical Colleges, 68*(3), 207–213. https://doi.org/10.1097/00001888-199303000-00013

Dolmans, D. H. J. M., Loyens, S. M. M., Marcq, H., & Gijbels, D. (2016). Deep and surface learning in problem-based learning: A review of the literature. *Advances in Health Sciences Education: Theory and Practice, 21*(5), 1087–1112. https://doi.org/10.1007/s10459-015-9645-6

Forbes, H. M., Syed, M. S., Flanagan, O. L., Forbes, H. M., Syed, M. S., & Flanagan, O. L. (2023). The role of problem-based learning in preparing medical students to work as community service-oriented primary care physicians: A systematic literature review. *Cureus, 15*(9). https://doi.org/10.7759/cureus.46074

Gao, J., Yang, L., Zhao, J., Wang, L., Zou, J., Wang, C., & Fan, X. (2020). Comparison of problem-based learning and traditional teaching methods in medical psychology education in China: A systematic review and meta-analysis. *PLoS One, 15*(12), e0243897. https://doi.org/10.1371/journal.pone.0243897

Hartling, L., Spooner, C., Tjosvold, L., & Oswald, A. (2010). Problem-based learning in pre-clinical medical education: 22 years of outcome research. *Medical Teacher, 32*(1), 28–35. https://doi.org/10.3109/01421590903200789

Hmelo-Silver, C. E. (2004). Problem-based learning: What and how do students learn? *Educational Psychology Review, 16*(3), 235–266. https://doi.org/10.1023/B:EDPR.0000034022.16470.f3

Holen, A., Manandhar, K., Pant, D. S., Karmacharya, B. M., Olson, L. M., Koju, R., & Mansur, D. I. (2015). Medical students' preferences for problem-based learning in relation to culture and personality: A multicultural study. *International Journal of Medical Education, 6*, 84–92. https://doi.org/10.5116/ijme.558e.6451

Jones, R. W. (2006). Problem-based learning: Description, advantages, disadvantages, scenarios and facilitation. *Anaesthesia and Intensive Care, 34*(4), 485–488. https://doi.org/10.1177/0310057X0603400417

Koh, G. C.-H., Khoo, H. E., Wong, M. L., & Koh, D. (2008). The effects of problem-based learning during medical school on physician competency: A systematic review. *Canadian Medical Association Journal (Journal de l'Association Medicale Canadienne), 178*(1), 34–41. https://doi.org/10.1503/cmaj.070565

Neufeld, V. R., & Barrows, H. S. (1974). The "McMaster Philosophy": An approach to medical education. *Academic Medicine, 49*(11), 1040–1050.

Norman, G. R., & Schmidt, H. G. (1992). The psychological basis of problem-based learning: A review of the evidence. *Academic Medicine: Journal of the Association of American Medical Colleges, 67*(9), 557–565. https://doi.org/10.1097/00001888-199209000-00002

Park, K.-W. (2012). Exploration of the difficulties in applying problem-based learning (PBL) to the class and the solution. *Journal of Curriculum and Evaluation, 15*, 81–102. https://doi.org/10.29221/jce.2012.15.1.81

Robinson, T. J., Fischer, L., Wiley, D., & Hilton, J. (2014). The impact of open textbooks on secondary science learning outcomes. *Educational Researcher, 43*, 341–351. https://doi.org/10.3102/0013189X14550275

Schmidt, H. G. (1983). Problem-based learning: Rationale and description. *Medical Education, 17*(1), 11–16. https://doi.org/10.1111/j.1365-2923.1983.tb01086.x

Schmidt, H. G., Loyens, S. M. M., Van Gog, T., & Paas, F. (2007). Problem-based learning is compatible with human cognitive architecture: Commentary on Kirschner, Sweller, and Clark (2006). *Educational Psychologist, 42*(2), 91–97. https://doi.org/10.1080/00461520701263350

Solomon, Y. (2020). Comparison between problem-based learning and lecture-based learning: Effect on nursing students' immediate knowledge retention. *Advances in Medical Education and Practice, 11*, 947–952. https://doi.org/10.2147/AMEP.S269207

Tsai, T.-I., Lee, S.-Y. D., & Yu, W.-R. (2018). Impact of a problem-based learning (PBL) health literacy program on immigrant women's health literacy, health empowerment, navigation efficacy, and health care utilization. *Journal of Health Communication, 23*(4), 340–349. https://doi.org/10.1080/10810730.2018.1445798

Vernon, D. T., & Blake, R. L. (1993). Does problem-based learning work? A meta-analysis of evaluative research. *Academic Medicine: Journal of the Association of American Medical Colleges, 68*(7), 550–563. https://doi.org/10.1097/00001888-199307000-00015

Walton, H. J., & Matthews, M. B. (1989). Essentials of problem-based learning. *Medical Education, 23*(6), 542–558. https://doi.org/10.1111/j.1365-2923.1989.tb01581.x

Zaveri, N., Coty, M., McCarver, V., Vidic, C., Nolan, T., Nath, S., & Vanier, C. (2019). Changes to an active learning curriculum in osteopathic medical education: Effects on exam outcomes and board scores. *Medical Science Educator, 29*(1), 1. https://doi.org/10.1007/s40670-018-00674-1

Zheng, Q.-M., Li, Y.-Y., Yin, Q., Zhang, N., Wang, Y.-P., Li, G.-X., & Sun, Z.-G. (2023). The effectiveness of problem-based learning compared with lecture-based learning in surgical education: A systematic review and meta-analysis. *BMC Medical Education, 23*, 546. https://doi.org/10.1186/s12909-023-04531-7

Chapter 2
Constructing Problem-Based Learning Cases

Mark A. Best

2.1 Introduction

The Problem-Based Learning (PBL) cases are the foundation of the PBL curriculum, providing the primary framework for students to discover, explore, and apply basic medical/health sciences in clinical decision-making. The PBL approach shares commonalities with other active learning strategies (Huggett & Jeffries, 2015). A well-designed PBL case consists of multiple components, including content, context, conceptual depth, and timeline. These elements work together to create a structured, yet dynamic learning experience. Key activities such as questioning, brainstorming, and clinical case discussions are essential to fostering active engagement and deeper understanding (Brown et al., 2014; Linsenmeyer, 2015). This chapter provides a comprehensive guide to developing new clinical cases, revising and updating existing cases, and preparing facilitator guides. It outlines essential principles for designing effective PBL cases and optimizing them to align with educational goals and learning objectives.

2.2 Learning Theories and Objectives of PBL Cases

The PBL case provides the context for identifying, exploring, and applying the basic medical/health sciences in an authentic, real-world clinical scenario. From the Greek philosophers to our current age, we try to understand how we learn. The teaching-learning methods used reflect philosophies such as rationalism, empiricism, and the following educational psychology learning theories: behaviorism, cognitive, constructivism, humanism, connectivism, transformative, social, and experiential

M. A. Best (✉)
Lake Erie College of Osteopathic Medicine, Bradenton, FL, USA
e-mail: mbest@lecom.edu

S. Lorenzo and B. Zhang (eds.), *Mastering Problem-Based Learning in Health Profession Programs*, https://doi.org/10.1007/978-3-032-05405-0_2

theories (Phillips, 2021). Considering these educational theories are important when designing the PBL cases and in the PBL tutorial process.

The two primary philosophical views of how humans gain knowledge are rationalism and empiricism. Rationalism is mainly defined by deductive reasoning, logic, math, and innate ideas. Empiricism is defined by inductive reasoning, experience, and sensory observation. The scientific method, predicting the day's weather by looking at the clouds, and learning to speak are examples of empiricism.

There are several theories of learning that apply to individuals, interactions with others, learning environment, and objectives. Behaviorism theory is one that focuses on repetition, increasing tasks in a progressive manner, along with positive reinforcement and conditioning. Learning new knowledge, improving collaborative learning, and optimizing classroom management are some applications of behaviorism.

Cognitive learning theory is another, and its key elements are focused on memory, attention, perception, and problem solving. It applies active learning and connects new knowledge to prior knowledge to increase understanding.

Constructivism is another learning theory. It uses experiences, self-reflection, and interactions with others to build understanding, and new knowledge via active learning that uses questioning, topic exploration, and problem-solving. Learners build on prior knowledge by sharing ideas and perspectives with others and thus creating a more meaningful understanding of the context.

Connectivism learning theory focuses on networks and connections in which learners interact with others to discuss ideas, and to help each other learn. Applying life-long learning and using diverse resources and perspectives allows for a more comprehensive understanding. Using technology and decision-making are addressed.

Humanism learning theory includes a focus on the whole person to develop emotional, social, and spiritual well-being, as well as learning. Other key elements include having a supportive environment for learning, such that learners feel safe, valued, and respected. Self-directed learning is a main component. Other key elements include working on problems together (collaborative learning), using a variety of materials (history, pictures, lab results, etc.) to learn, encouraging learner discussions, and having teachers that provide individual feedback.

Transformative learning theory is one that is used more often in adult education. It focuses on developing critical thinking by reflection, questioning assumptions, considering biases, and other explanations. It helps learners get a better understanding of themselves, their beliefs, and their behaviors.

Social learning theory is based on observing others. Seeing someone get rewarded or seeing a role model motivates one to imitate that person. New behavior is the result.

Experiential learning theory uses active engagement in real-world experiences, reflection, and application of the knowledge in a real-world context. This theory has a lot in common with constructivism learning theory.

Many of these learning theories overlap in several aspects. Constructivism seems to have the closest fit for PBL. The PBL facilitator prompts, mediates, and coaches learners to build and assess their understanding and learning. Learners work collaboratively to find solutions to real-world problems. Outside the classroom, learners

LEARNING THEORIES AND PBL CASE DESIGN PRINCIPLES

Learning Theories	Key Elements	Matched PBL Principles
Cognitive Learning	Memory, attention, perception and problem solving	Problem solving
Constructivism	Build on prior knowledge by questioning and problem-solving via interacting with others	Use prior knowledge as a foundation
Connectivism	Learners interact with others to discuss ideas and to help each other learn	Elaboration via discussion
Transformative Learning	Develop critical thinking by reflection, questioning assumptions, and considering biases and other explanations	Critical thinking
Experiential Learning	Engage in real-world experience, apply knowledge and reflect	Transfer knowledge grounded in a realistic context to future applications

Fig. 2.1 Learning theories applicable to PBL include cognitive, constructivist, connectivism, transformative, and experiential learning theories

apply more focus on self-directed learning. All of these learning theories provide some application in PBL (Fig. 2.1).

Dolmans et al. (1997) considered seven key principles for PBL case design. Des Marchais (1999) discussed nine criteria. In total, these are:

- using prior knowledge as a foundation to build new knowledge,
- elaboration via discussion,
- critical thinking,
- content that will transfer to future application, and be grounded in a realistic context that will transfer knowledge,
- integration of learning across disciplines,
- encouraging self-directed learning,
- stimulating interest and curiosity,
- discovering gaps in knowledge, and
- addressing the course objectives.

Thus, the goal of the series of PBL cases, as a whole (the gestalt), should require both revisiting and reinforcing knowledge, and discovering new gaps in knowledge that can be explored. The series of PBL cases allows for repeated exposure with interleaving and spaced retrieval practice, and the introduction of new content.

The PBL case is designed based on learning objectives. The case should be at the complexity level that is appropriate for the learner, as it relates to prior knowledge.

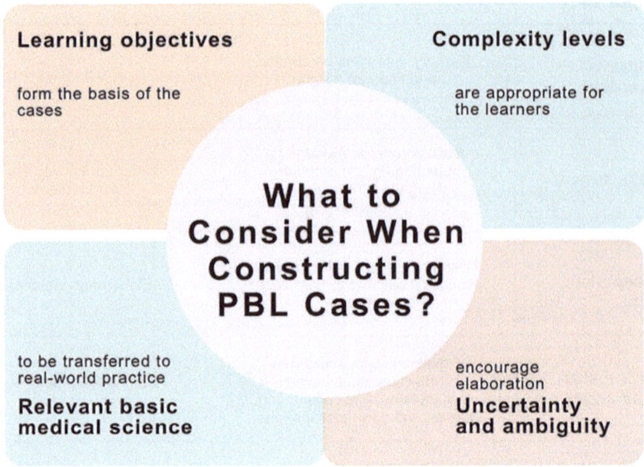

Fig. 2.2 Things to consider when constructing PBL cases include learning objectives, appropriate complexity levels, relevant basic medical sciences and elements of uncertainty and ambiguity

The PBL case provides cues for teams seeking explanations and clarifications via discussions, retrieval practice, elaboration, and collaborative learning. Each PBL case should have content relevant to the specific health profession so that knowledge will transfer, contextualize, and integrate basic medical/health sciences. The PBL case should avoid being overly structured or fully detailed. Instead, it should incorporate elements of uncertainty and ambiguity to encourage elaboration and active retrieval through teamwork (collaborative learning), prompt the generation of learning issues (self-directed learning), and facilitate the exploration of alternative explanations, fostering curiosity, interest, and motivation (Fig. 2.2).

2.3 Tools (Key Elements) for the PBL Case Design

The components and structure of the PBL case design include: the PBL case, the PBL case table of contents, and the facilitator guide. During PBL sessions, other tools, such as whiteboards, are used for learners to stay focused as a collaborative learning team for organization and expansion of learning issues and discussion of concepts (Fig. 2.3).

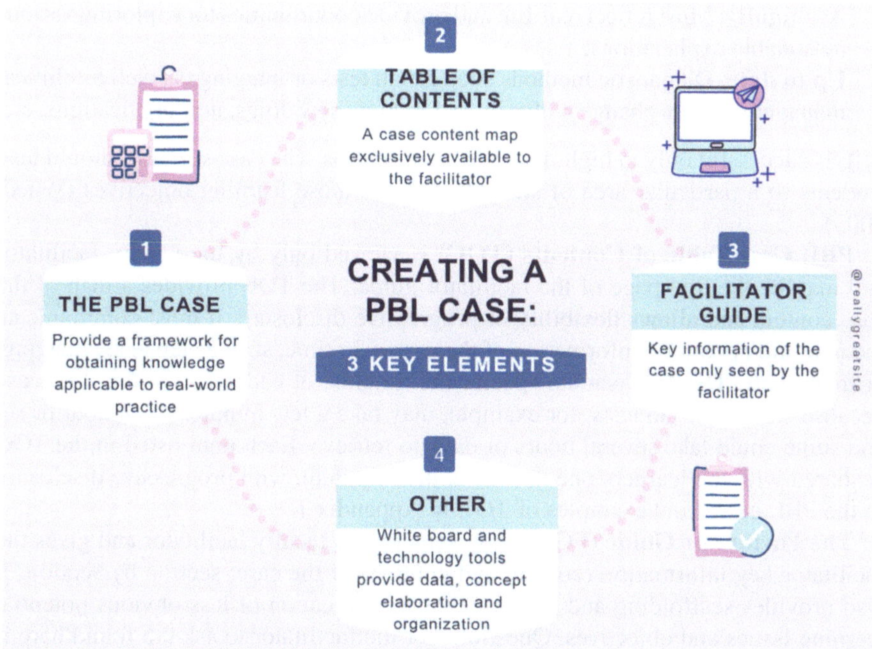

Fig. 2.3 The key elements of PBL case design include the PBL case itself, the PBL case table of contents, the facilitator guide and other tools

The **PBL Case** provides a framework for exploring the basic medical/health sciences applicable to the profession in the clinical **context**. The case may be paper or computer-based (e.g. simulated electronic medical record). It should contain a narrative (written or audio), images, reports, and video clips. The primary PBL case design considerations are:

1. **Structure**: The PBL case must reflect the real world in terms of the **context** and how information is obtained. For example: history, physical exam, patient management, lab tests, clinical update, additional lab tests, later clinical update, etc.
2. **Timeline**: The time frame of the PBL case should be adequate for the real-life context so that changes over time can be communicated. For example: minutes or hours for history and physical exam, minutes, hours, or days for lab test results, clinical updates as needed, etc.
3. **Uncertainty**: The PBL case should not read like a novel but instead have some details missing. Progressive disclosure may provide more detailed information after questions generated by elaboration and critical thinking. There is a difference between uncertainty and misinformation. The uncertainty that mirrors real-life is needed. Do not delete critical information that would be found in real life. Early-on in the PBL process (initial case or cases), the **level of material** should have less uncertainty since that would have fewer new concepts to explore.

4. **Ambiguity**: Must reflect real-life and provide opportunities for exploring various reasonable explanations.
5. **Up to date**: Diagnostic methods such as lab tests or imaging, as well as clinical management, can change with new technology, new drugs, new applications, etc.

PBL is successful only in high-quality case scenarios. The case scenario should lead students to a particular area of study to achieve those learning objectives (Wood, 2003).

PBL Case Table of Contents (TOC) is viewed only by the faculty facilitator and may be the first page of the facilitator guide. The TOC provides a map of the case content and allows flexibility of progressive disclosure. It must communicate the new and upcoming information of the case over time, such as lab tests, imaging, or treatments. The TOC should specify the timeline of each page in the PBL case because some new lab tests, for example, may take a few minutes or an hour or so, and some could take several hours or days to retrieve. Each item listed in the TOC is shared with the learners one at a time, item by item, with progressive disclosure of the PBL case. Find examples of TOC in Appendix 1.

The Facilitator Guide (FG) is only seen by the faculty facilitator and gives the facilitator key information (content and context) of the case, section by section. It also provides scaffolding and increases the identification of less-obvious potential learning issues and objectives. Questions for the facilitator to ask are found here if needed to stimulate discussion, elaboration, or identifying learning issues. Ideally, a mature functional PBL group is expected to ask all necessary questions themselves, which is not necessarily always the case. Examples of probing questions could be: What is the mechanism of action for the drug provided? What are some adverse side effects? What do the CBC results indicate? For more probing questions, see Appendix 3.

Other (e.g., whiteboards, technology tools, etc., more on this in Chap. 8) provides data, concept elaboration, and organization. It is used so that all the team members can keep focus on data, concepts, and questions for continued elaboration, and for listing the learning issues selected by the team members. Being "on the same page" will assist the learners to work as a team in collaborative learning. Cassara (2015) implies concept maps may be used to assist in integrating disciples and showing inter-relatedness of concepts and disciples.

2.4 Content of the PBL Case

The core element of a PBL case is the problem itself, whether it be signs, symptoms, disease, or disorder (Barrows & Tamblyn, 1980; Duch, 1996). PBL case content is designed to facilitate learning in the basic medical/health sciences within the context of a real-world clinical setting, ensuring that knowledge gained is transferable to professional practice. Contextualizing learning and applying knowledge to clinical scenarios enhances retention and reinforces experiential learning, making it applicable to future real cases (Kolb & Kolb, 2005). To be effective, the case inventory must comprehensively cover the topics outlined in the course objectives. These objectives, whether directly addressed (e.g., through diagnosis) or indirectly included (e.g., in differential diagnosis), serve as key themes across integrated disciplines, guiding the selection of learning issues for both collaborative and self-directed learning. Additionally, case content extends beyond medical knowledge, incorporating psychosocial factors such as living conditions, beliefs, education, social support, community, and culture, as well as workplace considerations like the healthcare system, patient care, and communication. These elements provide the broader context in which foundational health sciences are embedded, ensuring a well-rounded and clinically relevant learning experience.

In the initial stages, the PBL cases are designed to be more straightforward, focusing on just a few disciplines (e.g. anatomy, physiology, biochemistry). This gradual increase in case complexity aligns with cognitive load theory (Wissman, 2018; Young et al., 2014; Leppink & Duvivier, 2016), allowing learners to concentrate of mastering PBL process and developing teamwork skills essential for collaborative learning, particularly as PBL is new to them. As students gain a deeper understanding of the PBL approach, cases should become more complex incorporating additional disciplines such as pathology, microbiology, and pharmacology). These advanced cases may also introduce non-linear structures, where key information or steps in a cause-outcome relationship are intentionally omitted, challenging learners to integrate and apply knowledge more dynamically. For instance, an early case may focus primarily on basic anatomical concepts, such as a Pancoast tumor, whereas a later, more intricate case could involve multifactorial conditions like malignancy or hepatitis. Gooding et al. (2017) emphasizes the importance of structuring PBL cases progressively from simple to complex. This sequential approach supports learners in building their knowledge base by forming and refining cognitive schemas, ensuring a more effective and comprehensive learning experience.

All PBL cases should begin with some degree of strategic ambiguity, presenting data with multiple plausible explanations. This intentional uncertainty encourages learners to engage in critical thinking and reasoning by defining unfamiliar vocabulary and elaborating on concepts through collaborative learning. It also drives the identification of learning issues for self-directed learning, which individual team members can later introduce to the group for retrieval practice at spaced intervals. As the case progresses and students successfully gather data, the content should become more concrete, refining their understanding. Each PBL case should unfold over at least 3-h sessions, and at least two meetings, ensuring sufficient time for self-directed learning between meetings. This structure allows for the generation of new pre-class content, facilitates retrieval practice, and promotes deeper elaboration through in-class collaborative learning (Fig. 2.4).

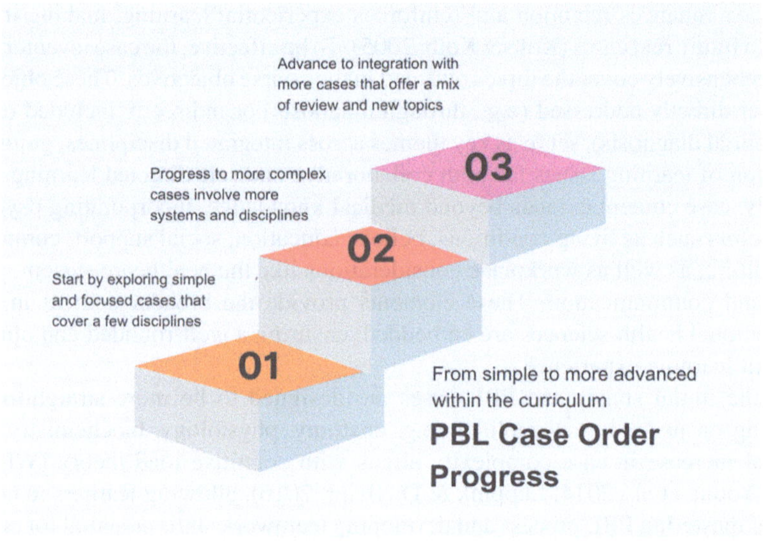

Fig. 2.4 The order of PBL cases progresses from simple to more advanced levels within the curriculum

The timeframe for exploring and processing PBL case content must accommodate both collaborative learning (discussion, elaboration, critical thinking and identifying learning issues within the classroom) and self-directed learning (researching questions, finding answers, and studying learning issues outside the classroom). Yardley et al. (2012) emphasize that learning is situated, meaning it is inherently tied to the context in which it occurs. Accordingly, PBL cases are structured as clinical case studies to provide an authentic and relevant learning experience.

The clinical science content of PBL cases typically includes:

- Basic medical/health sciences—Covering the majority of objectives and potential learning issues.
- Patient safety and quality improvement—Addressing topics such as medical errors, reliability, probability, and effective communication.
- Healthcare Systems—Exploring available resources, referrals, interprofessional communication, and the roles of various stakeholders.
- Epidemiology—Incorporating risk factors, social determinants of health, probability, and population health considerations.

By integrating these elements, PBL cases ensure a comprehensive, contextualized learning experience that fosters critical thinking and real-world application.

In conclusion, the case design provides the structure for achieving the outcome of the learning objectives and goals of PBL. The PBL case **content** includes basic medical/health science that reflects the course learning objectives, so that learners select the appropriate topics (e.g. textbook chapters) as learning issues. The PBL case **context** shall be authentic real-world scenarios (e.g. clinical setting) which allows

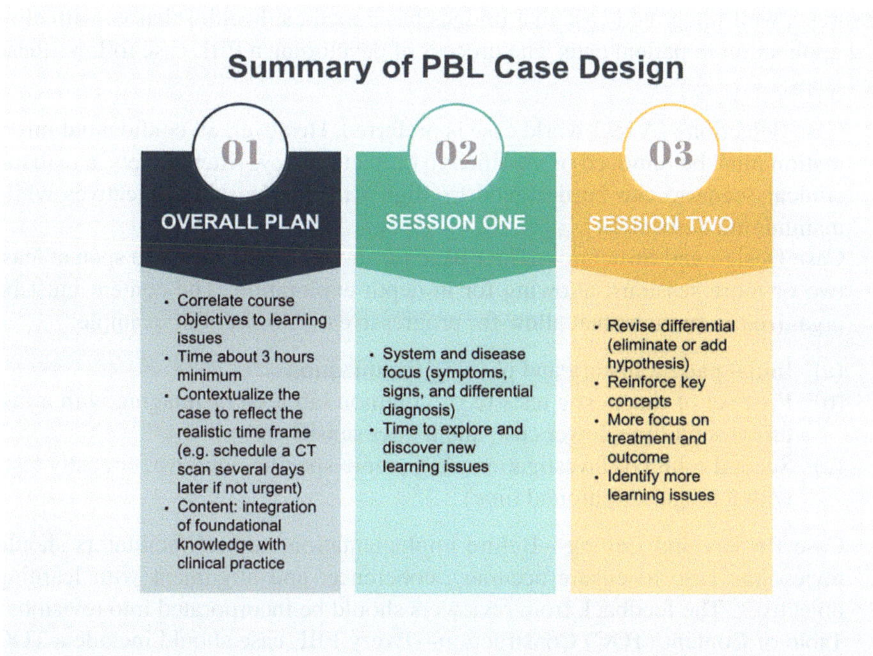

Fig. 2.5 Summary of PBL case design. When designing a PBL case, consider developing an overall plan and determining what to include in each of the two group discussions

contextualization and integration of basic medical/health science, and transfers to future goals. The PBL **case length and time allotted** for each case should be at least filled with enough meaningful content to explore for at least 1½ sessions that last 2 h each (3 h total), or at least 2 sessions with 3 h total. The PBL **case series and order** of cases should (Fig. 2.5):

- Cover all the learning objectives of the course
- Be arranged from simple to more complex
- Include some content from prior cases to encourage practicing active retrieval
- Be arranged from more basic to more advanced topics in the same discipline or system (e.g. heart anatomy → heart physiology → ECG → heart pathology)

2.5 Constructing New PBL Cases

The construction of a new PBL case should be a collaborative effort, ideally involving 3–5 educators with different expertise, such as clinicians, basic medical/health science faculty, and other relevant professionals. The interprofessional approach ensures a well-integrated case that bridges basic medical/health sciences with clinical application in patient care. The process of developing a PBL case follows these key steps:

1. Case Selection—A real-world case is preferred. However, all confidential information must be removed or modified to protect privacy. Alternatively, a realistic clinical scenario can be designed to align with the learning objectives while maintaining authenticity.
2. Case Design and Structure—The PBL case should be structured to span at least two or more sessions, allowing for in-depth exploration. The content must be organized in sections that allow for progressive disclosure. For example:
   (a) Initial patient history and physical examination
   (b) First set of diagnostic tests (e.g., common lab tests or imaging with a fast turnaround time, lower cost, and higher sensitivity)
   (c) Second round of investigations (e.g., more specific, invasive, or costly tests with a longer turnaround time)
3. Case Review and Editing—Before implementation, several facilitators should review the case to ensure accuracy, coherence, and alignment with learning objectives. The feedback from reviewers should be incorporated into revisions.
4. Table of Content (TOC) Construction—Every PBL case should include a TOC accessible only to facilitators. The TOC provides an overview of the case, outlining key sections such as the initial presentation, data gathering, diagnostic procedures, treatment plans, evolving patient conditions, and final outcome. An example of TOC in provided in Appendix 1.
5. Facilitator Guide Development—A detailed facilitator guide should accompany each PBL case to ensure consistency in delivery and alignment with best practices (see Sect. 2.7 below).

By following this structured approach, PBL cases can effectively foster problem-solving skills, critical thinking, and clinical reasoning in learners while ensuring a seamless integration of foundational and clinical sciences.

2.5.1 Common Data Elements in a Clinical PBL Case

In a PBL case, facilitators progressively provide clinical data to learners, one item at a time, simulating real-world patient management. Below are common examples of data that may be disclosed at different time points:

1. Initial Presentation
   - Chief complaint
   - Patient history
2. Physical Examination Findings

3. Immediate Diagnostic Tests (available within minutes, as requested)
   These tests have a rapid turn-around time (TAT) and can be provided in any order based on learner request:
   - Finger-stick glucose level
   - Arterial Blood Gas (ABG)
   - Dip-stick Urinalysis (UA)
   - Electrocardiogram (ECG)
   - Initial management decisions (e.g., hospital admission, IV line placement, etc.)
4. Results available within 1–3 h (as requested)
   - Basic Metabolic Panel-7 (BMP, also known as Chem-7)
   - Complete Blood Count (CBC)
   - Liver Function Tests (LFT)
   - Thyroid Function Tests (TFT)
   - Imaging studies (e.g., non-urgent chest X-ray obtained 4 h after initial presentation)
5. Follow-up information several hours later
   - Patient status update (e.g., improvement, no change, or worsening condition)
6. Additional testing 1–3 days later
   - Imaging studies (e.g., CT scan scheduled for day 3)
7. Case closure on day 4
   - Discharge plan (e.g., home discharge, follow-up appointment in 1 week, prescribed medications)

This structured approach to progressive disclosure allows learners to engage in clinical reasoning, prioritize diagnostic tests, and adapt their management plans in a realistic, stepwise manner (Fig. 2.6).

2.6 Revising and Updating Existing Cases

Revisions to existing PBL cases are primarily driven by feedback from facilitators, either before or after using the case with a team of learners. Minor revision can be handled by a small group of educators, such as the PBL director (course director) and PBL case manager (PBL case committee chair). However, more substantial changes require input from at least two additional educators with relevant expertise. Appendix 2 provides an example of a PBL case feedback form.

Key areas for revision include:

Educator's Progressive Disclosure	Learner's Response
1. History	Gather data (take notes), discuss primary organ system(s), request physical exam
2. Physical Exam (PE)	Gather data (take notes), discuss differential diagnosis, and request initial management steps (e.g., admission, IV access, finger-stick glucose, dipstick urine analysis). Identify individual and team learning issues.
3. Initial Findings (Admitted, IV started, glucose level 184, urine within normal limits)	Modify differential diagnosis if needed, request first round of tests (less invasive, lower cost, and higher sensitivity) such as lab tests or imaging studies
4. First Round of Tests (Available in Any Order as Requested (Complete Blood Count, Liver Function Tests, Basic Metabolic Panel, Thyroid-Stimulating Hormone, Chest X-ray)	Modify differential diagnosis if needed, request second round of tests (more invasive, higher cost, and higher specificity), such as ABG and CT scan of chest
5. New Clinical Information (Patient's respiratory status worsening, ABG shows hypoxia and acidosis, CT scan reveals a mass)	Request consult, identify new learning issues
6. Biopsy Report (consistent with malignancy)	Request referral to a specialist, identify additional learning issues
7. Follow-Up (Surgeon and oncologist initiate treatment, months later, primary care follow-up indicates patient recovering well	Select final learning issues and discuss case closure.

Fig. 2.6 Example of a PBL clinical case

- Quality of Images or Information—As technology advances, higher quality images may become available, allowing for improved visual representations in PBL cases.
- Updated Diagnostic Procedures—New diagnostics methods offering improved accuracy, sensitivity, specificity, faster turnaround time, or lower costs should replace outdated techniques to keep the PBL current.
- Updated Treatments—As medical advancements introduce new treatment options, including techniques, applications, and medications, these should be incorporated into the case in place of older methods.
- Expanding the Differential Diagnosis—To prevent premature closure in clinical reasoning, PBL cases should incorporate sufficient ambiguity and uncertainty, encouraging learners to explore a broader range of possibilities and explanations.
- Emphasizing Key Basic Medical/Healthscience Learning Objectives—Occasionally, an essential learning may be overlooked or underemphasized. When this occurs, the case should be adjusted to highlight the topic more effectively, ensuring all intended learning issues are addressed.

Regular updates to PBL cases help ensure their relevance, accuracy, and educational value, thereby enhancing the learning experience for students.

2.7 Facilitator Guide Design

The Facilitator Guide (FG) is an essential resource that only facilitators can access. It is a structured resource designed to support facilitators in leading PBL sessions effectively as it provides a comprehensive overview of the case, ensuring that facilitators can guide discussions, reinforce key learning objectives, and maintain alignment with the course curriculum.

Core Elements of Facilitator Guide Design:

1. Case learning objectives: Clearly defined objectives that align with the intended educational outcomes.
2. Annotations for Each Section in the Table of Contents (TOC): Each item in the PBL case's TOC should include facilitator notes highlighting the significance of new data, guiding discussions, and ensuring alignment with learning objectives.

The FG is designed to facilitate **active learning and integration** of clinical and basic medical/healthsciences. If students do not naturally address specific learning issues, facilitators can use **Socratic questioning** (Elkowitz, 2015) to encourage deeper exploration. The guide ensures that every clinical data point connects back to relevant physiological, biochemical, or pathological mechanisms.

For example, in the **initial presentation and history**, the FG may highlight how symptom duration helps distinguish between acute and chronic conditions, shaping the differential diagnosis. Similarly, during the **physical exam**, the FG may provide prompts to explore the underlying mechanisms of **edema formation in congestive heart failure**, such as hemodynamics and capillary pressure changes.

Maintaining and Updating the Facilitator Guide:

To ensure the FG remains relevant and effective, it undergoes regular updates through:

1. **Ongoing facilitator feedback** from real-time PBL sessions.
2. **Scheduled case review committee meetings** to incorporate advancements in medical knowledge and refine case-based discussions.

By following these design principles, the Facilitator Guide serves as a **valuable tool for structured case facilitation**, helping educators maintain a high standard of inquiry-based learning in PBL sessions.

The **Facilitator Guide** (*only for facilitators*) provides insight and support for facilitators to ask questions (Brown et al., 2014; Cassara, 2015), and creates opportunities for scaffolding to take place in terms of concept formation and growth, exploring interconnections of concepts and disciplines, and increasing awareness of potential learning issues. In conclusion, the Facilitator Guide supports the process of achieving the outcome of the learning objectives and goal of PBL.

2.8 PBL Case Table of Contents

The **Table of Contents** (*only for facilitators*) is the most important document for the process of PBL. Its structure allows for progressive disclosure of the sections of the PBL case, with enough time for collaborative learning to take place, and for the selection of learning issues for later self-directed learning endeavors. **Feedback** from facilitators should be an ongoing process for updating and improving both the PBL cases and the Facilitator Guides.

2.9 Summary of Learning Objectives

To summarize: the learning objectives of the PBL case include:

- identifying, defining, and learning basic medical/health sciences,
- expanding clinical reasoning and critical thinking skills,
- developing problem-solving skills,
- enhancing collaboration, and team-working skills,
- improving communication and interpersonal skills,
- stimulating curiosity, interest, and motivation,
- developing self-directed learning skills and life-long learning habits.

Appendix 1: Sample Case with TOC & Facilitator Guide

College Name

Problem-Based Learning
College Name
Course Name
For educational purposes only.
Case No. 001
Karen Carter

Medical Records (From 2 Days Ago)

Chief Complaint (CC) "bad cough for last few days"

History of present illness (HOPI): Karen Carter is a 62 year old who came to my office complaining of a cough for 6 days and that has worsened in the last 3 days. She describes it as coming on suddenly. It is worse at night and therefore she hasn't slept well. She has increased sputum over the last 3 days and it is yellow-brownish in color without any noticeable blood. She reported being short of breath but denies any pain. The cough is worse when being very active or laughing. She has had some relief with over-counter Robitussin cough syrup. She states that other people at work have had similar illness. She thinks she might have a slight fever but has not checked it.

Past Medical History (PMH)

1. Medications: 1200 mg calcium a day, vitamin pill a day, no herbal meds
2. Allergies: no drug, food or environmental allergies
3. Past illnesses: bronchitis 5 years ago, gallbladder stones 15 years ago, no history of heart disease, high blood pressure, or diabetes
4. Surgery: Gallbladder removed 15 years ago for gallstones
5. Hospitalizations: two times for child births, one time for concussion and broken arm after a motor vehicle accident (MVA)

Family History (FH)

1. Mother is alive and age 79, she has emphysema and is a smoker
2. Father deceased at age 62 from heart attack
3. Two sisters and a brother alive and healthy
4. No family history of cancer, tuberculosis (TB), diabetes or high blood pressure

Social History (SH)

1. Works at Nursing Home as receptionist
2. Married and has two adult sons
3. Smokes 1 pack per day $\times$ 40 years

4. Alcohol 2 drinks per evening with husband
5. No recreational drugs use
6. No travel out of country

Review of Systems (ROS):

General: wt. same, slight fever.

Skin: no rashes or skin problems.

HEENT: wears reading glasses, and last eye exam 6 months ago was unchanged.

No glaucoma or other visual problems. No hearing loss or ear problems, sore throats, or dysphagia or thyroid problems. Has had sinusitis.

Heart: No cardiovascular concerns of chest pain, or dysrhythmias. She has had a few elevated BP readings, but normal the past year.

Respiratory: Dry cough at times which she relates to smoking. No wheezing or SOB, No hemoptosis. She had a TB skin test 2 months ago because of employment requirement.

GI: Gallbladder removed, but no other dyspepsia or regurge. Stools are normal and no change in habits, no blood in stool.

GU: Voids once per night and if she coughs hard or laughs hard, she has some leakage. She had a urinary tract infection (UTI) about 10 years ago.

Gyn: Menarche age 13 years. normal periods with 5 day flow till 7 years ago and she gradually stopped. She has had some hot flashes. Had been on birth control pills (BCP) for 15 years in the past.

Neuro: Concussion and broken right arm after MVA, she recovered well.

MS: She has had some mild low back pain, she says after lifting heavy items, but only mild osteoarthritis on X-rays.

Psy: No history of depression, anxiety, or other mental illness.

Physical Exam Results

Vital signs:

Temp. 100.9 °F	Blood pressure 138/84 (left arm, while sitting)
Pulse 94	Respirations 18
Height 5′4″	Weight 144 lbs
Pulse OX 95%	

General: She is in no distress, but coughs several times while talking, and spits out some thick yellow or brownish sputum on a tissue paper. She is no respiratory distress, and is alert and oriented × 3.

HEENT: Eyes PERRLA, fundus appears normal, wears glasses for reading. Ear canals are clear, TM's are intact and hearing is normal. Nose has sight mucosal membrane erythema and swelling, septum is midline, and turbinate's are red and boggy. Throat appears normal. Tonsils are present and atrophied with no erythema noted. Oral cavity has no lesions present and patient is edentulous with both upper and lower dentures. Thyroid is not enlarged. Minimal anterior cervical adenopathy, bilaterally, is present and no posterior or supraclavicular nodes are palpable.

Pulmonary: Lungs reveal slight crackles in right basilar area and dullness to percussion below eighth rib in this area; pleural rub in right basilar area.
Heart: Normal PMI and normal S_1 & S_2. Apical rate is RR&R with a grade 1 systolic murmur best heard along left sternal border with no radiation. No rubs, gallops, or clicks. No bruits of neck audible.
Abdomen: Upper right quadrant scar. Audible bowel sounds in all four quadrants. Non tender to light and deep palpation. Nondistended. No organomegaly noted
Pelvic examination: GU and GYN deferred; she had pelvic exam 2 months ago and only thing noted was grade 1 cystocele. Pap smear was normal.
Neurological: Mental status is normal; CN's II-XII are grossly intact. DTR's are 2+/4 bilaterally in all four extremities. Normal sensation with light touch and pinprick. 5/5 strength bilaterally throughout upper and lower extremity. Gait is normal. Negative Romberg and Babinski signs.
Musculoskeletal: Range of motion within normal range

Laboratory Test Results

CBC			
Test (units of measurement)	Reference range	Within range	Out of range
RBC (million/mm^3)	M: 4.6–6.2 F: 4.2–5.4	4.3	
Hgb (g/dL)	12–16	14.5	
Hct (%)	37–47	44	
WBC (thousand/mm^3)	5.0–10.0		15.1
Differential			
Neutrophils (%)	50–70		81
Lymphocytes (%)	25–40		10
Bands (%)	1–8		9

Laboratory Test Results

Blood chemistry			
Test (units of measurement)	Reference range	Within range	Out of range
Na (mEq/L)	136–146	140	
K (mEq/L)	3.7–5.3	4.0	
Cl (mEq/L)	101–111	102	
CO_2 (mEq/L)	21–31	22	
BUN (mg/dL)	5–24	22	
Creatinine (mg/dL)	0.7–1.3	0.8	
Glucose (mg/dL)	65–115	96	

CXR reveals consolidation in right basal area (All images Optional: facilitator provides image 1)

EKG was normal.

Three sets of blood cultures and a sputum sample were sent for Gram stain, cultures and sensitivity. Urine was sent for Legionella antigen. Nasopharyngeal swabs were sent for influenza and respiratory viral cultures.

Mrs. Smith was placed on amoxicillin/clavulanate 875 mg p.o. bid for 10 days. She was advised to stop smoking. She was scheduled to return in 2 weeks. She was also told to get a pneumonia shot when this episode was over. She gets a skin test for TB yearly because of her job.

Microbiology results were received from the lab:

- Gram stain of sputum—remarkable (images 2 and 3)
- Cultures of sputum on blood agar—yielded significant results (images 4 and 5)
- Legionella urinary antigen—negative
- Direct DFA of NP swab for respiratory viruses (influenza, adeno, RSV and pneumovirus)—negative
- Respiratory virus cultures of NP swab—negative
- Blood culture results show no growth to date

Microscopic: Gram-positive diplococci

Organism cultured: *Streptococcus pneumoniae*

Susceptibility Results

MIC interpretation		MIC (μg/mL) for susceptible	
Azithromycin	0.25	Sensitive	(≤0.5)
Cefotaxime	0.025	Sensitive	(≤0.05)
Chloramphenicol	2	Sensitive	(≤4.0)
Clindamycin	0.25	Sensitive	(≤0.25)
Erythromycin	0.5	Resistant	(≤0.25)
Levofloxacin	0.5	Sensitive	(≤2.0)
TMP/SMX	0.5/9.5	Sensitive	(≤0.5/9.5)
Linezolid	1.0	Sensitive	(≤2.0)
Penicillin	2.0	Resistant	(≤0.06)
Rifampin	0.5	Sensitive	(≤1.0)
Tetracycline	2.0	Sensitive	(≤2.0)
Vancomycin	0.25	Sensitive	(≤1.0)

Two Days Later

1. **Chief Complaint**: A 62 year old female, Karen Carter is brought to the emergency room (ER) by her husband because of her worsening pneumonia.
2. **Patient History**:
Mr. Carter brings his wife to the ER because of her worsening pneumonia. He says "she is getting worse". She was seen in her family physician's office 2 days ago and diagnosed with pneumonia, and put on Augmentin 875 mg 2× per day. The physician called and said it was a resistant bug and because she was becoming worse to come to the ER. She is weak, coughing up sputum (yellow-brownish in color) and in larger amounts. She is very short of breath. She did have a chest X-ray showing pneumonia 2 days ago, but her husband did not see the film.

Mr. Carter is anxious about his wife's condition and questions why she has become worse.

When asked, he relates she is not allergic to any medications and not taking anything else except vitamins, calcium and the antibiotic.

He says she had her gallbladder out 15 years ago and was in hospital years ago for a fracture of her right arm and concussion.
3. **Physical Exam (in the ER)**:
Vital signs:

- T: 102.7 °F
- BP: 92/60

- HR: 118
- RR: 24
- Pulse oximetry: 89%

General: 62-year-old woman appears stated age. Her color is gray ashen. Her breathing is rapid and slightly labored. She is oriented to time but is confused as to place and situation.

HEENT: Eyes: PERRLA, EOMI, fundiscopic exam was normal. Ears: external auditory canals were clear. TM's show normal cone of light and landmarks bilaterally. Nose: mild mucosal swelling and little yellow discharge noted. Throat was irritated and injected. Edentulous gums normal with dentures removed. Neck: No lymphadenopathy, thyromegaly, masses, carotid bruits, or JVD.

Pulmonary: Tachypneic and using some accessory muscles. Crackles heard at right base with E to A changes present. Positive dullness to percussion at the right base. No wheezes or other abnormal breath sounds appreciated.

Cardiac: PMI slight left of MCL 5IS. Tachycardia with grade I/VI systolic murmur best heard at the left upper sternal border. No S3/S4. No radiation into neck.

Abdomen: RUQ well healed scar noted. Bowel sounds audible in all four quadrants. Nontender/nondistended. No guarding/rebound. Digital rectal exam normal and Guiac test negative.

GU and GYN: Deferred.

Neuro: Mental status altered. Alert but not oriented to place or situation. Her Glasgow Coma score = 14. Cranial nerves II-XII intact. Generalized weakness but no focal deficits in sensation or strength noted in upper and lower extremities. DTR's were 2+/4 bilaterally in upper and lower extremity. Negative Brudzinski and Kernig sign. She was not tested for gait or Romberg due to weakness.

Skin: Gray ashen in color. Warm to the touch, with clammy skin. No purpura, rashes, or other lesions noted, except scattered petechiae are present.

4. **Laboratory Test Results**:

CBC	**Reference range**	**Within range**	**Out of range**
WBC (thousand/mm^3)	(5000–10,000)		25,000
Hemoglobin (g/dL)	(12–16)		9
Hematocrit (%)	(37–47)		28
Differential			
Granulocytes (%)	(50–70)		79
Lymphocytes (%)	(25–40)		7.5
Bands (%)	(1–8)		13.5
Platelets (thousand/μL)	(150,000–400,000)		18,000

5.

Coagulation markers	Reference range	Within range	Out of range
PTT (s)	(23–35)		45 s
PT (s)	(9.5–12.5)		35 s
INR	(0.9–1.1)		1.6
C-reactive protein (mg/dL)	(<0.8)		12

6.

Blood chemistry	Reference range	Within range	Out of range
Na^+ (mmol/L)	(136–146)	144	
K^+ (mmol/L)	(3.7–5.3)		3.6
Cl^- (mmol/L)	(101–111)	102	
CO_2 (mmol/L)	(21–31)		16
BUN (mg/dL)	(5–24)	24	
Creatinine (mg/dL)	(0.7–1.3)		3.7
Glucose (mg/dL)	(65–115)		153

7.

Arterial blood gas	Reference range	Within range	Out of range
pH	(7.35–7.45)		7.21
pCO_2 (mmHg)	(35–45		30
pO_2 (mmHg)	(75–100		55
HCO_3 (mmol/L)	(22–28		11.6

8.

Liver function tests	Reference range	Within range	Out of range
Protein, total (g/dL)	(6.4–8.3)	6.4	
Albumin (g/dL)	(3.4–4.8)		2.8
Alkaline phosphatase (U/L)	(25–100)	77	
ALT	(7–30 U/L)		900
AST	(9–26 U/L)		840
LDH (U/L)	(208–378)		588
Bilirubin, total (mg/dL)	(0.3–1.2)		1.4

9. CXR revealed consolidation in the right basal area.
Head CT was done and showed no evidence of bleed, mass, or midline shift.
10. The ER physician admits Mrs. Carter to the hospital. Mrs. Carter has a consolidation in the right lower lobe with a Pneumonia Severity Index Risk class IV. Additionally, she has evidence of renal and liver failure, and her platelet levels are very low, and she has an oxygen requirement. Blood, sputum samples, and cerebrospinal fluid (CSF) were obtained for gram stain, culture, and antibiotic susceptibilities. The CSF was obtained by lumbar puncture (LP) after the CT of the head was reported as normal. Antimicrobial treatment with I.V. Ceftriaxone 1 g plus I.V. Azithromycin 500 mg was started as empiric treatment for presumed septicemia of pulmonary origin. The patient has also received 1 L of normal saline I.V. fluid.

You discuss this with the patient and her husband and indicate that she will need to be hospitalized for IV therapy and close monitoring. You explain that the situation is very serious and requires prompt action. You provide empathy for their situation. They wisely agree to the admission and thank you for taking the time to explain the situation and for your concern. You ask if durable medical attorney has been granted to anyone by Mrs. Carter. You also ask for a decision regarding "code status". They ask you to explain "code status".
11. The Carters explain that they previously had appointed each other as having durable medical power of attorney in case one of them became incapable of making medical decisions. The husband asks if he could use a phone to contact their sons to inform them of the situation and to have them bring in the legal paperwork pertaining to the power of attorney. You show him to a phone and politely let him know of the hospital's visitor policy.
12. You decide to admit her to the ICU because she clearly meets SIRS (systemic inflammatory response syndrome) criteria and likely has sepsis or severe sepsis. Her Acute Physiology and Chronic Health Evaluation (APACHE) II score is 37.
13. You order two 18-gauge intravenous lines to be placed. You continue aggressive fluid resuscitation with Lactated Ringers.

She is placed on none-rebreather face mask for oxygenation. Thirty minutes later her pulse oximeter reading is 88% with labored breathing.
14. You decide to intubate her via a rapid sequence intubation protocol. After giving her etomidate and succinylcholine, you successfully intubate her and connect her to the ventilator to take control of her airway.

Now that her breathing is under control, you must address the other urgent issues. After the fluid boluses her blood pressure seems stable at this time (100/70) but urine output is 20 cc/h. You order the lab tests for evaluating the hemostatic parameters and infectious status.

A Swan-Ganz catheter was placed to monitor left atrial filling pressures and guide fluid replacement. Original wedge pressure is 8. Fluid is at 200 cc/h. and IV rate was increased to try to increase urine output.

15. Test Results:

Hemostatic markers	Result	Normal range
Antithrombin	8 mg/dL	(17–39 mg/dL)[a]
D-dimer	3144 μg/L	(<500 ng/mL)[a]
Fibrinogen	122 mg/dL	(150–400 mg/dL)[a]
FDP	51 μg/mL	(0–10 μg/mL)[a]

FDP fibrinogen degradation products

Microbiology Lab Results:

Microscopic: Gram-positive diplococci in (blood and sputum); many PMNs in sputum
Organism cultured: *Streptococcus pneumoniae* (blood and sputum)

Culture of CSF yielded no growth.
Susceptibility Results:

MIC interpretation		MIC (μg/mL) for susceptible	
Azithromycin	0.25	Sensitive	(≤0.5)
Cefotaxime	0.025	Sensitive	(≤0.05)
Chloramphenicol	2	Sensitive	(≤4.0)
Clindamycin	0.25	Sensitive	(≤0.25)
Erythromycin	0.5	Resistant	(≤0.25)
Levofloxacin	0.5	Sensitive	(≤2.0)
TMP/SMX	0.5/9.5	Sensitive	(≤0.5/9.5)
Linezolid	1.0	Sensitive	(≤2.0)
Penicillin	4.0	Resistant	(≤0.06)
Rifampin	0.5	Sensitive	(≤1.0)
Tetracycline	2.0	Sensitive	(≤2.0)
Vancomycin	0.25	Sensitive	(≤1.0)

16. **Hospital Course:**

Based on sensitivities, antibiotics were changed to cefotaxime (2 g IV q4h) and vancomycin (1 g IV q12h). Her blood pressure (77/38) was now becoming difficult to control with just fluid resuscitation.

17. You place an arterial radial line, a triple lumen central line, and a foley catheter and begin treatment with norepinephrine at an initial dose of 2–3 mL (from 8 to 12 μg of base) per minute, adjusting the rate of flow to establish and maintain a low normal blood pressure (90–100 mmHg systolic) sufficient to maintain the circulation to vital organs. You would like to use drotrecogin-alpha IV, but realize that it would not be the best choice for this patient at this time. Since her hematocrit is not critically low, you decide to defer packed red blood cell transfusion at this

time and focus on replacement therapy to treat the DIC. After obtaining a type and screen, and getting a consult (hematologist, bloodbanking-transfusion medicine consult, and/or critical care consult), and getting a signed informed consent from the husband, 4 units of Fresh Frozen Plasma (FFP) and 6 units of platelets for transfusion was ordered. Additionally, hydrocortisone 50 mg IV q6h, IV insulin to maintain glucose between 80 to 110 mg/dL, IV Ranitidine 50 mg q8h, and TED hoses with Sequential Compression Device (SCD) was ordered. The following day, a nutritional consult is placed to obtain recommendations on enteral nutrition.
18. Over the next few days, Mrs. Carter clinical situation stabilizes and begins to improve. Her blood pressure remains stable in the 120s/70s despite discontinuing the norepinephrine. She has remained afebrile for >48 h. The most recent CBC shows:

WBC	11,000/mm^3	(5000–10,000)[a]
Hemoglobin	11.2 g/dL	(12–16)[a]
Hematocrit	33%	(37–47)[a]
Platelets	105,000/mL	(150,000–400,000)[a]

[a] represents Normal Range

The hemostatic parameters have normalized. Her kidney function has improved as reflected in a creatinine of 1.7 mg/dL and normal urine output. The liver function has nearly normalized.
On the fifth hospital day, she is extubated successfully. Shortly thereafter, she is transferred to the floor and has no further fevers and all subsequent blood cultures are negative. Physical therapy consultation is obtained to begin rehabilitation and get recommendations regarding long term rehab. A case manager/discharge planner is consulted to help the family choose a skilled nursing facility (SNF). She is then discharged to the SNF for continued IV antibiotic therapy to complete a 2-week course of treatment as well as for physical therapy. Antibiotics are continued IV for a total of 3 weeks.
Following her course of antibiotics, she is discharged to home from the SNF and told she could resume normal activity. She is instructed to monitor for fever and report any temp changes promptly to her local physician as well as any respiratory symptoms. She arranges to see her Family Physician for follow-up next week.

Table of Contents
Case 001—Karen Carter
NOT TO BE GIVEN OR READ TO STUDENTS

1. Medical Records
2. CC
3. History

4. PE
5. CBC
6. Coagulation markers
7. Blood Chemistry (chem 7)
8. ABG
9. Liver Function Tests
10. Chest X-ray
11. Admit to hospital
12. Power of Attorney
13. ICU
14. IV fluids and oxygen
15. Hemostatic & Microbiology studies
16. Hospital Course
17. Additional hospital course
18. Days later: recovery & discharge

FACILITATOR'S GUIDE
NOT TO BE GIVEN OR READ TO STUDENTS

This case traces the history of a patient who initially was evaluated and underwent community-acquired pneumonia (CAP). She failed to respond to the antibiotic (the cultured isolate was resistant to the antibiotic prescribed) and unfortunately developed sepsis.

As a result of this case, the student will be exposed to common causes of pneumonia, symptoms and signs, and the management of complications of pneumonia and severe sepsis due to bacteremia and over-reacting immune response. The students should address the following issues:

- Pulmonary **physiology**
- Normal defense (**immunology**) against lung and blood pathogens
- Epidemiology and risks of CAP
- The most common causes (i.e., **microbiology**) of CAP and virulence of bacteria that cause CAP
- Host immune response to systemic infection due to the invasive pathogens (especially, what causes the immune system to over react, leading to systemic inflammatory changes, coagulation defects, and multiorgan dysfunctions?)
- **Pathophysiology** of sepsis
- Diagnostic criteria to determine systemic inflammatory response syndrome
- Coverage of drugs to pneumonia and sepsis; **pharmacology** (i.e., pharmacokinetics and pharmacodynamics) of antibiotics of choice

First Presentation

The chief complaint is cough. The keys are fever and cough, raising yellow-brownish colored sputum and slight shortness of breath, in her HOPI. She is also a smoker. They did raise the point that people at her place of employment were ill which could lead to the other possibilities of influenza or viral illness but the fact that she works in a Nursing Home could include other diagnoses such as Legionnaires disease.

Her physical exam revealed that she had fever of 100.9 °F; no respiratory distress. Lungs revealed crackles and dullness to percussion in right basilar area. Her pulse oximetry was low but not alarming. She had a surgical scar on abdomen. Rest of exam was straight forward.

CBC showed increase in WBC's and neutrophils and decrease in lymphs which would indicate a bacterial infection.

Normal blood chemistry.

Pneumonia should be distinguished from infections of the airways such as bronchitis and from upper respiratory infections (URIs) such as laryngitis and sinusitis. Students must know that a chest X-ray is essential for confirming pneumonia and it helps to determine the location of pulmonary involvement (e.g. lobar, bronchial, interstitial), the nature of lung pathology (e.g., cavitary, necrotizing), whether a pleural effusion is present, and whether there is hilar adenopathy. Chest X-ray shows a consolidation in right basal area and would indicate pneumonia present. Students should ask if any underlying condition (i.e. lung cancer or TB) could be present. Follow up X-rays would be critical in considering these causes especially if she does not respond to antibiotic therapy as expected.

EKG was normal.

Pneumonia has many causes, but a few are responsible for the majority of infections seen clinically. *Haemophilus influenzae* and *Moraxella catarrhalis* are usually seen in patients with COPD, and *Klebsiella pneumoniae* is seen in alcoholics. *Staphylococcus aureus* is a likely pathogen in post-influenza pneumonia. *S. pneumoniae* often produces a sudden onset of symptoms and is the most common cause. *Legionella pneumophila* is an environmental pathogen that could cause a common source outbreak in a number of individuals in a nursing home setting.

A standard microbiologic lab approach to the confirmation of the bacterial etiology may include: Gram stain and cultures of sputum. Another useful approach for determination of the bacterial etiology is to do the blood culture. A significant (25–35%) percent of cases with typical pneumonia go on to develop bacteremia. In these cases, blood cultures in combination with sputum culture increase the sensitivity of detection of the pathogen.

At this juncture, students should be able to differentiate between typical and atypical pneumonia. The four most important characteristics of atypical pneumonia are

1. Nonproductive cough
2. Variable chest X-ray (patchy, diffuse infiltrates)
3. No bacteria on smear

4. No responses to β-lactam antibiotics (e.g., penicillins, cephalosporins)

To rule out atypical pneumonia in this case, urine was sent for Legionella antigen. Nasopharyngeal swabs were sent for direct fluorescence antibody staining and microscopy to demonstrate cells infected with respiratory viruses (e.g., adenovirus, influenza, RSV, pneumovirus).

She was started on amoxicillin/clavulanate which was one of the choices for community acquired pneumonia. She had a TB skin test for her job and received flu shot but not pneumonia immunization and that was recommended when she recovered.

Students should try to explain the Gram stain on the basis of presence of (1) inflammatory cells and (2) organisms. They should also be able to arrive at the presumptive identification of the pathogen based on the (a) Gram stain reactivity and (b) cellular arrangements (cocci in chains = streptococci, diplococci, cocci in bunch = staphylococci). Students should be able to describe the hemolytic characteristics of the isolated colonies on the blood agar growth plate. They should be able to characterize the colonies and arrive at the definitive identification (i.e., *Streptococcus pneumoniae*) based on (i) partial hemolysis and (ii) susceptibility to optochin. After a significant isolate has been identified, the organism may be tested against a battery of antibiotics to help determine appropriate therapy. Testing here included broth (antibiotic) dilution and after incubation with standard inoculums of organisms yielded quantitative results in the form of minimum inhibitory concentrations (MICs). Students should look up the definitions of MIC, MBC, and the role of such values in the determination of "susceptible", "intermediate", and "resistance". In this test, the isolate turned out to be resistant to penicillin.

End of First Presentation (2 Days Ago)

Second Presentation (Page by Page Breakdown)

1. Mrs. Carter was told that her culture showed bacteria that were resistant to the antibiotic she was currently taking. She was advised to go directly to the ER for possible admission so that IV therapy could begin immediately.
2. In the E.R., she is febrile, tachycardic, tachypneic, hypotensive, and has a low pulse oximetry. She appears pale and has altered mental status. It should be clear to the students that this patient is extremely ill and requires immediate intervention.
3. The CBC results are abnormal in all cell types. The WBC is elevated in response to bacteremia. The decreased hemoglobin and hematocrit (especially as compared to the previous result) suggests either rapid red blood cell losses or destruction. In combination with the extremely low platelet count and the overall clinical picture, it is becoming apparent that this patient is not only in septic shock but is in disseminated intravascular coagulation (DIC)—see Sects. 14, 15, & 16 for more info on DIC.

4. Prolonged PTT, PT, and INR (International Normalized Ratio) confirm that something has altered the body's ability to adequately clot. With this result, DIC moves to the top of the list. Students should understand that this progresses rapidly and is life threatening. They should be able to explain how sepsis can lead to DIC as well as the alterations that occur in the clotting cascade. The C-reactive protein is non-specific and is elevated in most infectious or inflammatory conditions. The degree of elevation suggests a very serious underlying process.
5. The chemistry panel reveals multiple abnormalities. The CO_2 is low resulting in an anion gap. This strongly suggests a metabolic acidosis that should be further evaluated with an arterial blood gas. Acute renal failure is present. The creatinine has increased dramatically from the previous value taken in the office. The underlying reason is probably multifactorial. That is, at the very minimum, a prerenal component (hypoperfusion secondary to volume depletion and hypotension) is present. Additionally, it is likely that an acute tubular necrosis has developed secondary to this severe persistent hypoperfusion. This would be confirmed by visualizing granular casts in the urine sediment; a fractional excretion of sodium (FeNa) would be helpful in distinguishing prerenal from renal causes. Prerenal changes in the creatinine respond favorably and generally quickly to fluid resuscitation and normalization of the blood pressure. As we see later, the creatinine improves with resuscitation and normalization of the blood pressure but does not completely return to baseline suggesting a combination of etiologies. These renal issues are not really explored in the clinical management outlined in the case. In this clinical situation, given the severity of the other issues, this would likely take a back seat until she is stabilized.
6. The arterial blood gas (ABG) suggests a high anion gap metabolic acidosis with compensated respiratory alkalosis. The most likely reason at this time is from lactic acidosis secondary to severe sepsis. Students should understand how to use the arterial blood gas results to determine the patient's acid-base status and how the clinical situation helps determine the interpretation of the ABG and conversely, how the ABG interpretation helps focus the differential diagnosis.
7. Multiple abnormalities are also present in the liver function tests. The albumin is low and may be result of recent malnutrition. The LDH and bilirubin are likely elevated secondary to ongoing red blood cell destruction. The elevated transaminases are secondary to "shock liver" or "ischemic hepatitis". The underlying pathophysiology involves changes in the portal and arterial blood supply as well as in microcirculation. Cross-talk between hepatocytes, Kupffer cells, and endothelial cells, leading to an inflammatory response mediated primarily by tumor necrosis factor-alpha (TNF-alpha). The hepatocyte undergoes dramatic alterations in synthetic activity, biliary transport, bile flow and glucose metabolism.

The management of shock liver is focused on the prevention of precipitating causes by controlling sepsis, circulation parameters and metabolism in addition to the cautious monitoring of therapeutic measures that can increase hepatic injury, which include intravenous nutrition, mechanical ventilation and catecholamine administration.

8. A chest X-ray confirms right lower lobe pneumonia. A CT of the head is obtained primarily to rule out intracranial pressure prior to performing a lumbar puncture (to obtain cerebrospinal fluid to evaluate for a CNS infection). Increased intracranial pressure can theoretically lead to cerebral herniation if a lumbar puncture is performed. It is controversial as to when this is necessary and there is little evidence supporting universal CT scans prior to LP although it is done routinely. Additionally, the patient has an altered mental status and therefore a CT can help evaluate for a subdural bleed or unknown mass as the etiology. Since the focus of this case is microbiology, students may want to pursue learning issues pertaining to infections of the CNS, common organisms, and CSF analysis.

9.–10. The Pneumonia Severity Index was developed to assist physicians in identifying patients at higher risk of complications and mortality and who are therefore more likely to benefit from hospitalization. It is a score based on patient characteristics pertaining to demographics, comorbid illness, physical examination findings, laboratory and radiologic findings. Class IV designates moderate risk with about 8% mortality and inpatient care is recommended.

She is treated by the ER physician for presumed septic shock secondary to bacteria originating in the respiratory tract. Empiric treatment is the appropriate approach here since early antibiotics are crucial in this situation. Use of Cefotaxime and Azithromycin allow for broad spectrum coverage. Students should be able to describe these medications' class, mechanism of action, pharmacokinetics, antimicrobial activity, etc.

The final section focuses on the importance of providing empathy when family members are faced with grave situations. Additionally, it becomes increasingly important to sort out the patient's end of life wishes and to clarify legal power of attorney for making life/death decisions.

11. The term *SIRS* is the clinical manifestation of the inflammatory response to a wide variety of insults, including infectious and noninfectious etiologies. The syndrome is recognized by the presence of two or more of the following clinical signs: (1) temp >38 °C or <36 °C; (2) heart rate >90 bpm; (3) respiratory rate >20/min or $PaCO_2$ <32 mmHg; and (4) a white blood cell count >12,000 or <4000 cells/mm^3. *Sepsis* describes when the process is from an infectious etiology and *severe sepsis* is used when it is also associated with organ dysfunction, hypotension, or hypoperfusion (manifested by lactic acidosis, oliguria, acute alteration of mental status, etc.). The students should be able to describe the pathophysiology of the body's response to septicemia.

Acute Physiology and Chronic Health Evaluation (APACHE) II score uses a point score based upon initial values of 12 routine physiologic measurements, age, and previous health status to provide a general measure of severity of disease. The newest scoring system (APACHE IV) includes additional parameters and is helpful in predicting mortality in ICU patients.

Because of her continued difficulty breathing, it is decided to electively take control of her airway rather than wait for an emergent situation. An induction agent and a depolarizing neuromuscular blocker are used. Why are these agents used prior to intubation?

12.–13. Since airway and breathing have been controlled (following the typical airway, breathing, and circulation) basic life support rules, it is time to focus on circulation. That includes blood pressure and in this case, further evaluation of hemostatic markers to confirm DIC
14. Since no single laboratory test or set of tests is sensitive or specific enough to allow a definite diagnosis of DIC, in most cases the diagnosis is based on the combination of results of laboratory investigations in a patient with a clinical condition known to be associated with DIC. The classical characteristic laboratory findings include prolonged clotting times (prothrombin time, activated partial thromboplastin time, thrombin time), increased levels of fibrin-related markers (fibrin degradation products, D-dimers), low platelet count and fibrinogen levels, and low plasma levels of coagulation factors (such as factors V and VII) and coagulation inhibitors (such as antithrombin and protein C). This patient clearly meets the criteria. How does DIC affect the clotting cascade?
15.–16. She is switched to Cefotaxime and to Vancomycin based on sensitivities (and resistance to erythromycin). Students should understand these drug classes, indications, mechanisms, etc.

Drotrecogin alpha or recombinant human activated protein C. It is a fairly new medication that has been shown to decrease overall mortality in patients with sepsis. It inhibits inflammation, neutrophil chemotaxis, endothelial activation, and thrombosis. Students should also incorporate study of this new drug when reading about treatments for sepsis. In this case, the patient is at significant risk of bleeding and will be receiving a platelet transfusion which is a contraindication to concurrent use of Xigris.

The patient is suffering from hemodynamic instability from the septic shock. Norepinephrine (Levophed) is needed temporarily to support this patient's blood pressure since she already shows evidence of vital organ hypoperfusion (kidney, liver, and brain). How does sepsis lead to hypotension?

Disseminated intravascular coagulation (DIC) is a very serious disorder characterized by massive systemic intravascular activation of coagulation, leading to widespread deposition of fibrin in the circulation which can compromise the blood supply to various organs, thus contributing to multiple organ failure. At the same time, the consumption of platelets and coagulation proteins resulting from the ongoing coagulation may induce severe bleeding. However, DIC is not a disease itself but is always secondary to an underlying disorder.

The aim of replacement therapy in DIC is to replace the deficiency due to the consumption of platelets, coagulation factors and inhibitors in order to prevent or arrest the hemorrhagic episodes. Platelet concentrates and fresh frozen plasma (FFP) is the mainstay of the treatment of patients with significant bleeding and coagulation parameters compatible with DIC. But the underlying cause has to be addressed, otherwise you are just "adding fuel to the fire." With DIC, a hematologist, bloodbanking-transfusion medicine doctor, or critical care consult is always needed if possible.

Corticosteroids and intensive insulin therapy have been shown to be beneficial in patients with septic shock on mechanical ventilation. There is apparent adrenal dysfunction in sepsis. This can be determined by a patient's response to a corticotrophin stimulation test. Students may want to try to understand this endocrine axis and how the stimulation test can determine the adrenal gland's ability to respond to stress. Stress hyperglycemia, if not controlled with insulin therapy, can have a detrimental effect on the development of nosocomial infections, multiple organ dysfunction, and mortality in critically ill patients. Additionally, an H2 blocker is used here to prevent stress ulcers.

17. After several days of supportive care and the interventions outlined above, the patient is able to recover and removal of all the tubes and lines commence (foley, central line, arterial radial line, endotracheal tube). Less intensity of care is required and she is transferred out of the ICU to the ward/floor. She is very weak and will require rehabilitation. A skilled nursing facility is an appropriate option for this patient to continue to receive the full course of IV antibiotics and to receive intensive physical therapy. Follow up with her primary care physician is crucial to maintain continuity and to assure that he/she is kept in the loop of her health care.

Appendix 2: Case Evaluation Form (Example)

For educational purposes only.

Facilitator: **Semester**_____

Yr_____

INSTRUCTIONS: Please answer each of the following questions relating to this case. When asked, please provide any additional information.

1. Were there any pages which were not requested at all? If so, which ones?

____
____
____
____
____
____

2. Was there any information which the students requested, which was not provided? If so, what was it?

____
____
____
____
____
____

3. If there is anything about this case that you feel requires more clarification in the Facilitator's Guide in order for you to better facilitate this case, list those items here.

4. List, by page (P), paragraph (¶), and line any typographic corrections that you find in this case.

5. If you have any other suggestions, technical, procedural or otherwise, please use the back of this page to make suggestions and to explain how or why you feel this would improve the PBL case.

THANK YOU FOR YOUR FEEDBACK.
Please return this form to the PBL Course Director.

Appendix 3: Potential Questions from Facilitator

1. Other than what you and your team have already discussed, can you think of any other possible causes for this patient history (or physical exam finding or clinical test result)?
2. Are the first medical tests or clinical studies that are requested (or ordered) considered less invasive, less costly, and/or more sensitive?

3. Are the later medical tests or clinical studies that are requested (or ordered) considered more invasive, more expensive, and/or more specific?
4. Are there any medical tests or clinical procedures that need to be done as soon as possible (ASAP)?
5. Compared to earlier patient status, is the patient now better, worse, or about the same?
6. What textbook chapters can you select to study in order to better understand the process reflected in this patient?
7. Are you satisfied with the team's list of learning issues (or selected textbook chapters) from this PBL session?
8. What other clinical data would you like to obtain? How can that information be obtained in the clinical setting?
9. What is the mechanism of action of that medication?
10. What is the most likely cause of that finding or observation?

During Feedback and Wrap-Up at End of PBL Session

1. What could have been better in this PBL session today?
2. What went well during this PBL session today?
3. What are some key take-away points from the PBL session today?

References

Barrows, H. S., & Tamblyn, R. N. (1980). *Problem-based learning: An approach to medical education*. Springer.

Brown, P. C., Roediger, H. L., & McDaniel, M. A. (2014). *Make it stick—The science of successful learning*. Belknap Press.

Cassara, M. (2015). Chapter 6: Concept mapping: An andragogy suited for facilitating education of the adult medical millennial learner. In A. Fornari & A. Poznanski (Eds.), *How-to guide for active learning* (IAMSE manuals). IAMSE.

Des Marchais, J. L. (1999). A Delphi technique to identify and evaluate criteria for construction of PBL problems. *Medical Education, 33*, 504–508.

Dolmans, D. H. J. M., Snellen-Balendong, H., Wolfhagen, I. H. A. P., & van der Vleuten, C. P. M. (1997). Seven principles of effective case design for a problem-based curriculum. *Medical Teacher, 19*, 185–189.

Duch, B. J. (1996). Problems: A key factor in PBL. *About Teaching, 50*, 7–8.

Elkowitz, D. E. (2015). Chapter 9: Socratic questioning to engage learners. In A. Fornari & A. Poznanski (Eds.), *How-to guide for active learning* (IAMSE manuals). IAMSE.

Gooding, H. C., Mann, K., & Armstrong, E. (2017). Twelve tips for applying the science of learning to health professions education. *Medical Teacher, 39*(1), 26–31.

Huggett, K. N., & Jeffries, W. B. (2015). Chapter 1: Overview of active learning research and rationale for active learning. In A. Fornari & A. Poznanski (Eds.), *How-to guide for active learning* (IAMSE manuals). IAMSE.

Kolb, A., & Kolb, D. (2005). Learning styles and learning spaces: Enhancing experiential learning in higher education. *Academy of Management Learning & Education, 4*(2), 193–212.

Leppink, J., & Duvivier, R. (2016). Twelve tips for medical curriculum design from a cognitive load theory perspective. *Medical Teacher, 38*(7), 669–674.

Linsenmeyer, M. (2015). Chapter 5: Brief activities: Questioning, brainstorming, think-pair share, jigsaw, and clinical case discussions. In A. Fornari & A. Poznanski (Eds.), *How-to guide for active learning* (IAMSE manuals). IAMSE.

Phillips, B. C. (2021). Chapter 3: Learning theories. In *Teaching in nursing and role of the educator* (3rd ed.). Springer.

Wissman, A. W. (2018). Cognitive load theory: Applications in medical education. *Technical Communication Capstone Course, 25*. Retrieved from https://cornerstone.lib.mnsu.edu/eng_comm_capstone_course/25

Wood, D. F. (2003). Problem based learning. *British Medical Journal, 326*, 326–330.

Yardley, S., Teunissen, P. W., & Dornan, T. (2012). Experiential learning: AMEE Guide No. 63. *Medical Teacher, 34*, e102–e115.

Young, J. Q., Van Merrienboer, J., Durning, S., & Ten Cate, O. (2014). Cognitive load theory: Implications for medical education: AMEE Guide No. 86. *Medical Teacher, 36*, 371–384.

Chapter 3
Facilitator Training for Problem-Based Learning

Todd A. Nolan

3.1 What Is a Facilitator? How Is a Facilitator Different from a Lecturer?

A facilitator, also known as a tutor in PBL, is typically a faculty member who helps groups of students explore case information in a problem-based learning course. They help students discover key information, make connections among various subjects, and encourage inquiry that leads to deep understanding and meaningful learning (Hmelo-Silver & Barrows, 2006). This differs significantly from that of a lecturer, as lectures are primarily about the unidirectional delivery of information from teacher to student. In contrast, facilitation promotes exploration, critical thinking, and self-directed learning among students (Azer, 2005).

At its most fundamental level, PBL facilitation is about helping students become self-directed, lifelong learners (Barrows & Tamblyn, 1980; Bridges et al., 2012; Callis et al., 2010) and nurturing the skills they will take with them throughout their careers (Neville & Norman, 2007). This contrasts starkly with the role of a lecturer whose purpose is to deliver content in an organized fashion and typically not stray far from the day's planned topic. While a facilitator encourages exploration with guidance, the lecturer requires the class to stay focused on the specific material with little room for variation in delivery style or adaptation to different ways of learning. The contrast between a facilitator and a lecturer underscores the unique and important role of a facilitator in student learning.

The role of the facilitator is complex and multifaceted. Key aspects include (Hmelo-Silver, 2004; Savery, 2006):

1. Modeling and coaching problem-solving and metacognitive processes
2. Encouraging student ownership of the learning process

T. A. Nolan (✉)
Lake Erie College of Osteopathic Medicine—School of Dental Medicine, Bradenton, FL, USA
e-mail: tnolan@lecom.edu

S. Lorenzo and B. Zhang (eds.), *Mastering Problem-Based Learning in Health Profession Programs*, https://doi.org/10.1007/978-3-032-05405-0_3

3. Facilitating collaborative knowledge construction
4. Providing scaffolding and guidance as needed
5. Monitoring group dynamics and individual participation
6. Assessing learning and providing constructive feedback

Facilitators must strike a careful balance between allowing students to grapple with problems independently and providing sufficient structure and support. They guide the PBL process but avoid directly giving answers, instead posing thought-provoking questions that spur students to think more deeply (Zhang et al., 2010). Facilitators also help regulate group dynamics, ensuring balanced participation and productive interactions (Hendry et al., 2003).

Becoming an effective facilitator requires developing a range of skills that go beyond traditional teaching. These include promoting inquiry, managing group processes, dealing with student difficulties, and flexibly adapting to the evolving needs of learners (Salinitri et al., 2015). Facilitators must be comfortable with ambiguity and not knowing all the answers. They need to resist their instinct to share their expertise and instead help draw out students' existing knowledge and reasoning abilities (Maudsley, 1999).

Ultimately, the facilitator's goal is to progressively fade their support so that students gain the skills to direct their learning (Hmelo-Silver et al., 2007). This requires patience, keen observation, and responsiveness to learners. Facilitators must continually monitor the group's progress and adjust their facilitation approach accordingly. It is a dynamic process that unfolds differently with each group of students.

In summary, facilitation and lecturing represent two distinct philosophies and approaches to teaching and learning. Lecturing efficiently transmits knowledge but leaves students in a passive role. In contrast, facilitation fosters active learning where students take the lead in the learning process and construct knowledge collaboratively with guidance and modeling from the facilitator. Transitioning from lecturer to facilitator is challenging but allows faculty to empower students as independent learners and problem-solvers.

3.2 Training the New Facilitator

Facilitator training is an ongoing, multi-dimensional process that blends short-term skill acquisition with long-term professional development. It emphasizes not only the cultivation of core competencies but also the confidence, adaptability, and reflective practice needed to guide student learning in PBL environments effectively. A well-trained facilitator fosters a learner-centered atmosphere where students feel empowered to explore complex problems, construct knowledge collaboratively, and develop self-directed learning habits.

Short-term skill development is typically the initial focus and centers on building a foundation for effective facilitation. These essential skills include:

1. **Formulating thought-provoking questions**: Facilitators must learn how to pose open-ended questions that stimulate analysis, synthesis, and evaluation rather than questions that elicit factual recall. For example, rather than asking, "What causes hypertension?" a skilled facilitator might ask, "How might lifestyle and genetic factors interact to influence a patient's blood pressure?"
2. **Asking probing questions about unfamiliar topics**: New facilitators often hesitate when topics stray beyond their own expertise. Training should emphasize techniques for asking clarifying or guiding questions that help students uncover assumptions and fill knowledge gaps without the facilitator needing to provide direct answers.
3. **Keenly observing group functioning and dynamics**: Facilitators must learn to monitor not just content discussions but also interpersonal interactions, group cohesion, and individual engagement. For instance, a facilitator might notice that one student dominates the conversation while others remain quiet and should be equipped to intervene subtly, perhaps by redirecting a question to a quieter student or inviting diverse perspectives.

Long-term skill development builds on this foundation and encompasses more advanced competencies such as:

1. **Case development and adaptation**: Experienced facilitators may contribute to designing or modifying PBL cases to suit the needs of specific cohorts, learning objectives, or curricular changes. Understanding how to craft authentic, complex, and relevant problems enhances the overall quality of student learning.
2. **Advanced group facilitation and management**: Over time, facilitators learn to navigate more nuanced group challenges, such as managing conflict, encouraging equitable participation, and supporting struggling learners without diminishing autonomy.
3. **Assessing individual and group learning**: Long-term development includes mastering formative assessment strategies, such as tracking learning issues, evaluating participation, and providing meaningful feedback on group processes and self-directed learning outcomes.

It is crucial to view facilitator training holistically as a combination of achieving short-term milestones and providing sustained institutional support. In the early stages, the primary objective is often to build facilitator confidence within the PBL context. One of the most common pitfalls for new facilitators, frequently highlighted in student evaluations, is the uncertainty about when to intervene or the tendency to over-facilitate (Haith-Cooper, 2003; Maudsley, 2002). These issues typically arise from insecurity or a misunderstanding of the facilitator's role, which ideally balances guidance with student autonomy.

Becoming a masterful facilitator is a career-long journey characterized by iterative practice, feedback, and self-reflection. Like clinical skills, facilitation techniques are honed over time through authentic practice and deliberate reflection. Facilitators must embrace a mindset of lifelong learning, continually seeking feedback from peers, students, and mentors to identify areas for growth and improvement (Salinitri et al., 2015; Maudsley, 2002). For example, reviewing video recordings of one's own sessions or participating in peer observations can provide valuable insights into facilitation style and impact.

Effective training programs extend beyond teaching basic techniques. They aim to foster deep pedagogical knowledge and reasoning that supports principled, theory-informed facilitation. This includes understanding the educational foundations of PBL, such as constructivism, adult learning theory, and metacognition (Savery & Duffy, 1995). Facilitators must also cultivate diagnostic reasoning, developing the ability to identify underlying causes of group dysfunction, cognitive stagnation, or disengagement, and select appropriate interventions that empower rather than direct students (Hmelo-Silver & Barrows, 2006). For example, if a group struggles with superficial reasoning, the facilitator might prompt deeper exploration by asking, "What mechanisms underlie this condition, and how might they differ in similar presentations?"

Facilitator development is significantly enriched through engagement with a community of practice (Wenger, 1998). These professional learning networks provide a collaborative space where facilitators can exchange ideas, share challenges, and celebrate successes. Regular interaction with peers fosters motivation, reduces isolation, and leads to collective knowledge building (Donnelly, 2010). For instance, monthly facilitator forums, interdisciplinary case discussion groups, or faculty learning communities can create valuable opportunities for growth. Institutions should prioritize the establishment of such communities by allocating protected time and providing administrative support.

Ultimately, facilitator development is not a finite process but a continuum of growth. With experience, facilitators not only become more adept at managing diverse learner needs and group dynamics but also evolve into mentors, case developers, curriculum designers, and educational leaders. Senior facilitators often play a crucial role in onboarding and coaching novice facilitators, creating a culture of continuous learning and shared responsibility (Dolmans et al., 2002). Moreover, the skills cultivated through facilitation, such as active listening, adaptive communication, and learner-centered teaching, have broad application across clinical, academic, and interprofessional settings.

Investing in robust facilitator development yields long-term dividends. It enhances the quality of PBL implementation, strengthens faculty engagement, and promotes a culture of teaching excellence. Ultimately, well-supported facilitators create ripple effects that elevate educational experience for students, colleagues, and the institution as a whole.

3.2.1 Breaking the Lecture Habit

One of the most significant challenges for faculty transitioning into the role of facilitator is stepping away from being the central figure in the classroom and the primary source of knowledge. In traditional lecture-based teaching, faculty members typically direct the learning experience by presenting information in a structured format. This places the instructor at the center of the learning process, often with students adopting a more passive role. In problem-based learning, however, the facilitator must adopt a different posture, acting as a guide who supports student inquiry and collaboration. This shift requires reorientation in both instructional technique and professional identity.

In problem-based learning environments, the most effective facilitators act as guides rather than lecturers. Their role is not to deliver content but to foster critical thinking, encourage student dialogue, and support exploration of complex problems. This is done primarily through the strategic use of questioning. Instead of providing information, facilitators prompt students to examine assumptions, articulate reasoning, and generate hypotheses. For example, rather than explaining a pathophysiological mechanism, a facilitator might ask, "What possible mechanisms could explain these symptoms, and how would we test those possibilities?" Such questions engage students in higher-order thinking and deepen their understanding (Hmelo-Silver et al., 2007).

Being an effective facilitator also means being present and responsive to the group's evolving needs. Presence involves attentiveness to student cues, group dynamics, and the intellectual flow of the session. Facilitators should allow space for students to express uncertainty, engage in collaborative reasoning, and link new information to prior knowledge (Silén, 2006). By doing so, facilitators help students develop ownership of their learning while reinforcing a supportive and inclusive learning environment (De Grave et al., 1999).

An essential aim of facilitation is the cultivation of self-directed learners. Skilled facilitators create conditions that enable students to independently identify learning issues, seek out resources, and integrate knowledge. Over time, students grow more confident in their ability to manage their learning, an outcome central to the goals of problem-based curricula (Hmelo-Silver et al., 2007). Facilitators can assist this transition by prompting students to reflect on their learning strategies and encouraging metacognitive awareness.

Despite its importance, refraining from over-directing student discussions can be difficult for new facilitators. Many struggle to resist the instinct to jump in with explanations or redirect conversations when students appear uncertain. These reactions are often shaped by years of experience in lecture-based teaching and reinforced by academic culture, where the instructor's expertise is expected to be on display (Azer, 2005). Letting go of that impulse requires intention, practice, and a willingness to embrace the ambiguity inherent in student-centered discussions.

Learning to tolerate that ambiguity is an important step in facilitator development. Unlike lectures, where the instructor controls the sequence and outcomes, problem-based learning sessions are unpredictable. Students may approach problems from unexpected angles or make errors as they reason through unfamiliar material. Skilled facilitators view these moments not as disruptions but as opportunities for learning. By holding back and allowing students to grapple with uncertainty, facilitators help them develop resilience and deeper understanding (Azer, 2005; Silén, 2006).

The topic of ongoing scholarly discussion is the role of content expertise in effective facilitation. Some argue that facilitators must possess deep knowledge of the subject matter in order to guide student reasoning, correct misconceptions, and ensure learning objectives are met (Leary et al., 2013). Others contend that strong facilitation skills can outweigh content knowledge and that non-expert facilitators, when properly trained, can be equally effective (Williams & Paltridge, 2017). Both perspectives have merit.

Content expertise can certainly enhance a facilitator's ability to understand student thinking and provide nuanced feedback. However, it can also lead to overparticipation if facilitators feel compelled to "teach" rather than guide. Research suggests that with robust training, clearly defined case objectives, and institutional support, facilitators without domain expertise can support student learning just as effectively as experts, particularly when the goal is to promote reasoning, inquiry, and collaboration rather than deliver facts (Hmelo-Silver et al., 2007).

In the author's experience, facilitators from a wide variety of disciplinary backgrounds can help students achieve strong learning outcomes when they are trained in facilitation principles and supported by high-quality cases. The key lies in the facilitator's ability to elicit student thinking, model curiosity, and create a safe environment for exploration. Content knowledge is beneficial but not essential. What is more critical is the facilitator's ability to foster student autonomy and encourage intellectual risk-taking.

Breaking the lecture habit does not mean discarding one's expertise. Rather, it involves learning to use that expertise strategically and sparingly. Facilitators must develop the discipline to support student exploration without steering it prematurely. They must also embrace the value of not knowing and model the kind of inquiry they want students to adopt. This shift, while challenging, is essential to creating learning environments that prepare students to think critically, work collaboratively, and engage in lifelong learning.

3.2.2 Learning from Experienced Facilitators

Observing experienced facilitators in action is an invaluable learning opportunity for those new to problem-based learning. Watching a skilled facilitator navigate the complex, dynamic nature of a PBL session provides novice facilitators with a concrete model of effective practice. It demystifies what facilitation looks like in real time and offers practical illustrations of theory in action. These live examples can help build a novice facilitator's mental framework for understanding group dynamics, questioning techniques, and facilitation strategies. By witnessing how experienced facilitators manage discussions, address confusion, and promote collaborative learning, newcomers are better able to envision what high-quality facilitation entails.

During observation, new facilitators should pay close attention to multiple aspects of the session. These include how the experienced facilitator sets the tone and communicates expectations for active engagement and respect within the group. Facilitators model inclusivity by encouraging broad participation, particularly by drawing out quieter students who may be hesitant to speak. Observers should also take note of how the facilitator frames and sequences questions to probe student thinking and promote deeper conceptual understanding. It is equally important to observe how the facilitator redirects conversations that stray off topic, guides students back to the central problem, and supports the group without dominating it. When students become stuck, effective facilitators provide appropriate scaffolding to move the discussion forward while preserving student agency. Finally, experienced facilitators typically end sessions with a structured debrief, during which they reflect on the process, highlight key insights, and offer constructive feedback to students.

While observation provides an important foundation, it is not sufficient on its own. Novice facilitators must also engage in deliberate debriefing sessions with the experienced facilitator after each observed session. These post-session conversations are critical for unpacking what occurred and understanding the rationale behind specific facilitation decisions. Debriefing serves as a reflective space where new facilitators can ask clarifying questions, express uncertainties, and begin to make sense of what they observed. Through this dialogue, the experienced facilitator can share the reasoning, decision-making strategies, and theoretical frameworks that inform their facilitation style. This allows new facilitators to move beyond surface-level imitation and begin building a deeper understanding of pedagogical intent.

Over time, experienced facilitators can also model the preparation and reflective processes that precede and follow each PBL session. This includes how to plan for sessions by reviewing the case in advance, anticipating potential student responses, and preparing open-ended guiding questions. New facilitators learn how to make in-the-moment decisions during a session, including when to intervene, how to balance student autonomy with support, and how to adapt their facilitation based on emerging group dynamics. They also see how experienced facilitators assess student learning through both informal observation and structured reflection, and how they provide feedback that is timely, specific, and constructive. Importantly, seasoned facilitators demonstrate the value of reflecting on one's own facilitation practice, identifying what went well and considering opportunities for improvement.

To maximize learning, debriefing sessions should go beyond a checklist of actions and delve into the pedagogical reasoning behind those actions. Novice facilitators should be encouraged to ask probing questions that uncover the facilitator's thought process. For example, questions such as "What student cues led you to intervene at that point?" or "What was your intended outcome when you posed that question?" help reveal the underlying intent behind facilitation moves. Other helpful inquiries include "How did you determine how much support to provide without taking over?" and "How would you handle that situation differently in a future session?" These types of questions help make tacit knowledge explicit and illuminate the often-invisible decision-making processes that define expert facilitation.

Through ongoing observation and reflective dialogue grounded in shared experiences, novice facilitators begin to internalize the habits of mind characteristic of effective facilitation. This apprenticeship model supports the development of pedagogical judgment, emotional intelligence, and adaptive expertise. Guided reflection enables new facilitators to connect theoretical concepts such as scaffolding, metacognition, and social constructivism to their practical application in the classroom. Ultimately, this process helps new facilitators move beyond simply mimicking observed behaviors and toward developing a facilitation style that aligns with their own strengths, values, and teaching philosophy.

3.2.3 Understanding Group Dynamics

To effectively facilitate PBL, facilitators must be deeply attuned to the complex and often subtle interpersonal dynamics that unfold within small groups. Group dynamics play a pivotal role in shaping the quality of collaboration, engagement, and learning. Healthy group dynamics promote mutual respect, active participation, shared responsibility, and a sense of belonging. In contrast, dysfunctional dynamics characterized by tension, mistrust, disengagement, or dominance by one or two individuals can significantly undermine the learning process. When group functioning is compromised, students may become frustrated, withdraw, or fail to develop the intended collaborative skills. Research has consistently shown that group interaction quality is closely linked to student satisfaction and achievement in PBL settings. Dysfunctional group dynamics marked by tension, unequal participation, or lack of cohesion can derail the PBL process (Hendry et al., 2003). Conversely, groups that gel well can achieve collective knowledge-building and problem-solving that surpasses what any individual learner could accomplish alone (Hmelo-Silver & Barrows, 2008).

Facilitators play a crucial role in catalyzing and sustaining productive group dynamics. From the first session, they help establish an environment where students feel safe asking questions, voicing half-formed ideas, and taking intellectual risks (Azer, 2005). This psychological safety is foundational for deep learning and authentic collaboration. Facilitators can model openness, curiosity, and humility to help normalize uncertainty and encourage students to do the same. Setting a tone of inclusiveness and mutual respect in the opening moments of the course can influence how students interact for the duration of the block.

Even seemingly simple moves on the part of the facilitator can significantly influence group cohesion. For example, beginning each session with a brief check-in question that invites students to share something from their lives outside of class helps ease the transition into learning, fosters rapport, and humanizes interactions. Facilitators can encourage students to learn and use each other's names, reinforcing peer recognition and accountability. These subtle practices help students see each other as collaborators rather than competitors and create a sense of shared ownership over the learning experience.

As PBL sessions progress, facilitators must monitor group interactions carefully and be ready to intervene when necessary to maintain a healthy and productive learning climate (Heron, 1999). Interventions might include drawing out quieter students who may be hesitant to speak, moderating dominating voices who unintentionally stifle contributions from others, or helping the group constructively navigate disagreements. When facilitators observe imbalances in participation, gently pointing them out can prompt the group to self-correct. For example, a facilitator might say, "I have noticed that we have not heard much from Ji-yoon or Marquis today. I wonder if they have thoughts to add." This kind of cue encourages students to reflect on their group process and reengage peers in a respectful and supportive way.

Facilitators also play an important role in helping students develop the collaboration skills needed for effective teamwork. Early in the PBL process, this may involve introducing students to concrete process structures, such as assigning rotating roles like timekeeper, scribe, or discussion leader. Facilitators can also support the development of group norms by inviting students to co-create agreements about participation, listening, and respectful dialogue. Additionally, they can model how to question ideas without questioning individuals, helping students learn how to challenge one another intellectually while maintaining a collegial tone (Azer, 2005). As students grow in their ability to manage their own group process, the facilitator gradually steps back, assuming more of a coaching role while allowing students to take greater responsibility for their interactions.

Facilitators must also be equipped to recognize and respond to common group challenges. Typical difficulties include unequal participation, dominance by one or two members, lack of cohesion or trust among group members, avoidance of conflict or critical discussion, rushing to conclusions without sufficient exploration, or getting stuck on a particular issue and losing forward momentum. These challenges are not unusual in collaborative learning environments and should not be interpreted as failure. Instead, they present opportunities for facilitators to guide the group in developing greater awareness and skill in managing group dynamics. When such issues arise repeatedly, the facilitator must help the group reflect on their process and identify ways to improve their collective functioning (Hmelo-Silver & Barrows, 2006). These conversations can be embedded within the session or held as focused reflections at the end of the meeting. Encouraging students to evaluate how they are working together is a step toward metacognitive growth and group maturity.

In addition to monitoring in-the-moment interactions, facilitators should take a longitudinal perspective on group development. This means observing how the group evolves across multiple sessions. Are patterns of exclusion, silence, or tension becoming entrenched? Or is the group demonstrating increased synergy, mutual support, and capacity to manage themselves effectively? Keeping brief notes after each session can help facilitators track group progress and identify areas of strength and concern. These notes can inform facilitation strategies for future sessions and provide a record to consult when issues persist. In cases where challenges are chronic or resistant to in-session interventions, it may be necessary to meet with individual students outside of class to better understand underlying issues and collaboratively develop strategies for resolution.

Ultimately, the ability to skillfully facilitate group dynamics is not innate. It is a professional competency that develops through reflective practice over time (Schön, 1983). Facilitators build this capacity by experimenting with different approaches, observing the effects of their interventions, and engaging in continuous self-assessment. Talking with colleagues, participating in professional development, and sharing case examples of challenging group situations can further enrich this learning process. With experience, facilitators cultivate a repertoire of strategies that allow them to both proactively create conditions for successful collaboration and respond flexibly to emerging issues. As facilitators grow in their ability to support productive group dynamics, they help students not only achieve deeper learning in the moment but also build essential skills for future collaborative work in professional and academic settings.

3.2.4 Asking Effective Questions

Asking questions that stimulate students' thinking and encourage deep exploration is at the heart of successful problem-based learning facilitation. The types of questions facilitators pose significantly impact the quality of student reasoning, the richness of group discussion, and the depth of conceptual understanding that emerges over time (Zhang et al., 2010). Developing the ability to craft and sequence effective questions is not merely a technique but a pedagogical art. It requires intentional practice, self-awareness, and iterative refinement based on feedback and reflection.

Many new facilitators struggle to move beyond the traditional pattern of posing closed, convergent questions that aim for a specific correct answer (Azer, 2005). This default mode, shaped by years of experience in conventional didactic teaching environments, tends to inhibit exploratory dialogue. In contrast, PBL thrives on questions that are open-ended, nuanced, and generative. These types of questions invite students to articulate their reasoning, consider multiple possibilities, examine evidence, and engage with complexity in meaningful ways.

Effective questions in PBL share several hallmark qualities (Hmelo-Silver & Barrows, 2006; Zhang et al., 2010). First, they are open-ended and thought-provoking, prompting a range of potential responses rather than a single right answer. Second, they are clearly worded, avoiding jargon and ambiguity that might derail comprehension. Third, they connect to students' prior knowledge and experiences, which helps ground new learning in familiar contexts. Fourth, they are strategically sequenced to support cognitive scaffolding, moving learners from surface-level understanding to deeper synthesis. Finally, effective questions are responsive as they evolve based on students' ideas, confusions, and discoveries.

This shift toward generative questioning can be challenging for new facilitators. Many are accustomed to guiding students toward predetermined outcomes rather than supporting exploratory processes. In PBL, however, the facilitator's role is to elicit student reasoning, not to deliver content. This entails asking questions that surface students' mental models, uncover assumptions, and encourage evidence-based reasoning (Torp & Sage, 2002). For example, instead of asking, "What is the most common cause of this patient's symptom?" a facilitator might ask:

- "What are some possible explanations for the patient's presentation based on the information we have so far?"

- "What do you think is happening pathophysiologically, and why?"
- "What additional data would help confirm or rule out our hypotheses?"

These types of questions stimulate dialogue, require justification of ideas, and promote critical thinking. They also invite students to engage with the uncertainty inherent in clinical reasoning, a key aspect of professional preparation.

Effective questioning also involves thoughtful sequencing. Facilitators must not only ask good questions but also ask the right kinds of questions at the right time (Azer, 2005; Zhang et al., 2010). Questions should guide students through a gradual deepening of understanding, moving from initial comprehension to higher-order analysis and synthesis. A well-sequenced questioning approach typically includes the following progression:

1. Clarifying questions that help the group identify what is known and unknown.
    - "What are the key facts presented in this case?"
    - "What assumptions might we be making without realizing it?"
2. Probing questions that encourage examination of mechanisms and relationships.
    - "What pathophysiological processes could explain these findings?"
    - "How does this symptom relate to what we know about the underlying system?"
3. Hypothesizing questions that prompt students to generate and evaluate possible explanations or diagnoses.
    - "What conditions might fit this clinical picture?"
    - "What patterns are emerging as we consider the evidence?"
4. Evaluating questions that help the group critically appraise their reasoning and evidence.
    - "How confident are we in this line of thinking, and why?"
    - "What would we do if our initial hypothesis is not supported?"
5. Synthesizing questions that encourage integration and abstraction.
    - "How does this case connect to other topics we have studied?"
    - "What broader principles can we take from this discussion?"

While this sequence provides a helpful scaffold, experienced facilitators understand that questioning in PBL is dynamic and nonlinear. They adapt based on students' responses and the emergent needs of the group (Hmelo-Silver & Barrows, 2006). This demands careful listening, patience, and a willingness to relinquish control over the direction of the discussion. Facilitators must read the room, notice when students are stuck or coasting, and respond in ways that either reframe the issue or push the group deeper.

Equally important is the facilitator's ability to model inquiry. Students often learn how to ask better questions by watching facilitators do so. This includes demonstrating curiosity, intellectual humility, and a comfort with uncertainty. When facilitators encounter a student comment or question they cannot immediately answer, they can use it as an opportunity to model collaborative problem-solving. Rather than feeling pressure to supply the answer, a facilitator might respond, "That's a great question, and I am not sure. What resources could we consult to explore that further?" In doing so, facilitators reinforce the idea that learning is a shared journey.

Developing expertise in questioning takes time and practice. Facilitators benefit from a range of professional development strategies, including:

- Observing experienced facilitators and noting how they pose and follow up on questions.
- Debriefing PBL sessions with peers or mentors, specifically analyzing which questions worked well and which fell flat.
- Recording one's facilitation and reviewing it with a focus on questioning techniques and student responses.
- Engaging in peer coaching, where facilitators support one another in experimenting with new questioning strategies.
- Participating in workshops or training sessions focused specifically on the art and science of questioning.

Reflection is also key. Facilitators should regularly ask themselves: What kinds of questions do I tend to ask? Do they promote exploration or shut it down? Are students doing most of the cognitive work, or am I? Where did the conversation spark, and what might have caused that? By engaging in metacognitive practices about their own facilitation, educators can improve not only the form but also the function of their questions (Schön, 1983).

Ultimately, asking effective questions is foundational to fostering self-directed learning, critical thinking, and collaborative inquiry. Questions serve not only as prompts for thought but also as scaffolds that support the construction of knowledge. Facilitators who master this skill help students develop the habits of mind needed to navigate complex problems and uncertain terrain, which are skills that are indispensable in professional practice. As students respond to well-crafted questions, they learn to formulate their own, further internalizing the processes of inquiry and reflection that define lifelong learning.

3.2.5 Gaining Confidence in PBL Facilitation

Building confidence as a PBL facilitator is a developmental journey marked by repeated cycles of experience, reflection, and growth. Unlike traditional teaching, where authority and knowledge delivery may feel more straightforward, PBL facilitation demands comfort with ambiguity, responsiveness to group dynamics, and trust in the students' capacity to take ownership of their learning. Developing these skills and the confidence to use them well takes time and deliberate support. New facilitators should be offered multiple opportunities to practice in low-stakes environments with the safety net of mentorship and timely feedback. Over time, as facilitators gain more experience and reflect on both their successes and challenges, they begin to develop their own facilitation style grounded in self-awareness, pedagogical clarity, and increasing self-assurance.

Many successful PBL training programs employ a scaffolded progression of learning experiences to support this confidence-building process (Salinitri et al., 2015). Typically, this training unfolds in four stages: observing experienced facilitators, co-facilitating with a mentor, facilitating independently while receiving close guidance, and eventually facilitating independently with periodic feedback and reflection. Each phase contributes incrementally to the facilitator's growth, allowing them to internalize essential strategies and principles in a supported environment (Fig. 3.1).

The early stages of observation and co-facilitation are particularly valuable. Watching an experienced facilitator in action allows new facilitators to see how theoretical knowledge about PBL translates into real-time instructional decisions. They witness how experienced facilitators set the tone for collaborative inquiry, manage group dynamics, and pose effective questions that guide student reasoning (Azer, 2005). During co-facilitation, novices take on partial responsibility for leading discussions while being supported by a more experienced colleague. This shared responsibility reduces pressure while still providing meaningful opportunities to engage with the facilitation process.

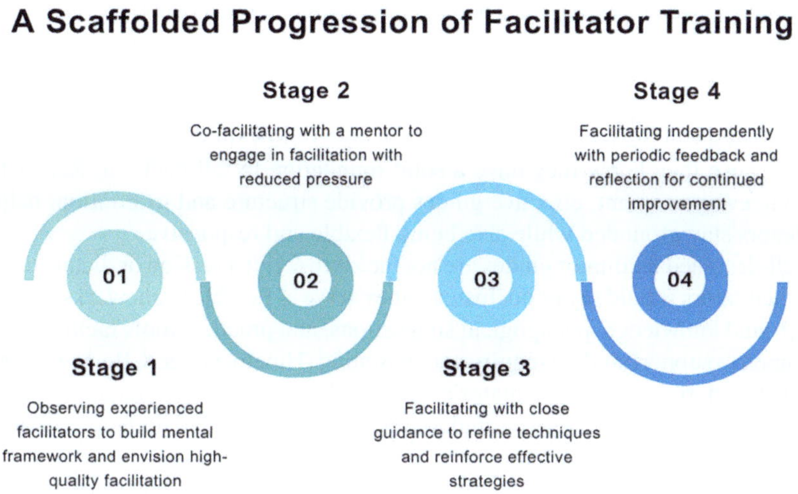

Fig. 3.1 A typical PBL facilitator training unfolds in four stages

Equally important are the debriefing conversations that follow each session. These reflective dialogues should occur as soon as possible after the session and serve several essential purposes. First, they allow the experienced facilitator to explain their decision-making in specific moments, thereby making tacit pedagogical knowledge visible to the novice. Second, they provide strengths-based feedback to reinforce the effective strategies the new facilitator used. Third, they create a space for brainstorming alternative approaches and refining techniques for future sessions. Finally, they normalize the emotional experience of facilitating by acknowledging that it is common to feel uncertain or overwhelmed at the beginning (Azer, 2005).

In these debriefs, experienced facilitators should be intentional in noticing and affirming moments when the novice facilitator made positive contributions, even if these were small or imperfectly executed. Drawing attention to early successes, such as a well-timed question, a thoughtful redirection, or an empathetic response to student uncertainty, can build the novice's sense of competence. According to Heath and Heath (2010), recognizing and amplifying bright spots helps individuals build on what works and sustain motivation during the learning process.

Throughout the training journey, it is also essential to cultivate a growth mindset among new facilitators. Based on the work of Dweck (2006), a growth mindset emphasizes the belief that abilities can be developed through effort, feedback, and learning. Facilitators who adopt this mindset are more likely to view challenges and mistakes as natural parts of the process rather than signs of failure. Phrases like "I am not yet comfortable with managing silence" or "I have not yet mastered questioning techniques" reflect a constructive orientation toward learning. Encouraging this kind of thinking fosters resilience and openness to feedback.

Another foundational support for building facilitator confidence is the availability of high-quality instructional tools and resources. One of the most effective resources is a thoughtfully developed facilitator guide. These guides often include learning objectives, key content knowledge, sample questions, anticipated misconceptions, and suggestions for guiding discussions (Watson et al., 2018). Facilitators who feel well prepared with such materials are more likely to allow students to take intellectual risks because they know they have a solid foundation to fall back on. Rather than scripting every moment, effective guides provide structure and inspiration, helping facilitators stay grounded while also being flexible and responsive.

Well-designed facilitator guides are not meant to script a session or dictate exactly what facilitators should say or do. Instead, they serve as flexible frameworks that offer background knowledge, pedagogical suggestions, and practical tools facilitators can draw upon to support student inquiry and reasoning (Hmelo-Silver & Barrows, 2006). Rather than narrowing the facilitator's options, these guides are intended to expand them, offering multiple ways to stimulate student thinking and maintain a productive, learner-centered discussion.

A well-constructed guide might include several key elements, such as the learning objectives for the case, the central concepts students are expected to explore, and suggested strategies for launching the discussion in an engaging way. It may also offer diagnostic questions that facilitators can use to check for student understanding, propose analogies or examples that clarify complex concepts if confusion arises, and recommend wrap-up questions to help students synthesize and reflect on what they have learned.

As facilitators gain experience and begin to internalize the underlying logic of these strategies, their reliance on facilitator guides typically decreases. Rather than using them as step-by-step instructions, confident facilitators come to view the guides as resources they can consult when faced with uncertainty or when preparing for particularly complex discussions. In this way, the guides evolve from being a lifeline to a source of inspiration and reassurance.

Ultimately, a facilitator's confidence stems from more than just familiarity with a guide. It is grounded in a well-developed philosophy of PBL and a robust set of facilitation strategies that are thoughtfully aligned with the goals of student-centered education (Torp & Sage, 2002). Confident facilitators can explain the reasoning behind their choices, link their in-the-moment decisions to broader learning outcomes, and maintain composure even in the midst of ambiguity. They recognize that intellectual struggle is a vital component of deep learning and can tolerate the discomfort that arises when students are working through difficult ideas. At the same time, they are skilled at identifying when scaffolding is needed and know how to provide timely support that moves students forward without taking over the learning process (Hmelo-Silver & Barrows, 2008).

This kind of nuanced professional judgment is not acquired overnight. It is developed through repeated cycles of deliberate practice, critical feedback, and reflective inquiry (Schön, 1983). Over time, facilitators evolve from following rigid protocols to demonstrating adaptive expertise, a hallmark of teaching professionals who can flexibly tailor their approach to meet the diverse and shifting needs of students. As Bransford et al. (2005) describe, these facilitators are able to creatively draw from a broad repertoire of facilitation moves and combine them in innovative ways to foster meaningful, context specific learning.

3.3 Informal and Formal Evaluation of the Facilitator

Ongoing facilitator evaluation is essential for promoting continuous growth and ensuring high-quality PBL experience for students. Evaluation offers facilitators meaningful feedback on their current practices and provides direction for their continued development.

An effective evaluation system should be multidimensional, combining both informal and formal approaches and incorporating input from multiple data sources (Salinitri et al., 2015). This comprehensive strategy helps build a more accurate and holistic understanding of each facilitator's strengths and areas for improvement. A well-rounded evaluation system typically includes (Fig. 3.2):

- Informal peer observations and follow-up conversation
- Formal performance reviews with a supervisor or PBL program director
- Student feedback surveys

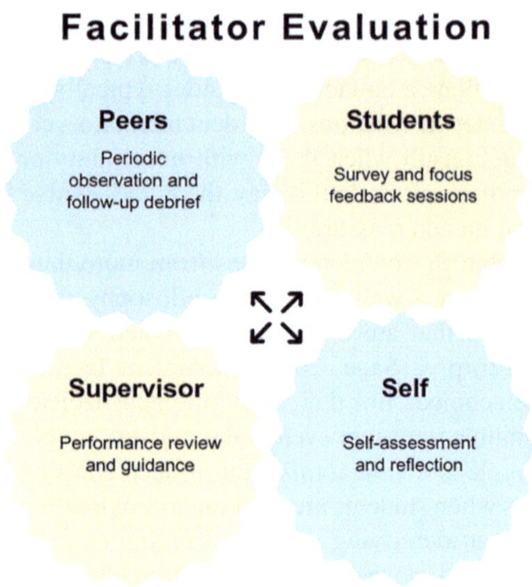

Fig. 3.2 A comprehensive facilitator evaluation system typically includes peer, student, supervisor and self-assessments

- Facilitator self-assessment and critical reflection

Informal peer observations should be scheduled periodically across the academic year. In these settings, facilitators observe each other's sessions and exchange formative, collegial feedback (Azer, 2005). These observations support facilitator development by exposing faculty to a variety of facilitation styles and strategies. Observing how a peer navigates a difficult group dynamic or poses an insightful, open-ended question can spark ideas that the observer can adapt for their own sessions.

The impact of peer observations is greatest when they occur in a climate of trust and psychological safety (Edmondson, 1999). Participants should begin by establishing shared agreements regarding the purpose of the observation, the areas of focus, and the norms for delivering and receiving feedback. Observations should be explicitly formative in nature, with feedback centered on facilitation practices rather than content expertise. Feedback conversations should begin with affirmations before moving into suggestions for improvement.

After the session, the observer and observed facilitator should meet promptly to debrief while the experience is still fresh (Salinitri et al., 2015). The facilitator being observed begins by offering a self-reflection, highlighting what they felt went well and noting any challenges they encountered. The observer can then provide specific feedback, pointing out examples of effective facilitation and suggesting alternative approaches. This debrief should be an open dialogue focused on learning, rather than a unidirectional critique.

On the formal side, facilitators should engage in annual performance reviews with their supervisor or the PBL program director (Azer, 2005). These reviews are an opportunity to reflect on the facilitator's growth over time and to set goals for continued development. Input should be gathered from various sources, including peer observation notes and student feedback to inform the review process.

Student feedback surveys are commonly used to gather learners' perspectives on facilitation quality (Salinitri et al., 2015). These surveys may assess areas such as:

- The facilitator's skill in asking effective questions
- The ability to promote critical thinking
- Responsiveness to student questions and needs
- Creation of a supportive learning environment
- Fairness in assessment and feedback

Although student feedback offers important insights, it should never serve as the sole data point in facilitator evaluation. Research shows that student evaluations can be influenced by extraneous variables such as a facilitator's gender, race, or personality traits and may not always correlate with actual teaching effectiveness (Fan et al., 2019). Therefore, student feedback should be viewed as one of several complementary sources of data.

Formal performance reviews should also include facilitator self-assessment and structured reflection (Torp & Sage, 2002). Facilitators should be prompted to critically examine their own practice, identify strengths and challenges, and articulate goals for the future. Supervisors can guide these reflections with targeted questions, such as:

- What aspects of your facilitation are you most proud of this year?
- What has been your most significant facilitation challenge, and how have you addressed it?
- How has your facilitation philosophy developed over time?
- What specific goals do you have for the upcoming year?
- What resources or support would help you achieve those goals?

The outcome of the annual review should be a personalized professional learning plan. This plan outlines the facilitator's goals, the steps they will take to reach them, and the resources or support they will need (Azer, 2005). This may include attending specific workshops, engaging in a peer observation cycle focused on a targeted skill, or partnering with a mentor for guidance and accountability.

Importantly, the annual review should not be treated as a standalone event. Supervisors and facilitators should meet periodically throughout the year to revisit goals, assess progress, and make adjustments as needed. Celebrating small wins and acknowledging growth along the way reinforces a culture of continuous improvement and reflection. In the long term, this approach cultivates habits of self-awareness and adaptability that facilitators carry throughout their professional journey.

3.4 Delivering Feedback for Improvement

Delivering constructive feedback is a core facilitator skill that plays a vital role in student growth. When done well, feedback helps learners recognize blind spots, affirm their progress, and gain the tools they need to advance their learning (Hattie & Timperley, 2007). Yet many facilitators find feedback conversations challenging, especially when trying to balance honesty with encouragement.

Effective feedback is (Fig. 3.3):

- Specific and actionable
- Timely and ongoing
- Based on observable behaviors
- Delivered with empathy and respect

Specificity is one of the most important features of helpful feedback (Wiggins, 2012). Vague comments like "nice job" or "this needs work" do not guide students toward improvement. In contrast, specific feedback names the exact behavior observed and suggests alternatives for future situations. For instance, rather than saying a student showed "strong critical thinking," a facilitator might offer: "I noticed how you asked the group several probing questions that led them to reexamine their assumptions. That shifted the conversation in a valuable direction. What if you made a habit of asking those kinds of questions earlier in our discussions?" This approach highlights an effective behavior, explains its impact, and encourages continued use.

Feedback should also be timely and closely connected to the learning experience (Brookhart, 2008). Immediate feedback helps students make adjustments while the context is still fresh. However, facilitators must also consider the learner's emotional readiness. If the feedback is sensitive or likely to trigger strong reactions, it may be better to wait and deliver it in a private, reflective setting. Timing is always a balance between urgency and the student's ability to receive the message.

Grounding feedback in observable data makes it more credible and helpful. Referencing specific student comments, behaviors, or trends over time strengthens the feedback and avoids generalizations. It helps students understand how their actions are perceived and connects feedback to shared experiences rather than subjective judgment (Brookhart, 2008).

At its heart, effective feedback is rooted in care and respect for the learner (Boud & Molloy, 2013). Facilitators must be attentive not only to the message itself but to how it is delivered. Students are far more open to feedback when they feel valued and supported. An empathetic approach helps create a climate of psychological safety that encourages growth and reflection.

Simple relational strategies can make a difference. These include expressing appreciation for the student's effort, asking permission to share feedback, and acknowledging the vulnerability that comes with being evaluated (Johnson & Johnson, 2009). Feedback should always be focused on behaviors rather than character, and it should be framed as an opportunity for development rather than a final

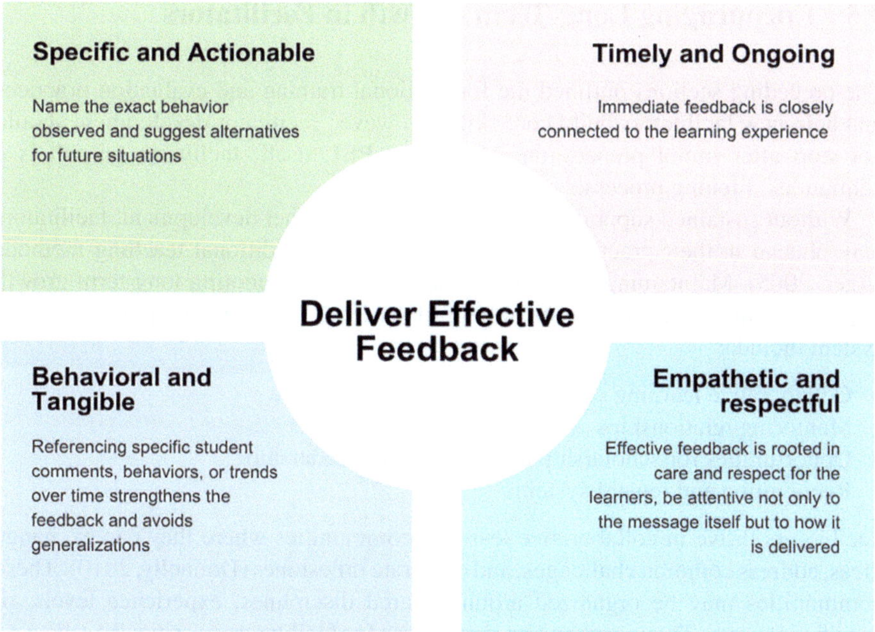

Fig. 3.3 Features of effective feedback include: specific and actionable, timely and ongoing, behavioral and tangible, empathetic and respectful

judgment. Embracing a growth mindset positions feedback as part of a continuous learning journey (Dweck, 2006).

Facilitators should also be sensitive to power dynamics and cultural influences that shape how feedback is interpreted (Ramani et al., 2019). In some cultures, feedback from authority figures carries significant weight, and even gently worded comments may be perceived as strong criticism. Learners who have experienced marginalization or bias may be particularly wary of feedback and concerned about fairness. Taking time to understand students' feedback histories and adapting communication accordingly is key.

Occasionally, facilitators must give feedback about sensitive issues, such as disruptive group behavior or unprofessional conduct (Bearman et al., 2013). In these situations, privacy and care are essential. These conversations should be unhurried and respectful, with facilitators using "I" statements to describe what they observed and how it affected the group. The goal is to invite the students' perspective, explore possible solutions, and collaboratively develop an action plan for moving forward.

Delivering feedback is a skill that takes time to master. Facilitators may not always get it exactly right, and that is part of the learning process. What matters most is approaching feedback with humility, empathy, and a sincere commitment to student growth. When facilitators model openness and reflection in these conversations, they help students do the same.

3.5 Encouraging Long-Term Growth in Facilitators

The preceding sections outlined the foundational training and evaluation practices that help new facilitators build core skills. However, facilitator development should not stop after initial preparation. Much like PBL itself, facilitator growth is a continuous, lifelong process.

Without sustained support and opportunities for further development, facilitators may plateau in their practice or even revert to more traditional teaching methods (Azer, 2005). Maintaining facilitator engagement and promoting long-term growth requires a multi-faceted institutional approach (Fig. 3.4). Key components of this system include:

- Collaborative learning communities
- Mentoring relationships
- Opportunities for scholarship and educational leadership
- Recognition and reward systems

Facilitators thrive in collaborative learning communities where they can exchange ideas, address common challenges, and celebrate milestones (Donnelly, 2010). These communities may be organized around shared disciplines, experience levels, or specific interests. They serve as ongoing spaces for facilitators to critically reflect on their practice and connect it to educational theory and evidence.

The most effective learning communities strike a balance between structure and flexibility. They may include regular meetings, shared readings, and protocols for discussion. At the same time, they remain responsive to participants' evolving needs. Experienced facilitators within the group often take on roles as conveners, posing thoughtful questions and guiding reflective dialogue.

Pairing facilitators with experienced mentors is another highly effective strategy for long-term professional growth (White et al., 2009). Mentoring offers individualized support, helping facilitators navigate complex situations, refine their approaches, and plan for future development. Mentors serve as thought partners, encouraging reflection, goal setting, and strategic action.

Trust is foundational to successful mentoring relationships. Both mentor and mentee must be committed to open and honest dialogue. Mentors should also be attuned to power dynamics and cultural influences that may shape the mentee's experiences and expectations (Ramani et al., 2019).

Beyond one-on-one support, institutions play a critical role in fostering a culture that values educational excellence. Facilitators should be encouraged to engage in the scholarship of teaching and learning by investigating questions about PBL and sharing their findings with broader audiences (Boyer, 1990). Activities such as presenting at conferences, publishing in educational journals, and leading workshops help raise the visibility and legitimacy of facilitation as a scholarly endeavor.

Institutions can further support facilitator development by creating clear pathways to educational leadership (Irby et al., 2020). Opportunities may include:

- Mentoring or coaching new facilitators

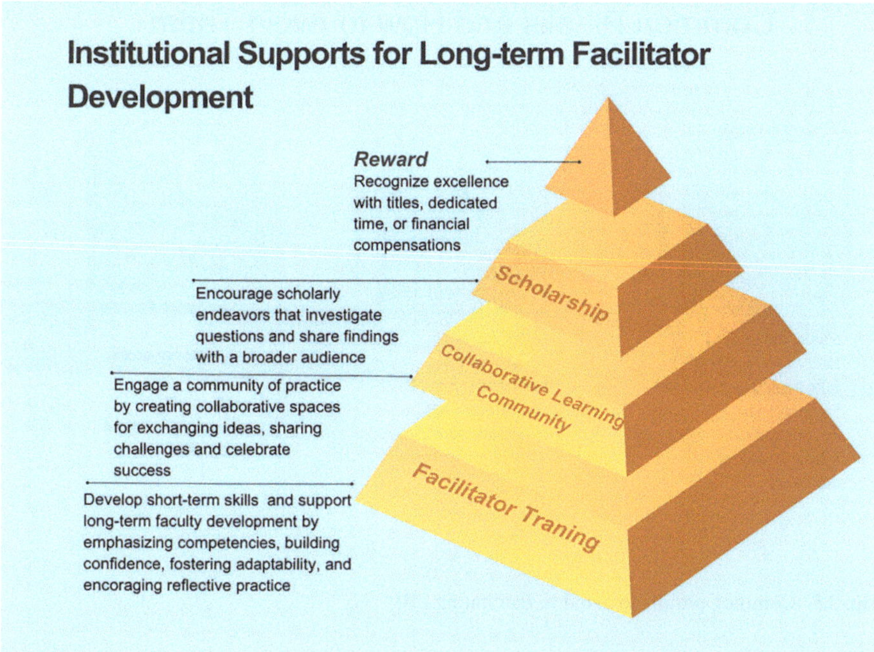

Fig. 3.4 Institutional support for long-term facilitator development is a multi-faceted system

- Leading the design or revision of PBL cases
- Coordinating facilitator development programs
- Participating in educational committees or working groups
- Leading scholarship of teaching and learning initiatives

When these roles come with formal recognition such as titles, dedicated time, or financial compensation, they send a strong signal that facilitation and educational leadership are valued contributions to the institution's mission.

Long-term facilitator development is essential for the sustainability and vitality of PBL programs. When facilitators are supported in their own learning, they are better positioned to create engaging, student-centered learning environments. Ultimately, investing in facilitator growth is an investment in educational excellence.

3.6 Pitfalls

Even the most experienced and skilled PBL facilitators can encounter challenges that hinder student learning. Surprisingly, several studies have observed that student learning outcomes may decline as facilitators gain experience (Leary et al., 2013; Azer, 2005). While the causes of this trend are not definitively known, several

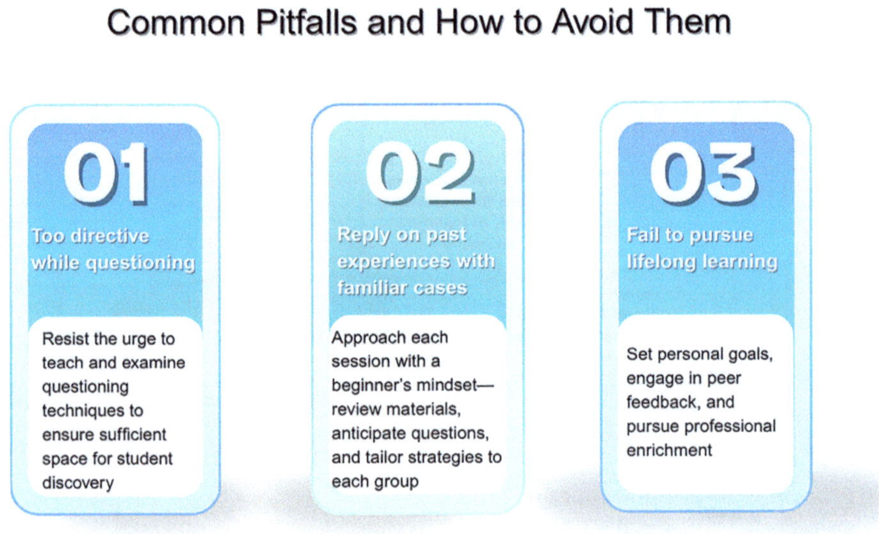

Fig. 3.5 Common pitfalls to avoid in facilitating PBL

plausible explanations have emerged, along with strategies facilitators can adopt to address them (Fig. 3.5).

One common pitfall is that as facilitators develop deeper content expertise, they may unintentionally become more directive in their facilitation (Leary et al., 2013). With greater subject matter knowledge, facilitators may be tempted to guide students toward "correct" answers or preferred lines of inquiry. This tendency can shift the dynamic from student-centered exploration to facilitator-led instruction, undermining the core principles of PBL.

To counteract this, experienced facilitators must stay grounded in the facilitative role, resisting the urge to teach content. Regular self-reflection is essential; facilitators should examine their questioning techniques and assess whether they are allowing sufficient space for student discovery. Reviewing video recordings of PBL sessions can be a valuable tool for identifying patterns in facilitation style, including the balance of facilitator versus student talk time.

Another helpful strategy is co-facilitation with novice facilitators (Leary et al., 2013). Observing and collaborating with less experienced colleagues can offer fresh perspectives and serve as a reminder of the importance of student autonomy. These partnerships can also spark meaningful reflection and help seasoned facilitators recalibrate their approach.

A second pitfall arises when facilitators become overly comfortable with the PBL process or familiar case materials (Azer, 2005). After guiding students through the same cases multiple times, facilitators may begin to rely on past experience rather than preparing thoughtfully for each new group. This complacency can reduce responsiveness and diminish the quality of the learning experience.

To maintain a high level of engagement, facilitators should approach each session with a beginner's mindset. This involves thoroughly reviewing the case materials, anticipating potential student questions, and tailoring strategies to the needs of each unique group. Getting to know each cohort and building strong relationships fosters trust and enhances the facilitator's ability to offer meaningful, personalized support.

A third challenge is the gradual erosion of facilitators' lifelong learning habits (Hmelo-Silver & Barrows, 2006). As facilitators become more experienced, they may be less likely to seek out new learning opportunities or engage in reflective practice. This can lead to stagnation and limit their capacity to model the curiosity, self-directed learning, and critical thinking that PBL is designed to cultivate.

Institutions play a vital role in mitigating this risk by providing ongoing professional development for facilitators (Fig. 3.2). Opportunities might include workshops on advanced facilitation strategies, journal clubs focused on emerging research, or collaborative educational scholarship projects. Facilitators themselves must also take responsibility for their continued growth by setting personal goals, engaging in peer feedback, and pursuing professional enrichment.

Ultimately, avoiding these pitfalls requires facilitators to stay anchored in the foundational values of PBL: humility, curiosity, continuous improvement, and a deep trust in students' ability to drive their own learning. By reflecting on their practice, soliciting feedback, and engaging in ongoing development, facilitators can continue to evolve and foster meaningful learning experiences.

Addressing these challenges also requires robust institutional support. Institutions must foster a culture that values educational excellence, providing facilitators with the resources, recognition, and time needed to reflect, innovate, and grow. This includes structured opportunities to learn from colleagues, explore new approaches, and engage with current research on PBL and student-centered learning.

By proactively addressing common pitfalls and cultivating supportive conditions for facilitator development, institutions can ensure that PBL remains a dynamic and transformative learning experience. Sustained investment in facilitator growth is an investment in the long-term success and impact of PBL programs and the future of inquiry-driven education.

References

Azer, S. A. (2005). Challenges facing PBL tutors: 12 tips for successful group facilitation. *Medical Teacher, 27*(8), 676–681.

Barrows, H. S., & Tamblyn, R. M. (1980). *Problem-based learning: An approach to medical education.* Springer Publishing Company.

Bearman, M., Molloy, E., Ajjawi, R., & Keating, J. (2013). 'Is there a Plan B?': Clinical educators supporting underperforming students in practice settings. *Teaching in Higher Education, 18*(5), 531–544.

Boud, D., & Molloy, E. (2013). Rethinking models of feedback for learning: The challenge of design. *Assessment & Evaluation in Higher Education, 38*(6), 698–712.

Boyer, E. L. (1990). *Scholarship reconsidered: Priorities of the professoriate*. Carnegie Foundation for the Advancement of Teaching.
Bransford, J. D., Brown, A. L., & Cocking, R. R. (2005). *How people learn: Brain, mind, experience, and school*. National Academies Press.
Bridges, S., Botelho, M., Green, J. L., & Chau, A. C. M. (2012). Multimodality in problem-based learning (PBL): An interactional ethnography. In S. Bridges, C. McGrath, & T. L. Whitehill (Eds.), *Problem-based learning in clinical education: The next generation* (pp. 99–120). Springer.
Brookhart, S. M. (2008). *How to give effective feedback to your students*. ASCD.
Callis, A. N., McCann, A. L., Schneiderman, E. D., Babler, W. J., Lacy, E. S., & Hale, D. S. (2010). Application of basic science to clinical problems: Traditional vs. hybrid problem-based learning. *Journal of Dental Education, 74*(10), 1113–1124.
De Grave, W. S., Dolmans, D. H., & van der Vleuten, C. P. (1999). Profiles of effective tutors in problem-based learning: Scaffolding student learning. *Medical Education, 33*(12), 901–906.
Dolmans, D. H., Gijselaers, W. H., Moust, J. H., de Grave, W. S., Wolfhagen, I. H., & van der Vleuten, C. P. (2002). Trends in research on the tutor in problem-based learning: Conclusions and implications for educational practice and research. *Medical Teacher, 24*(2), 173–180.
Donnelly, R. (2010). Interaction analysis in a 'learning by doing' problem-based professional development context. *Computers & Education, 55*(3), 1357–1366.
Dweck, C. S. (2006). *Mindset: The new psychology of success*. Random House.
Edmondson, A. (1999). Psychological safety and learning behavior in work teams. *Administrative Science Quarterly, 44*(2), 350–383.
Fan, Y., Shepherd, L. J., Slavich, E., Waters, D., Stone, M., Abel, R., & Johnston, E. L. (2019). Gender and cultural bias in student evaluations: Why representation matters. *PLoS One, 14*(2), e0209749.
Haith-Cooper, M. (2003). An exploration of tutors' experiences of facilitating problem-based learning. Part 2—Implications for the facilitation of problem based learning. *Nurse Education Today, 23*(1), 65–75.
Hattie, J., & Timperley, H. (2007). The power of feedback. *Review of Educational Research, 77*(1), 81–112.
Heath, C., & Heath, D. (2010). *Switch: How to change things when change is hard*. Broadway Books.
Hendry, G. D., Ryan, G., & Harris, J. (2003). Group problems in problem-based learning. *Medical Teacher, 25*(6), 609–616.
Heron, J. (1999). *The complete facilitator's handbook*. Kogan Page.
Hmelo-Silver, C. E. (2004). Problem-based learning: What and how do students learn? *Educational Psychology Review, 16*(3), 235–266.
Hmelo-Silver, C. E., & Barrows, H. S. (2006). Goals and strategies of a problem-based learning facilitator. *Interdisciplinary Journal of Problem-Based Learning, 1*(1), 21–39.
Hmelo-Silver, C. E., & Barrows, H. S. (2008). Facilitating collaborative knowledge building. *Cognition and Instruction, 26*(1), 48–94.
Hmelo-Silver, C. E., Duncan, R. G., & Chinn, C. A. (2007). Scaffolding and achievement in problem-based and inquiry learning: A response to Kirschner, Sweller, and Clark (2006). *Educational Psychologist, 42*(2), 99–107.
Irby, D. M., O'Sullivan, P. S., & Steinert, Y. (2020). Is it time to recognize excellence in faculty development programs? *Medical Teacher, 42*(8), 855–860.
Johnson, D. W., & Johnson, R. T. (2009). An educational psychology success story: Social interdependence theory and cooperative learning. *Educational Researcher, 38*(5), 365–379.
Leary, H., Walker, A., Shelton, B. E., & Fitt, M. H. (2013). Exploring the relationships between tutor background, tutor training, and student learning: A problem-based learning meta-analysis. *Interdisciplinary Journal of Problem-Based Learning, 7*(1), 40–66.
Maudsley, G. (1999). Roles and responsibilities of the problem based learning tutor in the undergraduate medical curriculum. *British Medical Journal (BMJ), 318*(7184), 657–661.

Maudsley, G. (2002). Making sense of trying not to teach: An interview study of tutors' ideas of problem-based learning. *Academic Medicine, 77*(2), 162–172.

Neville, A. J., & Norman, G. R. (2007). PBL in the undergraduate MD program at McMaster University: Three iterations in three decades. *Academic Medicine, 82*(4), 370–374.

Ramani, S., Könings, K. D., Ginsburg, S., & van der Vleuten, C. P. (2019). Twelve tips to promote a feedback culture with a growth mind-set: Swinging the feedback pendulum from recipes to relationships. *Medical Teacher, 41*(6), 625–631.

Salinitri, F. D., Wilhelm, S. M., & Crabtree, B. L. (2015). Facilitating facilitators: Enhancing PBL through a structured facilitator development program. *Interdisciplinary Journal of Problem-Based Learning, 9*(1), 73–82.

Savery, J. R. (2006). Overview of problem-based learning: Definitions and distinctions. *Interdisciplinary Journal of Problem-Based Learning, 1*(1), 9–20.

Savery, J. R., & Duffy, T. M. (1995). Problem based learning: An instructional model and its constructivist framework. *Educational Technology, 35*(5), 31–38.

Schön, D. A. (1983). *The reflective practitioner: How professionals think in action.* Basic Books.

Silén, C. (2006). The tutor's approach in base groups (PBL). *Higher Education, 51*(3), 373–385.

Torp, L., & Sage, S. (2002). *Problems as possibilities: Problem-based learning for K-16 education* (2nd ed.). ASCD.

Watson, S. L., Koehler, A. A., Ertmer, P. A., Kim, W. R., & Rico, R. (2018). Facilitation prompts and rubrics on higher-order thinking skill performance found in undergraduate asynchronous discussion boards. *British Journal of Educational Technology, 49*(5), 969–980.

Wenger, E. (1998). *Communities of practice: Learning, meaning, and identity.* Cambridge University Press.

White, C. B., Kumagai, A. K., Ross, P. T., & Fantone, J. C. (2009). A qualitative exploration of how the conflict between the formal and informal curriculum influences student values and behaviors. *Academic Medicine, 84*(5), 597–603.

Wiggins, G. (2012). Seven keys to effective feedback. *Educational Leadership, 70*(1), 10–16.

Williams, J. C., & Paltridge, D. J. (2017). What we think we know about the tutor in problem-based learning. *Health Professions Education, 3*(1), 26–31.

Zhang, M., Lundeberg, M., & Eberhardt, J. (2010). Strategic facilitation of problem-based discussion for teacher professional development. *Journal of the Learning Sciences, 19*(3), 342–394.

Chapter 4
Student Learning in Problem-Based Learning

Shaan Kunwar

4.1 Introducing the Student to PBL

When effectively implemented, PBL enhances student satisfaction and boosts measured test performance (Trullas et al., 2022). As ongoing performance evaluations yield positive results, educators in healthcare professions have increasingly adopted PBL (Cutrer et al., 2017a; Cabra-Torres et al., 2020).

At its beginning, we start with an introduction to PBL, where students will now be practicing an active form of learning by engaging with real-world problems. This provides the new students with clear expectations of their role (Fig. 4.1).

The introduction should advise students that they will use teamwork to understand the mechanisms of basic medical/health sciences and to uncover questions that will help guide them to the material they need to review to develop their understanding of the basic medical/health sciences. Not only will students be learning the basic medical/health sciences, but they will also learn interpersonal skills. It is beneficial to describe to them the value of developing good interpersonal skills for the future, and how the PBL approach can aid in developing such skills; this prepares them to assess their upcoming group participation. The act of cooperation is useful in allowing students to explore knowledge gaps they may have, both as individuals and as a group. Discussion and discord during group sessions can be used to help guide the individual to personal learning topics needed to understand the problem.

The students should be advised that this is a self-directed form of learning where they are in control of what material they wish to learn and review. They can be advised that being effective in identifying the pertinent material to learn is the essence of PBL.

The students will be introduced to the value of developing the ability to self-assess and identify personal knowledge gaps, an essential skill that will need refinement once group sessions begin. Self-assessment is a skill that, once cultivated, will lead to

S. Kunwar (✉)
Lake Erie College of Osteopathic Medicine, Bradenton, FL, USA
e-mail: skunwar@lecom.edu

S. Lorenzo and B. Zhang (eds.), *Mastering Problem-Based Learning in Health Profession Programs*, https://doi.org/10.1007/978-3-032-05405-0_4

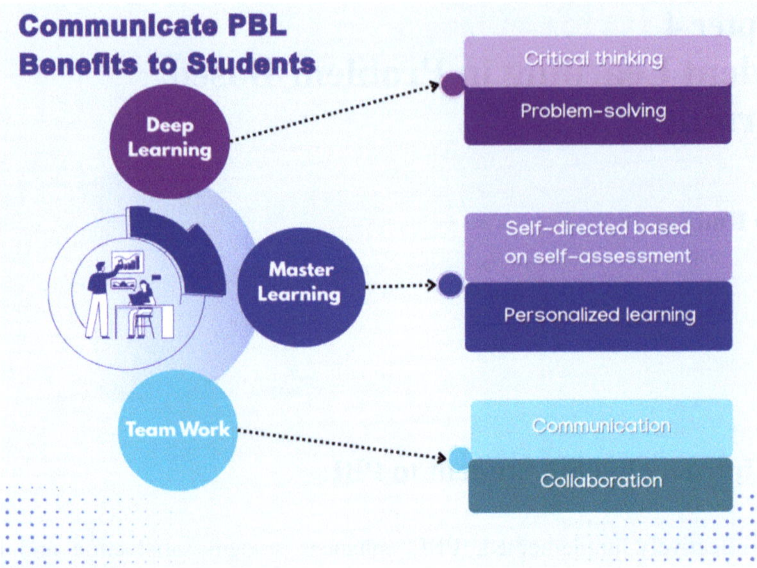

Fig. 4.1 Clearly communicate the benefits of PBL to students when introducing it. Through PBL, students develop a wide range of skills such as deep learning and teamwork

mastering adaptive learning techniques and promote lifelong effective learning. The master adaptive learner employs self-assessment to pinpoint knowledge gaps and then utilizes planning to learn the relevant material from credible, evidence-based resources effectively. They should be informed that this skill will facilitate effective application in clinical practice in the future.

In traditional lecture-based programs, teaching is instructor-centered, where the teacher delivers content through lectures, resulting in passive learning for students who primarily listen and take notes. The curriculum is standardized, with a focus on covering specific content (Hmelo-Silver, 2004). Student learning in this model is limited, as students are often passive recipients of information, focusing on memorization and reviewing material without question, with assignments and exams typically completed individually. Assessment in lecture-based programs is primarily through standardized testing, with summative assessments evaluating learning at the end of a unit or course and providing limited feedback, often focused on grades rather than detailed improvement suggestions.

In contrast, PBL programs place students at the center of their learning experience, with clinical scenarios driving active, hands-on engagement. The curriculum is flexible and often interdisciplinary, allowing it to adapt to students' interests. Collaboration is integral, as students work in groups, fostering communication and teamwork skills. Assessment in PBL programs is performance-based, involving presentations, Facilitator Assessment of Student Performance (FASP) scores, and test performance. Students will be guided towards developing assessment skills for and receiving continuous feedback to guide learning (Reznich & Werner, 2004). This approach provides useful information on both the students' learning process and mastery of basic medical/health sciences as the sessions proceed.

Learning outcomes in lecture-based programs emphasize knowledge retention, with limited focus on developing practical skills. Conversely, PBL programs aim for a deep understanding of concepts, strong skill development in critical thinking, problem-solving, and collaboration, with personalized learning outcomes based on individual learning objectives (Jost et al., 1998).

Classroom environments also differ significantly between lecture-based and PBL programs. Lecture-based programs typically feature a structured setting with fixed seating focused on the teacher, creating a predictable routine of lectures and exams. In these traditional programs, student autonomy is low, as students follow a prescribed curriculum and rely heavily on the teacher. Subjects are treated separately, with focused learning on each, emphasizing direct instruction and standardized knowledge retention. In contrast, PBL sessions are dynamic, following the progression of clinical cases and prompting students to give brief presentations on basic science mechanisms at the start of a session. PBL offers a high level of student autonomy, where students take significant control over their learning. They are responsible for setting learning objectives, making decisions about what to learn, and independently filling knowledge gaps. As will be discussed later, developing a rigorous self-assessment instrument and habit allows the learner to gain insight into what topics the individual needs to learn.

PBL also integrates multiple subjects for a holistic learning experience, connecting concepts across disciplines. Overall, PBL provides an interactive, student-centered approach, emphasizing the application of real-world clinical scenarios and the development of a wide range of skills needed in clinical practice, including problem-solving and interpersonal skills.

Perhaps under-emphasized to students enrolling in a basic medical/health science PBL program is the idea that the students are active stakeholders, along with the administration, in their joint aim to promote active learning for both students and administrators. Further, a partnership exists between the facilitator and the students to foster metacognitive thought and self-analysis. The administration can introduce these concepts to students and, by increasing the awareness of these concepts, will do well to employ what the current research suggests is an underutilized method of increased performance by way of self-assessment. At this level of university training, there is much opportunity to easily introduce students to these concepts they may not be aware of. All PBL facilitators should be interested in coupling metacognitive self-analysis to effectively drive learning guided by the clinical scenarios. To develop the skill of formulating questions and extracting correct pertinent information out of a large volume of similar background information, while budgeting time. A thorough understanding of the student's assessment of the PBL learning process and their engagement in this process will offer a continuous opportunity to promote active learning.

Students and administration share a common goal of promoting active learning, with both acting as key stakeholders in this endeavor. PBL represents a shift from the traditional didactic learning styles that students may be more familiar with. Instead of faculty-led lectures, students will now participate in a PBL group, where they will actively learn both independently and collaboratively, with minimal oversight. Although students may have only a vague understanding of this approach when they enter the program, research has shown that students generally develop positive attitudes toward PBL compared to the traditional format (Cutrer et al., 2017a). This growing preference for PBL explains its increasing adoption in educational settings. Students need to recognize that they are now engaging in a form of collaborative learning that requires active participation.

An important new concept that applies to PBL learning is that students should be made aware of the effort needed to identify personal knowledge gaps in the basic medical/health sciences through questions and self-assessment. Students should use these questions to guide them to the right learning material effectively. The students have 2 years to develop a comprehensive understanding of the basic medical/health sciences for their board exams and given the freedom to self-direct their own learning, they will need to be effective at covering all the testable material. The students understanding must be able to stand up to the heavy testing of biochemistry, physiology, pathology, and pharmacology.

4.1.1 The Importance of a Question

Generating questions is a fundamental component of PBL, it plays a critical role in guiding and advancing the active learning process. It requires curiosity and motivation on the part of the student and drives further inquiry as the students strive to identify and fill knowledge gaps. The process of generating questions about the problem presented promotes critical thinking in the individual and can assist other members of the group to form new questions. Questions can challenge one's assumptions and lead to a more accurate understanding of the topics surrounding the problem. Question asking is also the propellant of the self-directed learning process discussed above. It gives the student direction on what material matters to them most at that moment. When students formulate their own questions, they become invested in finding the answers, fostering critical thinking, and problem-solving skills. These questions provide a clear direction for learning and inquiry, helping students focus their efforts on relevant areas and explore topics more deeply.

Collaboration is further fostered through the practice of question generation, which encourages discussion and the exchange of ideas among team members, drawing on their diverse perspectives and insights (Savin-Baden & Major, 2013). This approach not only supports autonomy and ownership by empowering students to take control of their learning process but also ensures that the questions are personally meaningful, thereby enhancing motivation. Additionally, the act of generating questions promotes reflection and metacognition, as it prompts students to assess their current knowledge, identify gaps, and develop strategies for improvement (Fig. 4.2).

For many students, PBL will be a new experience with little to no prior exposure. As PBL sessions commence and students participate in group activities, facilitators

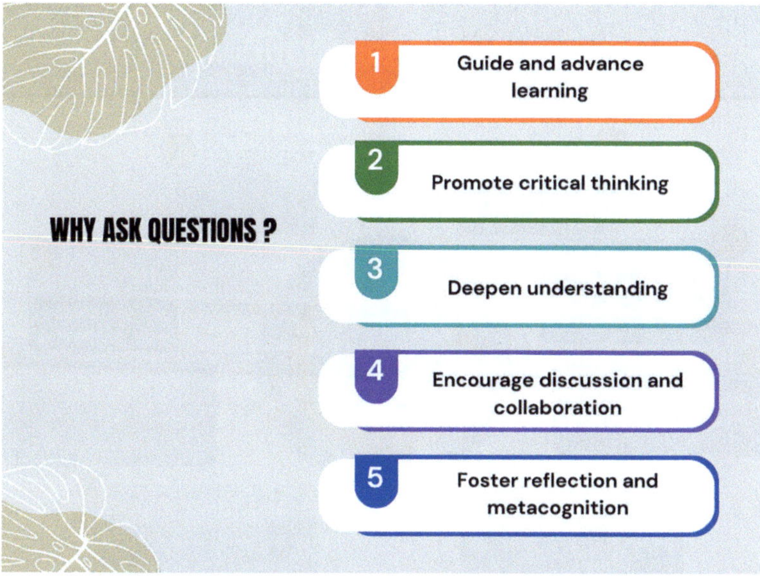

Fig. 4.2 The importance of asking questions in PBL includes guiding and advancing learning, promoting critical thinking, deepening understanding, encouraging discussion and collaboration, and fostering reflection and metacognition

should be mindful of the common challenges that have historically arisen in PBL environments (Al-Shaikh et al., 2015).

4.2 The PBL Learning Journey

The cyclical process of mastering problem-based learning aligns with master adaptive learning (Fig. 4.3).

PBL fosters a cycle of continuous improvement, guiding students to refine their skills and knowledge through repeated practice. This iterative process, often referred to as the "master adaptive learner" (MAL) model, helps students identify, address, and reassess their understanding and performance over time. The steps outlined below illustrate this adaptive learning cycle (Vernon & Blake, 1993; Kolmos et al., 2008):

1. **Planning**: Establishing clear objectives for each case or learning session.
2. **Identifying Performance Gaps**: Recognizing areas requiring improvement, whether in knowledge, skill, or attitude.
3. **Prioritizing Gaps**: Determining which gaps need immediate attention and are most crucial to address.
4. **Searching for Resources**: Identifying credible sources to fill the knowledge gaps.

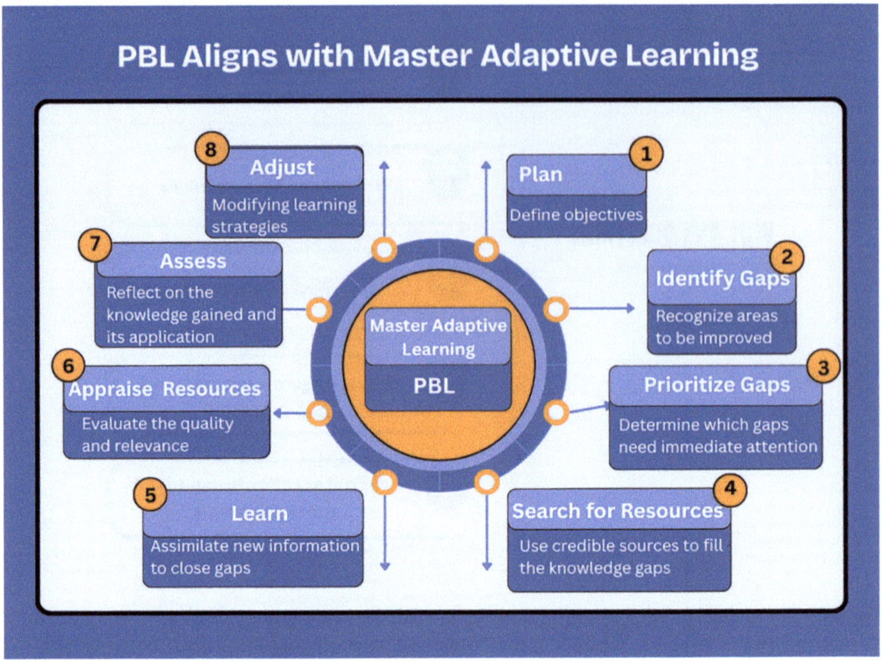

Fig. 4.3 PBL aligns well with the framework of master adaptive learning, as both involve planning, identifying gaps, learning, assessing, and adjusting

5. **Learning**: Assimilating new information to expand understanding and close gaps in knowledge.
6. **Critical Appraisal of Learning Resources**: Evaluating the quality and relevance of the chosen resources to ensure they effectively meet learning needs.
7. **Assessing**: Reflecting on the knowledge gained and its application to the case or broader understanding.
8. **Adjusting**: Modifying learning strategies based on reflection and assessment.
9. **Repeating the Cycle**: Revisiting these steps continuously to build expertise and deepen comprehension.

The above phases represent the core processes of the Master Adaptive Learning cycle, demonstrating adaptive learning in practice. While students in a PBL program are encouraged to seek appraised learning resources through structured recommendations, they still retain the flexibility to explore additional resources independently. The focus is on the active process of learning, particularly on understanding how learning occurs. By refining these strategies, students acquire the foundational skills necessary for lifelong learning—essential for healthcare providers who regularly face new information, evolving medical practices, and complex challenges. Developing these skills—critical thinking, self-direction, adaptability, effective communication, collaboration, and information literacy—requires motivation, curiosity, time, and effort. Mastery of this adaptive cycle equips students to remain flexible and responsive in real-world settings, where effective problem-solving is essential to everyday practice.

4.3 Overcoming Challenges in Student Learning

4.3.1 Challenges Students Face in PBL

4.3.1.1 Student Engagement

Historically, challenges have been identified in PBL that can impact student learning (Dolmans et al., 2005). The first challenge encountered is getting students to engage in active learning. In PBL, the learning process begins with a question. The question serves as a guide and motivation to acquire new information. Students need to learn how to ask these questions, as they will drive their learning forward. The questions generated during a PBL session become the key to understanding basic sciences. While students may be accustomed to reading assigned material passively, learning to ask questions is crucial for transforming passive learning into an active, self-directed process. The case scenario presented in a PBL session provides the material for the group to engage with and question.

4.3.1.2 Self-Reliance and the Role of the Facilitator

During these first encounters, students find themselves searching for answers without their regular support structure, which is the teacher. With the facilitator available only to provide questions when necessary, students must rely on themselves and their group to explore the problem presented. This is often a slow process at first, and the first session's closing remarks by each member can provide valuable feedback to the new students. This feedback reassures them that self-reliance is being evaluated, and emphasizes that this skill will develop over time and with repetition.

4.3.1.3 Selecting Learning Materials and Group Collaboration

In the initial PBL sessions, students often identify the selection of learning material as a challenge. The autonomy of self-directed learning comes with the challenge of lacking direct guidance from a teacher or faculty. Students may struggle with finding where to start when learning material pertinent to a new problem is presented or may have doubts about the context of the materials they've chosen. To address this, students are encouraged to work together to find common ground on relevant topics and knowledge gaps. The curriculum itself is often organized into blocks or themes that can provide further direction. In these early phases, students should be advised that broad learning of basic medical/health sciences is appropriate, and that the role of the facilitator is to prevent valuable time from being lost in sessions. This guidance reassures students and enhances their performance.

4.3.1.4 Navigating the Transition from Traditional Learning

Paradoxically, this independence is both a strength of PBL and a source of anxiety for many students. In traditional learning environments, students typically attend lectures where they are provided with all the required materials. However, in PBL, they must independently navigate their learning. Students will need to identify their personal basic medical/health science knowledge gaps. This can be a challenge for those accustomed to more traditional learning methods. It's important to note that there is no single "correct" sequence for learning basic medical/health science concepts. Each student will have a unique knowledge base and distinct gaps to address. As students develop the skill of asking questions, they will drive their acquisition of the foundational knowledge necessary for understanding the basic sciences. Students who struggle with self-direction may benefit from focusing on the content covered in group sessions, which can serve as a guide for further study. The robust list of questions and learning topics, when recorded and shared, provides direction while allowing students the flexibility to choose their study materials. During sessions, students can support each other by generating questions and collaboratively finding answers.

4.3.1.5 The Impact of Group Dynamics

Apart from the selection of learning materials and question generation, another challenge is the group dynamic. Students will vary in their degree of engagement due to factors such as personality types, personal experiences, and work habits. Some students may engage more actively than others, which can cause distractions from the clinical scenario being discussed. To address this, students are given time at the end of each session to reflect on how the session has progressed. Facilitators can also discuss strategies to improve the group's dynamics. Additionally, students should be reminded that working with a group is a skill to develop, one that will be essential in their future professions.

4.3.1.6 Choosing and Citing Reliable Learning Resources

A further challenge in PBL is the selection of appropriate learning resources. As students discuss the case and share information, they have access to a variety of sources. Students are encouraged to cite credible academic resources, such as textbooks, to strengthen the credibility of their contributions. A common issue arises when students reference non-approved sources, and sometimes disagreements emerge over what constitutes acceptable material. To address this, students are reminded that their performance in citing evidence-based sources is assessed in their FASP grade. They are encouraged to use reliable resources, and access to the internet, though useful, must be approached with caution, as it can lead to the use of information of varying quality. Students entering a basic medical/health science program learn at this time that evidence-based references are obligatory, and they usually do well to adapt to this demand early on in PBL, when prompted to.

4.3.1.7 Focusing on the Basics, Not Just the Diagnosis

Another challenge met in PBL is overlooking the essence of PBL itself. Students in this pre-clinical phase are often motivated to 'solve' the PBL case at a clinical level, and that can often lead to missed opportunities to explore pertinent basic science mechanisms that are unknown to the student or group. Or the assumption that a normal set of labs does not contain basic medical/health science knowledge gaps within it. In addition, they may be incentivized to complete the case so that learning topics can be selected and confirmed. To overcome this challenge, the students should ask open-ended questions to redirect attention back to the basic medical/health science. For example, in the clinical scenarios provided, there may be an abnormal finding that the students foresaw, for example, thrombocytopenia. Rather than proceed, the question can be asked, "Why are the platelets low?" or "How is platelet formation affected?" Students may feel the urge to compete for providing correct answers, a natural and prevalent behavior observed in session, this can lead to overlooking the exercise of exploration of the topic, and analysis of the problem. Students should be reminded that their performance evaluations specifically assess their understanding of basic medical/health sciences rather than just arriving at a correct diagnosis. This encourages deeper exploration of the subject rather than rushing to the solution.

4.3.1.8 Managing Student Biases and Work Experience Diversity

Students entering a basic science PBL program come from a variety of backgrounds, which can influence group dynamics. For instance, students may have prior workforce experience working as an RN, an ER clerk, or in a doctor's office, while others may not. This difference in experience can shape the interactions within the group. Typically, students with clinical experience are recognized by their peers, either during sessions or through informal conversations outside of class, and are often viewed as credible resources. While facilitators generally don't need to intervene directly, it is important to be aware of these dynamics and consider how they might impact the group. Raising awareness of this influence can help maintain a balanced and collaborative environment. In addition to varied work experiences, students will also differ in their prior learning experiences, which can further shape their approach to PBL. These learning experiences are often influenced by their home and work environments, contributing to their beliefs, values, and attachments (Cutrer et al., 2017a). The relationship between past learning and these environments can affect how students engage with the material and interact with their peers, potentially influencing group dynamics. It's important to recognize that these factors play a role in shaping each student's perspective and approach to problem-solving within the group.

4.3.1.9 The Influence of Student Habits on Learning

Student habits are another important factor that will emerge in PBL learning. As reflected in the learner profiles, personal biases can influence how students approach learning. For instance, students often express preferences for certain subjects over others, which can lead to imbalanced learning. A common example is when students say, "I enjoy genetics, I can't stand pharmacology!" Upon reviewing their study choices, we often find they avoid subjects they dislike or find too difficult, which can lead to knowledge gaps. These gaps are a concern for the program, especially as we strive to ensure more uniform learning across groups. Left unchecked, this bias toward favored subjects can create self-imposed limitations. Early detection and intervention are key to addressing these gaps and ensuring students engage fully with all areas of the curriculum.

4.3.1.10 Supporting Learning with Additional Resources

Numerous resources are available to support the learning of basic medical/health sciences in PBL, such as flashcards (Anki, Quizzlet, etc.), videos (YouTube, Sketchy, Pathoma, etc.), and review questions. Every student has a unique learning style, and these online tools can serve as a valuable complement and potentiate the learning that occurs via the reading of basic science textbooks. However, students in PBL may be tempted to rely solely on these alternative resources. The PBL facilitator plays a crucial role in guiding students away from this approach as exclusive use of these resources often leads to a superficial grasp of concepts and is based on memorization of isolated facts. In contrast, the process of reading and learning from the basic medical/health science textbooks enables students to have a broader and deeper understanding of the basic medical/health science concepts and mechanisms that are discussed during the PBL session.

4.3.1.11 Time and Resource Management Challenges

While PBL offers numerous advantages, it also brings challenges that can impact student learning. Time and resource management are major obstacles, as students often struggle with multiple tasks, managing time effectively, and meeting deadlines, which can lead to stress and incomplete learning. Limited access to essential resources, such as learning materials, technology, or expert support, can further hinder the progress and quality of their learning.

4.3.1.12 Communication and Collaboration Within Groups

Collaboration within PBL groups can be challenging as well. Differences in personalities, work habits, and skill levels may lead to conflicts or unequal contributions. Effective communication is essential to PBL success, yet students may face challenges in expressing ideas clearly, giving and receiving feedback, and coordinating efforts within their teams. It is easy for students to lose focus on the exercise of uncovering knowledge gaps with the aid of the clinical scenario and focus on their contributions to the group. This motivation is often based on the assumption that their FASP grade assesses this. The students should be provided with feedback that actively exploring the basic science concepts and learning what they don't know is more important than being right or making a point to the group. An example of this can be found with lab values often provided from the clinical scenario. Students may at times find differing values of what is normal from different sources, which can often lead to discussion and even confusion. It will serve the students well if they learn that this variance is often encountered depending on the referent they use, and is part of the larger picture.

4.3.1.13 Self-Direction and Motivation in PBL

Self-direction and motivation are also essential for successful learning in a PBL setting. Some students may struggle to take initiative and work independently without constant guidance from the facilitator, which can hinder both their progress and motivation. Maintaining interest and motivation throughout the study of complex basic medical/health science topics can be challenging, especially when students meet obstacles or feel frustrated.

4.3.1.14 The Role of Self-Assessment in PBL

Self-assessment is the next component that all students will need to become effective at PBL. Knowing what the student does not know is an exercise, and it can be challenging to develop this into an on-demand skill. Students' ability to self-assess is developed by the post-meeting wrap-up report, where each student and the facilitator can voice post-session comments and their overall sentiment of the preceding PBL group session. This offers students the ability to self-assess and hear from other students how they assess themselves; this provides experience and prepares the students for employing this more routinely. Once self-assessed students continue the cycle of generating questions and directing themselves to the pertinent information. The information then begins the process of integration into the students' understanding of the human body. As mentioned before, this process should begin broadly with a large overview of basic science concepts that become more detailed as time progresses.

4.3.1.15 Assessment and Feedback in PBL

Assessment and feedback in PBL are complex tasks, as they require evaluating both the learning process and the outcome, which often do not align with traditional grading systems. Facilitators and peers alike face the challenge of delivering timely and constructive feedback that guides improvement while maintaining student motivation. Striking this balance is essential to support students' growth without discouraging it and requires careful attention to both content and tone of feedback provided in PBL settings.

4.3.1.16 Ensuring Equity and Inclusion in PBL

Creating clinical scenarios in PBL cases that are relevant, realistic, and applicable to real-world practice can be challenging, particularly in fields focused on abstract concepts. Collaborating with external experts to provide real-world context and mentorship can be difficult to arrange. Additionally, promoting equity and inclusion within PBL requires ensuring that all students, regardless of background or ability, have equal opportunities to participate and contribute. This goal calls for tailored instructional approaches and additional support to meet diverse learning needs and styles.

These challenges have historically been part of the PBL experience (Fig. 4.4). By anticipating how students adapt to active, self-directed learning, program directors and facilitators can offer targeted guidance and support, helping students to navigate and overcome these obstacles.

4.3.2 Defining and Encouraging Student Engagement in PBL

Program directors closely monitor how and to what extent students engage in PBL sessions, as effective engagement is essential for achieving the educational goals of PBL. But what constitutes "good" student engagement? The program primarily gauges success through test performance; high scores often reflect strong engagement and learning outcomes. Achieving these scores requires students to critically analyze clinical case scenarios, identify key basic medical/health science questions, conduct thorough self-assessments, and actively share information within the group to address knowledge gaps (Fig. 4.5).

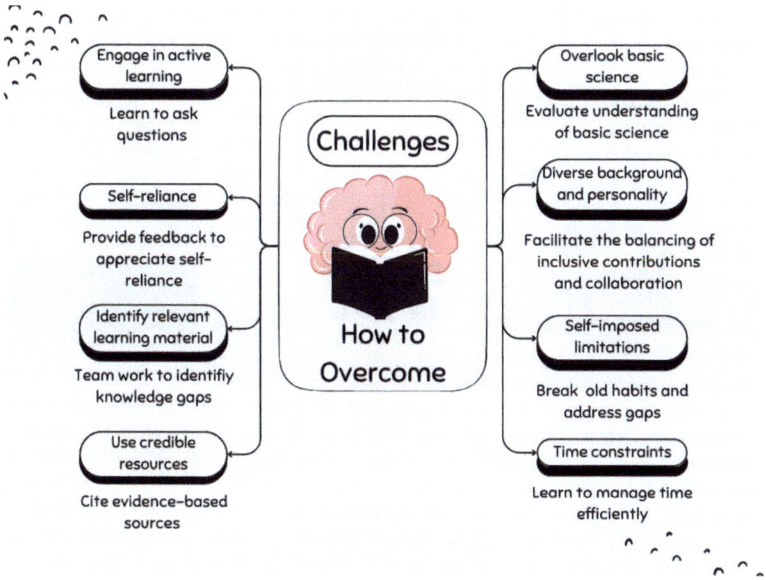

Fig. 4.4 Challenges faced by students in PBL and how to address them

Various factors, including facilitator assessments, personal goals, and group dynamics, can enhance engagement. The Facilitator Assessment of Student Performance (FASP) score is a key metric, in which facilitators evaluate students' engagement based on medical knowledge, interpersonal skills, and contributions to patient care (Reznich & Werner, 2004). These assessments encourage students to come prepared, actively participate in discussions, and effectively collaborate as a team. To foster transparency, facilitators should provide students with FASP criteria in advance, helping them understand the traits and behaviors associated with successful PBL engagement.

The collaborative nature of PBL presents students with opportunities beyond those in lecture-based settings. In doing PBL, students are not only developing their understanding of the basic sciences but also honing teamwork, communication, and delegation skills as they work through cases together. FASP forms highlight these aspects and discussing them before the sessions begin can reinforce the importance of mutual goals and shared responsibilities.

Personal goals also shape how students engage in PBL. While many prioritize high test scores, some students have other objectives, such as board exam preparation or developing specific competencies (Bransford et al., 2001). The FASP score, although valuable, has historically held less weight in the overall course grading scale due to its subjective nature. Therefore, students may demonstrate ambivalence towards it. Additionally, students with board exams on the horizon may divert their attention from group work to pursue individual study paths, potentially affecting group contributions. Facilitators can address this by reinforcing the value of the FASP assessment

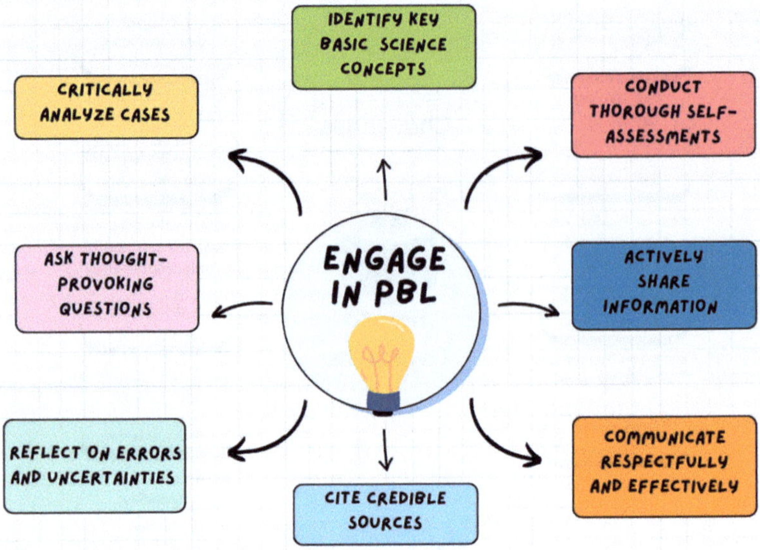

Fig. 4.5 Signes of student engagement in PBL include critically analyzing cases, identifying basic science concepts, thoroughly self-assessing, actively sharing information, communicating respectfully and effectively, cite credible sources, reflecting on errs and uncertainties, and asking thought-provoking questions

in promoting best practices and holding individual meetings to discuss ways students can balance personal goals with group engagement.

Interpersonal relationships within the PBL group also play a significant role in student engagement. As a collaborative and discussion-based learning approach, PBL naturally fosters both alliances and occasional disagreements. These interactions can either enhance or hinder group dynamics, depending on how they are managed. Students should understand that disagreements are a normal and productive part of the learning process. If discussions become obstructive, facilitators can step in, emphasizing the value of communication skills and using the situation to help students build consensus and improve their ability to communicate effectively.

Through structured assessments, clear communication, and supportive guidance, PBL programs aim to cultivate a strong foundation in the basic sciences while also preparing students to thrive in collaborative, real-world healthcare environments.

For students in a basic medical/health science PBL curriculum, it's essential to view their knowledge base as a sturdy foundation: a structure that, by the end of the pre-clerkship years, should be complete, accurate, and uniformly solid. This foundational understanding will support their future clinical learning. Gaps in this foundation, like cracks in a building's base, can weaken the structure, so continuous efforts to fill knowledge gaps are necessary for long-term success. To help students achieve this, the following strategies offer ways to identify and address these gaps effectively.

4.3.3 Enhancing Performance

A regular, honest assessment of knowledge can reveal specific areas needing attention. Pre-tests, quizzes, or practice exams are effective in exposing weak spots in understanding. Conceptual checklists, outlines, and self-testing strategies such as flashcards help students assess their familiarity with key topics, guiding their review process.

Reflecting on errors and uncertainties enhances learning by pinpointing areas of confusion. Students can use reflective journals to log moments of uncertainty in assignments or tests, helping them track and address recurring issues in their understanding.

Engaging in peer discussions enables students to see topics from multiple perspectives. Explaining concepts to each other and tackling complex problems together can reveal individual gaps in understanding, making study groups a powerful tool for reinforcing and expanding knowledge.

Working through diverse practice problems and diagnostic exercises highlights specific weaknesses, while creating concept maps allows students to visualize relationships between ideas and identify gaps in their mental model of the human body.

Feedback is crucial in identifying misunderstandings. Reviewing feedback on presentations, assignments, exams, or PBL sessions helps students recognize knowledge gaps, while peer evaluations can offer insights into areas where they may be lacking foundational understanding.

4.4 Strategies for Student Success in PBL

See Fig. 4.6.

4.4.1 Reading with Purpose

In the context of PBL, reading is not a passive activity but an active process driven by inquiry. When students approach reading with specific questions in mind, it transforms into a purposeful endeavor that not only fills existing knowledge gaps but also stimulates further questions, thereby deepening understanding. This approach

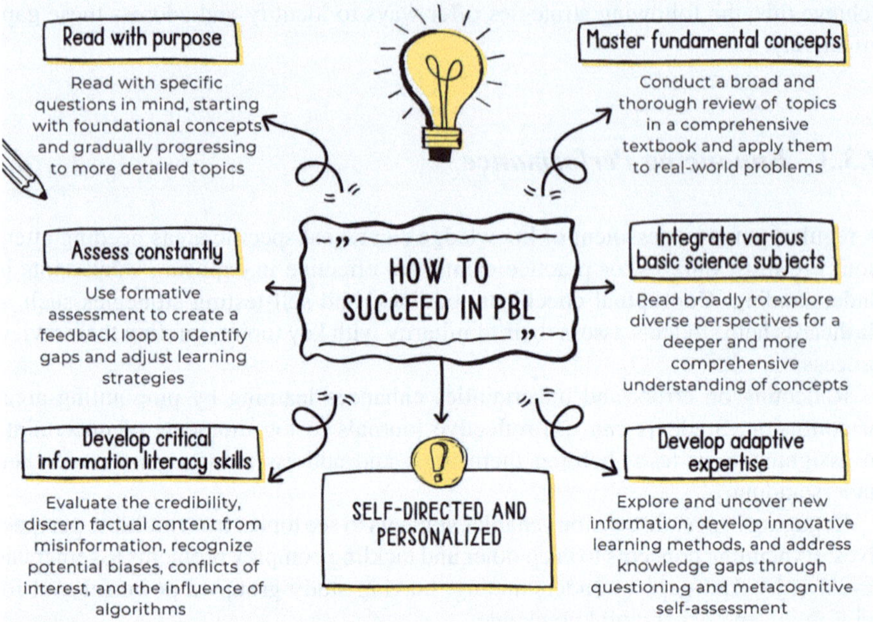

Fig. 4.6 Strategies for success in PBL include reading with purpose, continuous assessment, developing critical information literacy skills, mastering fundamental concepts, integrating various subjects, and cultivating adaptive expertise

aligns with the constructivist learning theory, which posits that learners build new knowledge upon the foundation of their existing knowledge base.

Beginning with foundational concepts and progressively delving into more specific details enables students to construct a coherent mental framework. This structured approach minimizes the likelihood of misconceptions and ensures a comprehensive understanding of complex topics. Such a strategy is particularly beneficial in medical education, where the integration of various physiological, biochemical, and anatomical principles is essential for understanding human health and disease.

While PBL students in a pre-clerkship phase may not engage in direct patient interactions, they can develop a conceptual model of the human body. This model serves as a mental construct that aids in comprehending the basic medical/health sciences. By utilizing PBL cases and the broader curriculum, students can generate targeted questions that challenge their current understanding. These questions act as triggers for further exploration and self-directed learning, fostering a deeper engagement with the material.

Through this iterative process of questioning and exploration, students can identify and address gaps in their knowledge. Moreover, this approach encourages critical thinking and problem-solving skills, as students learn to analyze complex scenarios, synthesize information from various sources, and apply their knowledge to novel situations. Such skills are indispensable for future healthcare professionals who must navigate the complexities of patient care and medical decision-making.

Reading with purpose in a PBL framework is a dynamic and interactive process. It transforms reading from a passive activity into an engaging learning experience that promotes deep understanding, critical thinking, and lifelong learning. By cultivating these skills early in medical education, students are better prepared to meet the challenges of clinical practice and contribute effectively to patient care..

4.4.2 Recognize Checkpoints

In the PBL framework, assessments are strategically placed throughout the curriculum to serve as critical checkpoints in the learning process. These assessments are not merely evaluative tools but integral components that guide students' learning journeys. By informing students of upcoming PBL written examinations, the program ensures that learners are aware of these pivotal moments, allowing them to prepare effectively and engage meaningfully with the material.

These assessments function as formative evaluations, providing students with timely feedback on their understanding of the basic medical sciences. This feedback loop is essential for quality control and quality assurance within the educational process. It enables students to identify areas where their knowledge may be lacking and make necessary adjustments to their study strategies. Such adjustments are crucial for continuous improvement and mastery of the subject matter.

Moreover, these checkpoints foster a sense of accountability and self-regulation among students. Knowing that assessments are embedded within the learning process encourages students to take ownership of their learning, engage in self-assessment, and seek resources to address knowledge gaps. This proactive approach to learning not only enhances academic performance but also cultivates lifelong learning habits essential for medical practice.

4.4.3 Quality of Information

In 2025, approximately 402.74 million TB of data are generated daily across the globe (Piaget & Inhelder, 2008). This vast digital landscape encompasses a multitude of information sources, including academic journals, news outlets, social media platforms, and personal blogs. However, with the sheer volume of content produced, the prevalence of misinformation has escalated, posing significant challenges to information integrity. As the size of a network grows, so does the potential for misinformation to proliferate, often outpacing the dissemination of accurate information (Cutrer et al., 2017b). Recognizing the importance of this issue, the program emphasizes the development of critical information literacy skills among students. This initiative aims to equip students with the tools necessary to evaluate the credibility of information sources, discern factual content from misinformation, and make informed decisions based on reliable data. By fostering these skills, the program seeks to mitigate the impact of misinformation and promote a culture of informed inquiry.

Students are introduced to various frameworks and methodologies for assessing information quality. One such approach is the CRAAP test, which evaluates sources based on Currency, Relevance, Authority, Accuracy, and Purpose. This tool serves as a guide for students to critically analyze sources and determine their reliability. Additionally, students are encouraged to consider the source's origin, the author's credentials, the intended audience, and the presence of supporting evidence when evaluating information.

The program also emphasizes the importance of understanding the broader context in which information is produced and consumed. Students are taught to recognize potential biases, conflicts of interest, and the influence of algorithms on information dissemination. By developing a nuanced understanding of these factors, students can better navigate the complexities of the digital information landscape.

Furthermore, the program encourages students to engage in discussions about the ethical implications of information sharing and consumption. Students are prompted to consider the consequences of spreading unverified information and the responsibilities they bear as consumers and disseminators of information. This holistic approach aims to cultivate a sense of accountability and ethical awareness in students, preparing them to contribute positively to the information ecosystem.

4.4.4 Building the Knowledge Base

In PBL, approaching the basic medical sciences through a broad overview is an effective strategy. Students begin by exploring major topics, akin to reviewing the table of contents in a comprehensive textbook. This method provides a holistic understanding of the subject matter and allows students to identify specific areas of interest for deeper exploration.

Establishing a strong foundation in fundamental concepts and recurring themes, such as homeostasis, is crucial. These core principles serve as the building blocks for understanding more complex mechanisms and systems within the human body. By grasping these basics early on, students can more effectively integrate new information and apply it to clinical scenarios.

PBL encourages students to actively engage with the material, fostering critical thinking and self-directed learning. Through the analysis of clinical cases, students learn to apply their foundational knowledge to real-world problems, enhancing their problem-solving skills and preparing them for future clinical practice. This approach not only aids in knowledge retention but also promotes a deeper understanding of the interconnectedness of various medical disciplines. By continuously building upon their knowledge base, students develop a comprehensive and integrated perspective of the medical sciences, essential for effective patient care.

4.4.5 Overlapping Chapters from Multiple Textbooks on the Same Topics

When it comes to mastering the basic medical/health science s, PBL is mostly effective when students engage in broad reading across multiple sources. This approach ensures a comprehensive understanding of fundamental concepts by integrating knowledge from various disciplines. For example, if the patient in the PBL case presents with edema, students should study fluid dynamics, capillary and hydrostatic pressures, and membrane channels from diverse textbooks, including those focused on physiology, pathology, biochemistry, and histology. By reading overlapping chapters from these different resources, students approach the same concept from different perspectives, enhancing their overall comprehension, which will provide the students with a much more in-depth understanding of the concept that can apply to a variety of clinical cases.

The integration of information from various basic medical/health science textbooks allows students to build a multidimensional understanding of concepts. This method aligns with educational theories that emphasize the importance of multiple representations and the integration of knowledge for deeper learning (Bransford et al., 2001). For example, studying fluid dynamics in a physiology textbook might provide a foundational understanding of the principles, while a pathology textbook could offer insights into how these principles apply to disease processes. A biochemistry textbook might explore into the molecular mechanisms underlying fluid dynamics, and a histology textbook could illustrate how these mechanisms manifest in the context of specific tissues.

Such a broad reading strategy aligns with the constructivist learning theory, which suggests that knowledge is constructed through the integration of new information with existing cognitive structures (Piaget & Inhelder, 2008). By encountering the same concept in different contexts, students are more likely to form robust mental models and transfer their knowledge to clinical practice effectively. Additionally, this approach supports the development of critical thinking and problem-solving skills, as students must synthesize information from various sources and apply it to clinical scenarios (Hmelo-Silver, 2004).

Broad reading across multiple basic medical/health science textbooks and resources is crucial for mastering health-related concepts in a PBL curriculum. This approach provides students with a more in-depth and integrated understanding of concepts, facilitating their application to clinical cases and solidifying their grasp of basic medical/health science principles. By engaging with diverse perspectives and integrating knowledge from various disciplines, students can achieve a more comprehensive and practical understanding of health science, potentially enhancing their clinical competence.

4.4.6 Developing Adaptive Expertise Through Metacognitive Self-Assessment

4.4.6.1 The Importance of Metacognition in Learning

The process of acquiring high-quality data and constructing a sound understanding of the basic medical/health science s as they apply to the human body requires a robust ability to assess one's own learning. Metacognition, or the ability to think about how one learns, is central to this process. It involves exploring and uncovering new information, as well as developing new methods for learning and filling knowledge gaps. Through metacognitive self-assessment, students gain the ability to monitor their learning, identify weaknesses, and adjust their strategies to enhance understanding and performance.

4.4.6.2 The Cycle of Questioning and Knowledge Integration

In basic medical/health science education, the goal is to guide students through a repeated process of questioning, extracting data, integrating credible information, converting it into knowledge, and applying it to practice. With each cycle, students progress from initial attempts to practiced skills, eventually achieving mastery. As students generate questions and find answers, they uncover new questions, which lead them deeper into interconnected subjects within the basic medical/health sciences. This process requires students to build connections across disciplines, developing an integrated understanding of the human body. Over time, these repeated cycles help students form a mental model of the human body that unifies key concepts from the basic medical/health science s, laying the foundation for clinical practice.

4.4.6.3 Personalizing the Learning Process in PBL

Traditional learning programs often offer students material that follows a fixed sequence of themes, which may not be optimal for each student's personal knowledge base. PBL, however, encourages students to tailor their learning process, focusing on identifying and addressing their individual knowledge gaps efficiently. This personalized approach may involve reading chapters or sections out of order, allowing each student to determine the most logical and beneficial sequence for their learning. While this flexibility has advantages, it may pose challenges for students with no prior experience in the basic medical/health sciences. In such cases, the logical progression of the textbook can provide a more structured foundation for learning fundamental concepts.

4.4.6.4 Evaluating Learning Through Time and Endurance

Effective learning in PBL must also be evaluated in terms of time and endurance, as students must manage the large volumes of dense, high-quality information required to master the basic medical/health sciences. Best practices in PBL include setting learning goals based on content mastery rather than time spent. Students are encouraged to ask themselves reflective questions: How many of my questions were resolved? How much deeper is my understanding of the case theme? What parts of my mental construct of the human body were strengthened? What gaps remain? By answering these questions, students assess their progress and adjust their learning strategies to ensure continued development.

4.4.6.5 The Role of Preparation and Proactive Learning

As we examine student behavior and outcomes in PBL health science programs, certain practices emerge as beneficial. One such practice is preparation. Students who come to class ready to discuss expected topics demonstrate responsibility and a strong grasp of their research. Historically, students tend to underestimate the session tempo, which can lead to struggles in keeping pace as the case unfolds. Encouraging advanced preparation supports in-session learning and simulates the forward-thinking approach essential for healthcare practice. Facilitators often rely on interval feedback from facilitator-student evaluations to gauge students' progress and encourage this proactive learning habit.

4.4.6.6 Building Mastery Through Repeated Learning Cycles

Historically, strong-performing students demonstrate familiarity with the case's history, a thorough understanding of the basic medical and health science concepts introduced, and a readiness to ask insightful questions. In pharmaceutical discussions, for example, students who know each compound's mechanism of action reinforce their mastery through repeated cycles of PBL learning. This repetition strengthens their understanding, ensuring the retention of key concepts that form the foundation for future learning.

4.4.6.7 Autonomy in Learning and Identifying Biases

In PBL, the curriculum and case scenarios offer a framework to guide relevant study, but students have the autonomy to pursue learning in personalized ways. From the first sentence of a clinical scenario, students begin prioritizing their lines of questioning and selecting their individual learning paths based on their unique literacy profiles. This autonomy offers valuable insights into potential biases students may face, which could affect their learning and progress. The cases presented in PBL encourage curiosity and personal inquiry, helping students develop critical thinking skills that will serve them well in clinical practice.

4.4.6.8 Personalized Learning Paths and Diverse Learning Strategies

Although PBL provides a structured framework, students often choose to engage with topics out of sequence if it better aligns with their current understanding. Effective learners in PBL employ various methods, from collaborative discussions with peers to independent study. These diverse learning strategies help build a comprehensive foundation in basic sciences, akin to constructing a solid, gap-free base that supports more complex learning as students' education advances.

4.4.6.9 Master Adaptive Learning Through Metacognitive Skills

Historically, the PBL curriculum has focused primarily on learning the basic medical/health sciences. Recently, facilitators have emphasized the development of master adaptive learners who utilize metacognitive skills to self-assess and adapt (Stringer et al., 2022). Early introduction of these skills prepares students to become self-sustaining learners. These students learn to identify gaps in their knowledge and competencies and adjust their approach accordingly, which are skills that are critical for their future roles as healthcare providers.

4.4.6.10 Evaluating the Quality of Learning Resources

With abundant information sources now available both in and outside of PBL sessions, one of the challenges of PBL programs is guiding students on how to assess the quality of these resources. While traditional peer-reviewed sources remain the gold standard, students often gravitate toward quicker, more accessible formats like videos or online courses, which may lack rigorous verification. PBL programs recognize this trend and are implementing policies to help students critically evaluate each resource, reinforcing the need for discernment and evaluation.

4.4.6.11 Applying Scrutiny to Scientific Information

Encouraging students to assess their sources for credibility mirrors the discernment they might naturally apply to news or media. However, it is essential for them to apply this same scrutiny to scientific information. For instance, students might implicitly trust an online video on biochemical pathways without questioning its accuracy. PBL programs can play a pivotal role by raising awareness about the variability in information quality and empowering students to practice discernment in all areas of their study. This approach not only reinforces their growth as independent learners but also prepares them for continuous self-directed learning in their professional careers.

4.4.6.12 Learning Resources to Support Adaptive Expertise

Using a variety of materials, such as textbooks, review guides, and high-quality educational videos, can deepen understanding and fill in gaps. These resources offer explanations that may differ from primary course textbooks, allowing students to see familiar concepts from new perspectives. Quizzes, flashcards, and online learning platforms with self-testing tools make it easier for students to spot areas that require additional study. Regular formative assessments provide timely feedback and help students track their progress in meeting their learning goals.

4.4.6.13 Structured Learning Assessments

Structured learning assessments, such as diagnostic tests, can provide students with a clear view of their progress against expected learning outcomes. Curriculum mapping helps students measure their current understanding against the program's objectives, making it easier to target areas that need reinforcement. By incorporating these strategies, students can work toward a thorough, unified understanding of the basic medical/health science s, preparing them for the advanced demands of clinical learning. This proactive approach supports their journey toward mastering the PBL curriculum and establishing a durable knowledge base in the foundational sciences.

4.5 The Progression of Student Learning

As students embark on their PBL journey, they face a significant learning curve as they adapt to collaborative learning, self-directed study, and critical questioning within the group context. Ideally, PBL group performance follows a sigmoid curve when plotted over time, with performance measured by the quantity and quality of basic medical/health science questions generated and the students' engagement in the self-assessment process. This curve reflects the progression of group productivity, moving through three primary phases: latent, exponential, and plateau (Fig. 4.7).

4.5.1 Early Stage (Latent Phase)

At the outset of PBL, students primarily focus on becoming acquainted with the overall structure, format, and expectations that govern their group discussions. This initial phase is often characterized by a slower pace of productivity, particularly in

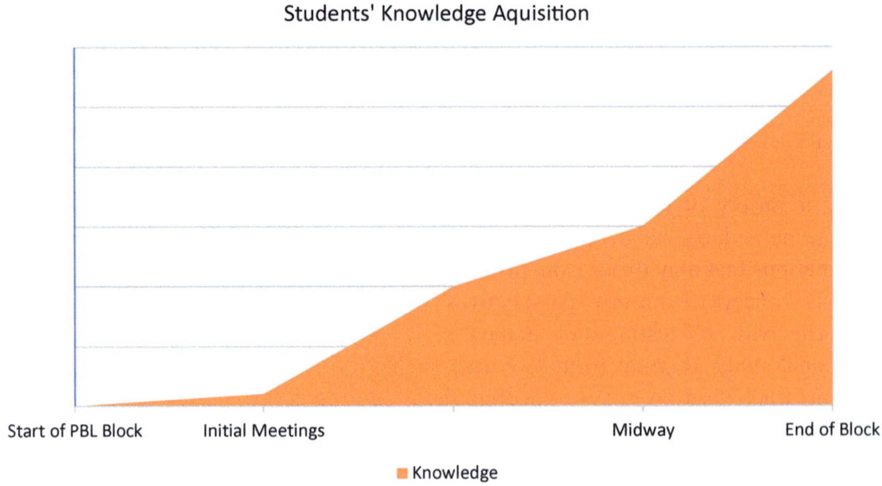

Fig. 4.7 The progression of PBL group productivity occurs through three primary phases: latent, exponential, and plateau

terms of generating thoughtful questions and acquiring foundational knowledge in the basic medical/health sciences. Many students are still learning how to systematically organize their approach to tackling PBL cases, how to effectively navigate the interpersonal dynamics within their group, and how to efficiently locate and reference appropriate learning materials. Because they are adapting to this new way of learning, students tend to be more preoccupied with the logistical and procedural elements of PBL sessions, such as understanding roles, managing time, and balancing participation, rather than immediately delving deeply into the scientific content itself. This early latent phase requires considerable patience and encouragement from both facilitators and students alike, as everyone adjusts to the unique demands and opportunities presented by the PBL framework. It is important to recognize that this period is a critical foundational stage where the skills for effective collaboration, communication, and self-directed learning begin to develop even if immediate content mastery is limited.

4.5.2 Growth Phase (Exponential Phase)

As students progress through several PBL sessions, a noticeable shift typically occurs. Comfort with the PBL process increases, and students begin to show a greater ease with group collaboration and case analysis. This stage is often described as the exponential or growth phase, where the volume and quality of question generation increase rapidly. Students become more adept at identifying gaps in their knowledge and are eager to explore these areas through inquiry and research. There is a marked improvement in both the efficiency and productivity of the group as members engage more actively, sharing insights, resources, and critical thinking perspectives. The collective understanding of the group grows significantly, allowing students to leverage one another's strengths to address complex questions more effectively. Facilitators will often observe increased group cohesiveness, with more balanced participation among members and a higher rate of engagement driven by student curiosity. The discussions become more dynamic, and study topics tend to be rich, diverse, and driven by well-formulated questions that push the group toward deeper learning. This growth phase is essential because it fosters both cognitive and social development, strengthening the students' capacity for teamwork, critical analysis, and lifelong learning skills.

4.5.3 Maturity Phase (Plateau Phase)

After a sustained period of active participation and consistent engagement, usually spanning several months, the PBL group typically reaches what is known as the maturity or plateau phase. At this stage, the group's productivity stabilizes at a high level, reflecting the maximum capacity for effective question generation, topic coverage, and collaborative problem-solving within the allotted session time. The productivity curve reaches an asymptote, signifying that the group has achieved peak efficiency and is able to conduct highly focused and productive learning sessions. Members have developed a rhythm and familiarity with each other's learning styles, which facilitates smooth communication and constructive dialogue. The group is less likely to experience major disruptions or declines in participation, and discussions tend to be rich in content and critical thinking. Facilitators can view this plateau as evidence that the students have mastered not only the subject matter but also the processes and interpersonal skills necessary for optimal group function. When this PBL cycle concludes, and if the group composition changes for a new set of cases or students, the learning curve typically resets and follows a similar sigmoid pattern of latent, growth, and maturity phases as the new group acclimates to the PBL process.

4.5.4 Facilitator Evaluation, Encouragement, and the PBL Learning Journey

In the PBL process, student learning is at the forefront, and facilitators play a key role in supporting and guiding this learning journey. Effective PBL group performance can be measured by the volume and relevance of questions generated by students, the quality and efficiency of information exchange, and the depth and speed with which students identify and address gaps in their understanding of basic medical/health sciences. Unlike traditional lecture formats, where students may passively absorb information, a productive PBL session thrives on active discussion, collaborative problem-solving, and mutual engagement. Facilitators actively monitor student participation, recognizing that some students may contribute more than others. To foster equitable participation, facilitators emphasize the value of active involvement, not just for enhancing personal learning but also for influencing their evaluations, such as facilitator assessment scores (FASP). By helping students understand the connection between engagement and their learning outcomes, facilitators can encourage even the more reserved students to participate more fully.

The essence of PBL lies in helping students appreciate that the learning process itself is as important as the end goal. Each case study and interaction with peers is a step in building critical thinking, problem-solving, and collaborative skills that are crucial for success in health sciences. Facilitators support this by guiding students to view each PBL session as an opportunity to deepen their understanding, not merely a task to complete. By engaging in this reflective learning process, students are encouraged to connect theoretical knowledge with practical application, which reinforces their understanding of the basic medical/health sciences. This continuous cycle of inquiry, discussion, and self-reflection helps students build a comprehensive and interconnected mental model of the human body. Over time, they develop not only a deeper grasp of scientific concepts but also the adaptive learning skills necessary for lifelong learning and professional practice.

4.5.5 Building a Foundation for Advanced Learning

The structured, phased approach of PBL allows students to build a solid foundation in basic medical/health sciences while simultaneously refining essential skills for effective teamwork and clinical problem-solving. As students progress through these stages, they become better equipped to handle more complex clinical scenarios and engage in interdisciplinary collaboration in future learning phases. This integration of knowledge acquisition with interpersonal skill development ensures that students not only master scientific concepts but also develop collaborative and problem-solving abilities crucial for their future careers. The synergy of these skills fosters a comprehensive foundation that extends well beyond the classroom, preparing students for the dynamic challenges they will face in their professional practice.

4.6 Self-Assessment and Adaptive Learning

As PBL sessions begin, the focus shifts toward establishing a productive learning environment where students engage in collaborative learning through clinical scenarios. Students work together to formulate questions, identify knowledge gaps, and integrate new information into a comprehensive model of human health. This process is critical in building an interconnected understanding of basic medical and health science concepts.

For many students, the metacognitive processes underlying PBL are initially invisible. Debriefing sessions or post-session wrap-ups are vital moments to explicitly introduce these skills, encouraging students to become Master Adaptive Learners (MALs). The MAL framework, focusing on Planning, Learning, Resilience, and Motivation, offers a structured approach to fostering adaptability and lifelong learning, which are vital qualities for future healthcare providers (Piaget & Inhelder, 2008). As students develop these skills, they begin to appreciate the value of reflecting on their learning process and identifying areas for growth.

The introduction of metacognitive concepts within PBL is an evolving process, and interest in developing adaptive learners is growing steadily (Cutrer et al., 2019). To support this, students are encouraged to engage in rigorous self-assessment and continuously identify their knowledge gaps. By evaluating their understanding and seeking answers, students not only expand their knowledge but also gain insight into the learning process itself. This metacognitive shift allows students to become more effective in their approach to problem-solving and critical thinking. By citing credible references and sources as part of their learning practice, students reinforce their knowledge while honing the critical thinking skills essential for professional growth.

Our existing subjective assessment tool for PBL performance, the Facilitator Assessment of Student Performance (FASP), has shown that students often prioritize receiving positive feedback over actively engaging in the case to generate questions and guide targeted information gathering. Educating students on the importance of engaging deeply with the material at the start of the course may help foster a more collaborative mindset, encouraging them to explore the basic science themes presented and develop strong questioning skills. This approach promotes deeper learning, ultimately benefiting their overall development as healthcare professionals.

Effective assessment in PBL requires insight into students' thought processes during sessions. Understanding how students approach problem-solving, generate questions, and integrate new information provides a richer perspective on their learning. To capture this insight, assessment tools are evolving through questionnaires and accepted cognitive frameworks, such as the correlation between a positive attitude and active engagement in PBL, which is believed to improve test performance. Facilitators who understand these cognitive processes can more effectively guide students toward critical thinking and deeper comprehension, ensuring the learning process is both meaningful and comprehensive.

After the PBL session concludes, students continue their learning journey by searching for answers to the questions they generated and often generate additional questions on their own. During independent study time, students may engage in discussions with peers from other groups who may be at different stages in the case progression. This interaction is often driven by anxiety as students may fear neglecting important topics or may be seeking a preview of what's coming next. While these inter-group discussions can offer insights into the clinical case, they do not always contribute to building a strong foundation in basic medical/health sciences. This challenge can distract students from learning material in a sequence that works best for them. To address this, we emphasize the importance of developing a comprehensive individual understanding of the foundational sciences. Students are reminded that while sharing insights can be helpful, their learning path is unique, and a steady, focused approach to mastering the basics will best support their long-term success.

In the broader context of the program, even an introductory understanding of metacognitive strategies is valuable. PBL provides students with opportunities to encounter challenges, conflicts, and diverse perspectives, which in turn fosters self-reliance and adaptability. These are skills crucial for their careers, where learning will continue outside academic environments and must keep pace with evolving medical knowledge.

As students progress through PBL's thematic blocks, group dynamics evolve as well. Under optimal conditions, collaboration becomes more effective, with students efficiently sharing information, identifying knowledge gaps, and consistently building on each other's contributions. This environment not only supports knowledge acquisition but also helps students refine the adaptive learning skills they will rely on in their future medical practice.

Ultimately, PBL helps students transition from structured learning to self-directed inquiry. By instilling the tools necessary for lifelong learning, PBL prepares students to continually expand their knowledge base, equipping them to keep pace with ongoing advancements in medical science. Through this process, students develop into independent, adaptive learners, which are skills essential for their future roles as healthcare providers.

4.7 Conclusion

Student learning in a PBL environment represents a significant shift from passive absorption to the active construction of knowledge. As discussed throughout this chapter, successful learning in PBL is about more than just content mastery, it involves the development of adaptive expertise, metacognitive awareness, collaborative competence, and disciplined self-direction.

PBL enables students to ask meaningful questions, identify and address knowledge gaps, and build a comprehensive understanding of human biology through repeated learning cycles. These cycles, driven by curiosity, critical thinking, and self-assessment, serve as the foundation for becoming a master adaptive learner. In contrast to traditional lecture-based education, which often encourages rote memorization of isolated facts, PBL promotes a deeper, transferable understanding by tying learning to real-world clinical problems and collaborative dialogue.

However, PBL also presents distinct challenges, including navigating uncertainty without prescriptive guidance, managing group dynamics, and evaluating the credibility of information in an age of overwhelming digital content. Students must cultivate the ability to discern reliable sources, assess their own progress, and build a solid knowledge base in a deliberate and progressive manner. While this process requires time and patience, it ultimately nurtures resilience, autonomy, and the lifelong learning habits essential for professional development.

Facilitators are integral to guiding students through these challenges. By providing structured orientation, thoughtful feedback, and adaptive support, facilitators help students move through the latent, growth, and maturity phases of PBL learning. Their encouragement fosters an environment of psychological safety, promotes productive discourse, and encourages a culture of continuous improvement.

The ultimate goal for students is to create a solid, gap-free foundation in the basic medical/health science s that will support their future clinical learning and practice. As future healthcare professionals, they must not only understand the science but also learn how to learn, unlearn, and relearn as necessary. PBL offers an ideal platform for this ongoing professional formation.

This chapter underscores that the value of PBL lies not just in what students learn, but in how they learn and who they become through the process. The skills developed in PBL are not only vital for academic success but also essential for practicing compassionate, informed, and adaptable healthcare in an ever-evolving medical landscape.

References

Al-Shaikh, G., et al. (2015). Perception of medical students regarding problem based learning. *Kuwait Medical Journal, 47*, 133.

Bransford, J. D., Brown, A. L., & Cocking, R. R. (2001). How people learn brain, mind, experience, and school. In *Early childhood development and learning: New knowledge for policy*. National Academies Press. Retrieved from https://www.ncbi.nlm.nih.gov/books/NBK223290/

Cabra-Torres, F., et al. (2020). Information literacy profiles of university students. In *Information literacy in higher education* (SpringerBriefs in education). Springer.

Cutrer, W. B., et al. (2017a). Fostering the development of master adaptive learners: A conceptual model to guide skill acquisition in medical education. *Academic Medicine, 92*, 1.

Cutrer, W. B., Miller, B., Pusic, M. V., Mejicano, G., Mangrulkar, R. S., Gruppen, L. D., & Burk-Rafel, J. (2017b). Fostering the development of master adaptive learners: A framework for medical education. *Academic Medicine, 92*(9), 1208–1214.

Cutrer, W. B., Jain, V., & Walz, A. (2019). *Who is the master adaptive learner?*

Dolmans, D. H. J. M., De Grave, W., Wolfhagen, I. H. A. P., & van der Vleuten, C. P. M. (2005). Problem-based learning: Future challenges for educational practice and research. *Medical Education, 39*(7), 732–741. https://doi.org/10.1111/j.1365-2929.2005.02205.x

Hmelo-Silver, C. E. (2004). Problem-based learning: What and how do students learn? *Educational Psychology Review, 16*(3), 235–266. https://doi.org/10.1023/B:EDPR.0000034022.16470.f3

Jost, J. T., Kruglanski, A. W., & Nelson, T. O. (1998). Social metacognition: An expansionist review. *Personality and Social Psychology Review, 2*, 137.

Kolmos, A., Du, X., Holgaard, J. E., & Jensen, L. P. (2008). *Facilitation in a PBL environment*. UCPBL UNESCO Chair in Problem Based Learning, Aalborg University.

Piaget, J., & Inhelder, B. (2008). *The psychology of the child*. Basic Books. Retrieved from https://books.google.com/books?hl=en&lr=&id=-Dpz05-rJ4gC&oi=fnd&pg=PR9&dq=Piaget,+J.+(1972).+The+psychology+of+the+child.+Basic+Books.&ots=qv5aGV_3vD&sig=lC48ooqxWcBT_IOA2IcFQ9XJyGg

Reznich, C. B., & Werner, E. (2004). Facilitators' influence on student PBL small group session online information resource use: A survey. *BMC Medical Education, 4*, 9.

Savin-Baden, M., & Major, C. H. (2013). *Exploring the principles of problem-based learning*. McGraw-Hill Education. Retrieved from https://www.mheducation.com/highered/product/foundations-problem-based-learning-savin-baden-major/M9780335215317.html

Stringer, J. K., Gruppen, L. D., Ryan, M. S., Ginzburg, S. B., Cutrer, W. B., Wolff, M., & Santen, S. A. (2022). Measuring the master adaptive learner: Development and internal structure validity evidence for a new instrument. *Medical Science Educator, 32*, 183–193.

Trullas, J. C., et al. (2022). Effectiveness of PBL methodology in undergraduate education: A scoping review. *BMC Medical Education, 22*, 104.

Vernon, D. T., & Blake, R. L. (1993). Does problem-based learning work? A meta-analysis of evaluative research. *Academic Medicine, 68*, 550.

Chapter 5
Facilitate a Problem-Based Learning Session

Teresa M. Hunter-Pettersen and Bei Zhang

5.1 Facilitator Role

In PBL facilitation, facilitators must thoughtfully reflect on their role to effectively run a session. They oversee group dynamics to foster a cohesive and high-quality exchange of information. The ultimate goal is to create an environment that engages students emotionally, enabling them to develop competencies through analyzing complex concepts and clinical scenarios (Salinitri et al., 2015).

To facilitate a PBL session, the facilitator aims to assist the students to:

- take personal responsibility for learning, both during and after healthcare professional school,
- attain a relevant knowledge base with essential depth, breadth, and flexibility,
- obtain and critically assess new knowledge as it is applied to the clinical case,
- develop proficiency in clinical reasoning through repeated exposure to clinical cases,
- formulate diagnostic hypotheses based on identified problems and reliable resources,
- work in a team effectively through communication, cooperation, commitment, and mutual support and respect,
- adequately prepare for entry into clinical clerkships.

During a PBL session, the facilitator actively listens to students' discussions (Hmelo-Silver, 2004). They utilize strong listening skills, share relevant case information, and ask well-timed questions to guide the group. It's essential for the facilitator to

T. M. Hunter-Pettersen
Lake Erie College of Osteopathic Medicine, Bradenton, FL, USA
e-mail: tpettersen@lecom.edu

B. Zhang (✉)
Robert Larner, M.D. College of Medicine at the University of Vermont, Burlington, VT, USA
e-mail: bei.zhang@med.uvm.edu

S. Lorenzo and B. Zhang (eds.), *Mastering Problem-Based Learning in Health Profession Programs*, https://doi.org/10.1007/978-3-032-05405-0_5

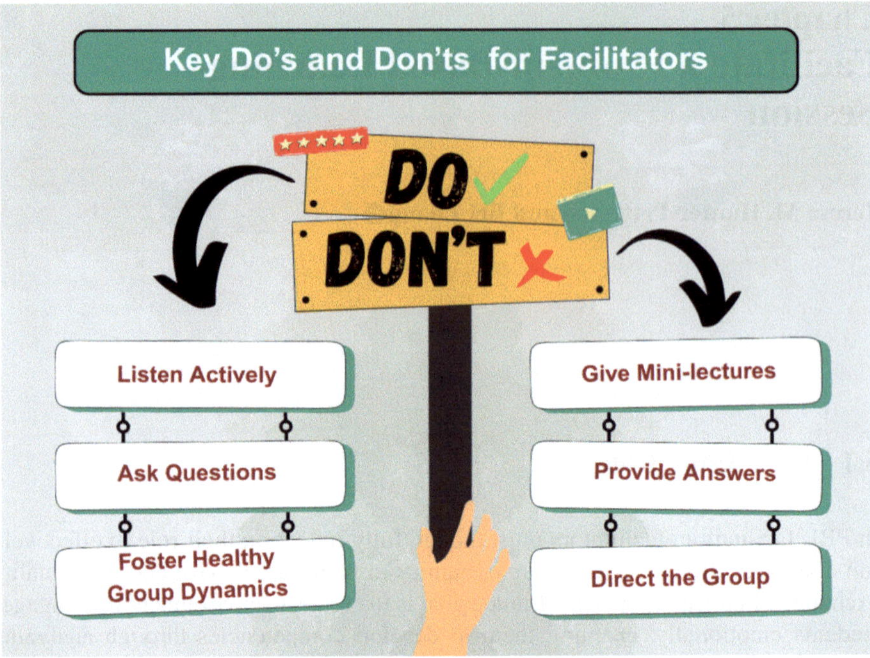
Key Do's and Don'ts for Facilitators
DO
DON'T
Listen Actively
Ask Questions
Foster Healthy Group Dynamics
Give Mini-lectures
Provide Answers
Direct the Group

Fig. 5.1 What to do and what not to do when facilitating a PBL session, shifting from traditional didactic teaching

stay attentive throughout the 2-hour session, knowing when to step in with a question and when to hold back to avoid disrupting the active learning process (Fig. 5.1).

The facilitators disclose the case progressively during the PBL session. Effective facilitators do not try to mini-lecture or "teach." Instead, they have the students take the lead on the case and mostly only disclose the case information when requested. According to Salinitri et al. (2015), facilitators utilize a learning methodology grounded in constructivist philosophy and function as guides or coaches. In PBL, the role of the facilitator contrasts significantly with traditional lecturing methods. Rather than delivering content through direct instruction, a PBL facilitator adopts a guiding, supportive approach that encourages students to explore, question, and collaboratively solve problems. The facilitator does not provide answers or lectures on the material; instead, they create an environment where students take an active role in their own learning. This shift from instructor-centered to student-centered learning enables students to develop critical thinking, problem-solving, and self-directed learning skills, which are core to the PBL model.

A skilled facilitator asks thought-provoking and appropriate questions, which encourage students to take personal responsibility for learning and strive to get relevant knowledge referenced in all basic medical/health science subjects. A seasoned facilitator develops flexible strategies through open-ended questioning that encourages learning and promotes the development of metacognitive skills in students.

Facilitators use open-ended and metacognitive questioning to embolden students to seek explanations and recognize knowledge deficiencies they may not have discovered before the PBL session. Newly discovered learning deficiencies might remain undetected and unaccounted for if the facilitator does not push for explanations while guiding and facilitating the students through the case. Facilitators are encouraged to listen carefully to a wide range of responses to help confirm or rule out possible causes related to the chief complaint and symptoms associated with the case. During the discussion, explanations offered by students can generate numerous potential sources to support or exclude possible causes for the chief complaint. Progress is maintained by continuously mapping correlations through open-ended questions, exploring connections within the case details, history, physical exam findings, lab results, and imaging data to identify likely causes. These possible causes should be validated through cross-referencing with key concepts and mechanisms found in the literature provided in the curriculum. The facilitator should remain in active listening mode throughout the session, fostering understanding of key concepts, maintaining student focus, identifying knowledge gaps, and ensuring that mechanisms of action are clearly connected to causal facts. The facilitator's goal is to foster a group dynamic that nurtures active learning and ensures fluent flow through the 2-hour PBL session. This approach allows students to assess the depth of their understanding, encouraging individual accountability within group dynamics and preparing them for the next PBL session, typically held within a day or two. Both the facilitator and the students recognize the importance of time management in this curriculum, ensuring that discussions are productive and aligned with learning goals.

The facilitator plays a critical role in maintaining healthy and safe group dynamics during PBL sessions. In this student-centered, problem-solving-focused learning environment, key elements such as collaboration, re-evaluation, and reformulation of ideas are fostered through critical thinking, self-reflection, and peer feedback. An effective facilitator creates a collaborative atmosphere by encouraging all students to actively participate, whether by asking questions, sharing knowledge, or researching references. Attentive facilitators monitor students' engagement and track the group's progress over multiple sessions.

They also observe and document the varying roles students assume, such as student doctor, reader, or board scribe. Additionally, facilitators note individuals who explain concepts, reference required textbooks, or demonstrate exceptional levels of civility and courtesy (Table 5.1).

5.2 Self-Directed Learning

Facilitators play a pivotal role in setting the stage for self-directed learning at the beginning of each curriculum block during PBL group sessions. They ensure that the group maintains collaboration, continuous re-evaluation, and the reformulation of ideas throughout the learning process. By doing so, facilitators foster a learning environment that cultivates and enhances clinical critical thinking skills (Fig. 5.2).

Table 5.1 Facilitator note table for documenting students' participation

PBL CLASS NOTES DAY/DATE: ______________ TIME Class Held: ______________ GROUP : ROOM #: CLASS YEAR:				
STUDENT NAME	**ROLE (Presenter, Scribe, Reader)**	**Present (P) Absent (A) Tardy (T)**	**Participation Level (√+, √, √-)**	**Facilitator Observations/Comments:**

(continued)

Table 5.1 (continued)

General Group Observations:				
Material Reviewed: **CASE #1:** **Case #:_____________Case Name: ____________________** **CASE SEGMENTS COMPLETED:** CC HX PE CDs: 1, 2, 3, 4, 5, 6, 7, 8, 9, 10 DX TX OUTCOME Clinical Course CDs: 11, 12, 13, 14, 15 DX TX OUTCOME OTHER:				
NEW Learning Issues Identified:				
Exam Topics/Chapters Voted On and Submitted:				
WRAP-UP DISCUSSION:				
ADMINISTRATIVE INFO/ACTION TAKEN:				
FACILITATOR SIGNATURE: ____ ________				

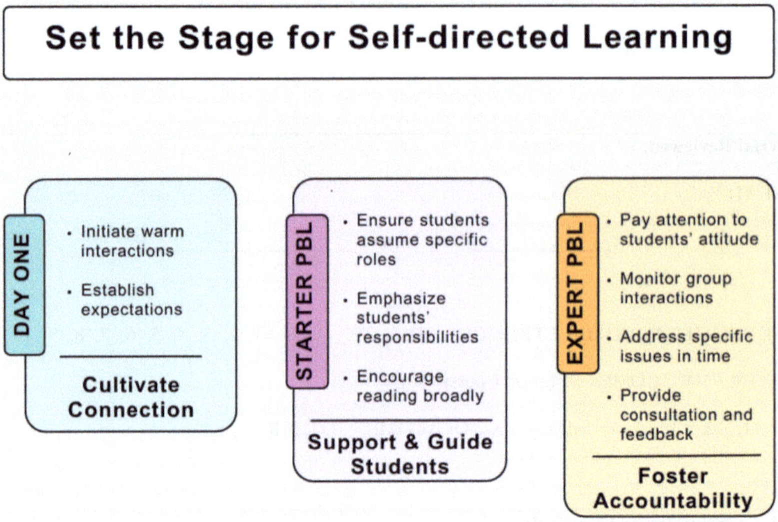

Fig. 5.2 Facilitators play a pivotal role in setting the stage for self-directed learning by employing various strategies tailored to each stage of the PBL process

5.2.1 Fostering Connection and Responsibility from Day One

Warm and welcoming initial interactions are crucial for building rapport and helping students feel comfortable with one another. Both facilitators and students should participate in introductions, allowing the group to uncover shared backgrounds, areas of strength, and commonalities (Barrows, 1998). These introductions promote self-awareness, productivity, and courtesy, which are essential for fostering an effective, healthy, and dynamic group environment. When group discussions are conducted with civility, self-control, and attentiveness, the quality of the verbal climate is enhanced, ultimately maximizing learning outcomes (Fonteijn & Dolmans, 2019).

Facilitators establish expectations at the beginning of each PBL session, emphasizing the importance of active participation and accountability in the learning process. They empower students to become valuable contributors by encouraging them to read foundational medical and health science texts, cite references accurately, explore a wide range of topics, and pose challenging, integrative questions that connect basic medical/health science concepts and mechanisms. Through this approach, students quickly recognize that independent learning and collaboration are fundamental skills for success in the PBL curriculum.

5.2.2 Structuring Roles and Promoting Early Critical Thinking

Facilitators play a crucial role in supporting and guiding students throughout the PBL process (L'Ecuyer et al., 2015). A key responsibility is ensuring that students assume specific roles at the beginning of each session. One student should take on the role of the reader, who reads the case aloud to focus the group's attention. At the same time, another assumes the role of the board scribe, who is responsible for outlining key information and compiling a list of learning issues on the board. In subsequent sessions, a different student should serve as the presenter, delivering a progress report to the group. This rotational system ensures equitable participation and allows students to develop a range of skills by sharing the PBL group roles each time the group convenes.

From the very beginning, facilitators play a pivotal role in fostering and promoting critical thinking, a cornerstone for students to become active learners in a PBL environment (Hung et al., 2008). In the early stages of PBL learning within a curriculum, facilitators should emphasize that students must integrate and extrapolate facts from a broad spectrum of basic medical and health science disciplines, including anatomy, histology, embryology, genetics, nutrition, physiology, biochemistry, pharmacology, pathology, behavioral science, microbiology, and immunology. Facilitators must consistently prioritize the process of self-directed learning within a collaborative team framework, reinforcing that students are ultimately responsible for the depth and breadth of their learning. For example, during sessions, the group's reader begins by verbally working through the case, starting with the chief complaint and progressing through the case history, physical examination, and lab and imaging data until the session concludes with a wrap-up. Concurrently, the scribe captures key points discussed by the group on the whiteboard, ensuring a structured and organized flow of thought. This practice of reading aloud and scribing fosters group focus and clarity while supporting collaborative learning. Students can refer to the allowed resources to expand their understanding. Facilitators should track role assignments, including which students have acted as readers, presenters, or scribes, ensuring that every participant has the opportunity to perform each role by the end of the semester. This rotation ensures equitable participation and skill development across the group.

5.2.3 Fostering Accountability and Group Cohesion Through Proactive Facilitation

Facilitators must remain attentive to students' attitudes, as they can significantly impact group dynamics and the overall learning process. Negative attitudes within the group such as tardiness, lack of enthusiasm or curiosity, poor concentration, hostility toward peers, the unfair delegation of responsibilities, timidity, dominance, or lack of interest, can disrupt cohesion and hinder productivity. To address these challenges, facilitators should encourage the group to tackle open-ended questions early on to promote focus and redirection. Establishing clear guidelines and expectations, such as punctuality, active participation, and respectful communication, can help mitigate many poor behaviors. Open and honest discussions provide an opportunity to foster shared responsibility and ensure tasks are equitably distributed among group members. Regular check-ins, both group-wide and individual, are essential for addressing specific issues such as timidity, dominance, or lack of interest, allowing facilitators to provide tailored support and interventions. Facilitators also monitor interactions within the group using tools such as the tracking record sheet (Fig. 5.1), which helps document and evaluate each student's participation and behaviors during PBL sessions. By actively supervising and addressing these dynamics, facilitators promote a positive and productive group environment.

Students quickly learn that staying on top of the workload requires consistent effort and preparation for each session to contribute meaningfully to the group's learning process. When a student fails to adopt this mindset and falls behind, their lack of engagement becomes evident to the group, raising questions about their commitment to the group's success. During the wrap-up portion of the session, students reflect on their performance, often commenting on whether they met expectations and, in some cases, explaining any shortcomings. Wrap-up serves as a structured opportunity for participants to provide feedback on the session's quality, both individually and collectively. This reflection allows the group to evaluate their progress toward achieving the stated objectives, fostering accountability, and promoting productivity.

According to Gibbon and Marcangelo (2012), students develop mutual respect and a sense of partnership essential for fostering healthy interprofessional relationships, which are crucial for achieving successful outcomes in clinical settings. PBL sessions are perceived by students as high-stakes learning experiences, where time is valuable and cannot be regained once the session concludes. Facilitators play a vital role by observing the group's dynamics, including the quality and tempo of interactions. In a well-functioning and cohesive PBL group, students share a common goal of striving for excellence. This mindset drives them to work efficiently and make the most of their time together. Each PBL group collaborates for 20 weeks (i.e., one semester) before participants are reassigned to new groups by the PBL Director. Student commitment to maximizing efficiency and productivity is largely determined by the group's participants. Recognizing the rarity of working with the same peers in subsequent groups, students place significant value on self-directed learning, which hinges on sharing, validating, and collectively understanding information to optimize learning potential. In such an environment, the facilitator serves primarily as an observer and guide, consistently asking questions to stimulate critical thinking and ensure progress toward case completion. Typically, facilitators are assigned to oversee two PBL groups per semester, supporting their development and maintaining group cohesion.

5.3 Performance Outcomes

Successful facilitation requires effective communication of expectations for PBL group performance, along with consistency in guiding the group and maintaining the proper structure for the roles of presenter, board scribe, and reader. Facilitators must also ensure that the group stays on track to complete the case within the time frame set by the PBL Director. This approach helps maintain focus and ensures the learning objectives are met efficiently.

5.3.1 Balancing Preparation and Responsiveness: Supporting Student Learning Without Teaching the Content

Facilitators undergo formal and extensive training to ensure they are fully prepared to perform optimally (see details in Chap. 3). After observing and learning from an experienced mentor facilitator, novice facilitators gain a conceptual understanding of PBL goals and the roles of facilitation. By the time they begin facilitating their first PBL session, they are well-equipped to guide the group effectively (Salinitri et al., 2015).

To effectively facilitate a PBL session, facilitators must first understand the case and the flow of educational information to guide student learning. Preparation involves studying the facilitator guide, which outlines key concepts or mechanisms to be discussed during the session. Occasionally, facilitators may refer to textbooks to probe students' understanding. Each case-specific guide provides an overview of the subject matter and includes page-by-page annotations, helping facilitators stay on track. These guides are carefully structured to ensure a smooth session within the designated time limit, allowing facilitators to manage the learning process without being content experts.

The facilitator guides are regularly updated by the PBL Director to maintain consistency and cohesiveness across all PBL groups, especially in large classes of up to 200 students. Facilitators must adhere to the guide to ensure uniformity in learning outcomes and progression across groups throughout the semester. The time spent reviewing the facilitator guide varies depending on the facilitator's background and experience. The guide's purpose is to prepare facilitators to support student learning without directly teaching the content. PBL is not about the facilitator being a case expert. Regardless of their level of expertise, facilitators need to be familiar with the case content to assist students in recalling, integrating, analyzing, and problem-solving (Azer, 2011).

During each 2-hour session, the PBL group works together to identify key learning issues and potential test topics. The facilitator observes how the group's dynamics evolve from session to session based on student preparedness across various basic medical/health care science disciplines such as anatomy, histology, embryology, genetics, nutrition, physiology, biochemistry, pharmacology, pathology, behavioral science, microbiology, and immunology. Facilitators must stay alert to identify moments where questions can stimulate further exploration and prevent stagnation or the overlooking of key concepts in the learning process.

5.3.2 Structuring Roles for Deep Learning: Practical Frameworks That Elevate PBL Engagement

Each semester, facilitators are typically assigned to two PBL groups for 10 weeks and then switch to another two groups for the following 10 weeks. While most facilitators work with two PBL groups during the academic year, there may be some variation, with some facilitators assigned to just one group or as many as three.

Effective PBL sessions are structured and highly regulated. In a typical PBL session, students take on specific roles such as reader, scribe (on the whiteboard or in a shared electronic document), and physician/case presenter. The facilitator assigns these roles throughout the 10-week session, ensuring that each student has the opportunity to perform each task. This approach allows the facilitator to track each student's performance and provide feedback. The facilitator explains the roles to be played in the session and oversees how students assign these roles among themselves, ensuring consistency and an even distribution of tasks throughout the block. The roles and responsibilities should be clearly outlined by the facilitator from the start, with students rotating through different roles to maximize their learning experience. According to Gibbon and Marcangelo (2012), role-playing enhances healthcare profession students' reasoning abilities by enabling them to learn through problem-solving rather than rote memorization. This approach creates a practical, hands-on way for students to apply their knowledge in patient care. By experiencing different roles, reader, board scribe, and physician/case presenter, students gain valuable perspectives from each vantage point. This process fosters critical thinking, communication, and the ability to evaluate, reformulate, and refine ideas. The roles facilitate information processing, enhance knowledge acquisition, and provide a structured foundation for case discussions and the identification of key learning issues.

It is essential for the facilitator to track student performance in each role to provide specific, targeted feedback. In a typical PBL session, the reader communicates the information disclosed by the facilitator, ensuring that the group maintains focus and progresses through the case. The board scribe organizes and records information clearly, often using a systematic strategy such as the SOAP note approach:

- **S (Subjective)**: Gathering the patient's history
- **O (Objective)**: Recording physical examination findings
- **A (Assessment)**: Formulating a differential diagnosis
- **P (Plan)**: Creating a plan for further action, including tests, referrals, and patient education

Using the SOAP format helps students organize their learning systematically, incorporating patient history, physical examination, lab tests, imaging, and holistic patient needs. The board scribe ensures all aspects of the case are captured, which are then used to identify learning issues or test topics.

In the second PBL session for the same case, the presenter shares a progress note that summarizes the case development up to that point, outlining what has been accomplished and what remains to be done. Each student has the opportunity to present the case, contributing to their performance evaluation. This presentation sets the tone for the session, starting with the chief complaint, followed by the history and physical examination, and progressing through clinical data that reveals both subtle and crucial information. All case information is related to basic medical/health science concepts and mechanisms, which students review and discuss.

Towards the end of the session, the group votes on the learning issues and test topics, helping to guide the direction of further study. This structured approach ensures that all students actively engage in the learning process and develop a comprehensive understanding of the clinical case.

5.4 Facilitator as Inquiry Catalyst

The facilitator plays a key role in understanding and engaging with the PBL group. Each PBL group develops its own dynamic, which is shaped through introductions and interactions among group members, including the facilitator. The facilitator integrates into this dynamic, fostering a collaborative and cohesive learning environment that directly influences the group's PBL performance. As a keen observer and listener, the facilitator anticipates discussions, interjects questions at appropriate moments, and monitors student participation. By actively listening to content and assessing the levels of engagement, the facilitator knows when to guide the group to keep discussions on track and manage time effectively. According to Gibbon and Marcangelo (2012), educational evaluation in PBL is rooted in the facilitator's intrapersonal behavior. This behavior contributes to an active, self-directed, contextual, and collaborative learning process, ensuring that students remain engaged and productive throughout the session.

5.4.1 Guiding the Flow of Clinical Reasoning

In a PBL curriculum, cases are designed to simulate the clinical encounters students will experience during clerkship rounds. Each case begins with the presentation of a chief complaint. Students then generate a comprehensive list of differential diagnoses based on the initial information. Once all reasonable possibilities have been explored, they may request additional details, such as the patient's medical history and physical examination findings, which the facilitator provides. Laboratory test results are shared only when students explicitly request them, mirroring the clinical process of ordering tests.

As students work through the case, they consult required textbooks, analyze the information provided, and engage in discussions to deepen their understanding. This process helps them identify knowledge gaps, clarify unclear mechanisms, and address conflicting interpretations from various resources. These insights emerge rapidly through verbal discourse within the group, driving collaborative problem-solving.

Facilitators play a pivotal role in guiding this process. They actively listen to group discussions, monitor dynamics, and follow the facilitator guide to ensure consistency across sessions. While doing so, they balance staying engaged with knowing when to step back to allow the group to take ownership of their learning. The facilitator guide is carefully constructed to outline the learning objectives for each case, allowing facilitators to focus on listening rather than reading during sessions. Most cases are disclosed in a logical sequence dictated by the students. Occasionally, discussions may deviate from this sequence as students dive deeply into a particular concept or mechanism. However, because the facilitator has been thoroughly prepared in advance, such deviations do not disrupt the session's flow. This flexibility in presenting clinical data stimulates critical thinking and active questioning. As Tai and Yuen (2007) note, this approach reflects the authentic, non-linear nature of real-world clinical situations.

Frequent practice enables facilitators to become comfortable and adept at managing these dynamics. They can seamlessly provide clinical data and guidance without disrupting the quality or tempo of the students' learning process. Facilitators also manage the unique pace, flow, and flexibility of each group's discussions, ensuring alignment with the case's learning objectives while fostering a collaborative and engaging environment.

To prepare effectively, facilitators plan both before and during PBL sessions and reflect afterward to refine their approach. The PBL Program Director ensures that facilitators and groups stay aligned with case pacing and meet the semester's goals and objectives. Regular facilitator meetings, led by the PBL Director, provide updates, allow for questions, and offer a forum for sharing insights and making curriculum recommendations. These meetings promote consistency and contribute to the continuous improvement of PBL experience.

During each case, facilitators observe and support students as they engage in a seven-step cognitive critical thinking process (Fig. 5.3). This process is repeated two to three times per week over 10 weeks, with each group consisting of 8–9 healthcare profession students. Facilitators focus on how groups negotiate, build consensus, and scaffold information while ensuring that discussions align with the case's learning objectives.

As Salinitri et al. (2015) emphasize, facilitators also play a critical role in fostering metacognition. Metacognition involves planning, monitoring, and evaluating one's intellectual capabilities and strategies. By encouraging this reflective process, facilitators help students refine their critical thinking and problem-solving skills, empowering them to become more effective learners.

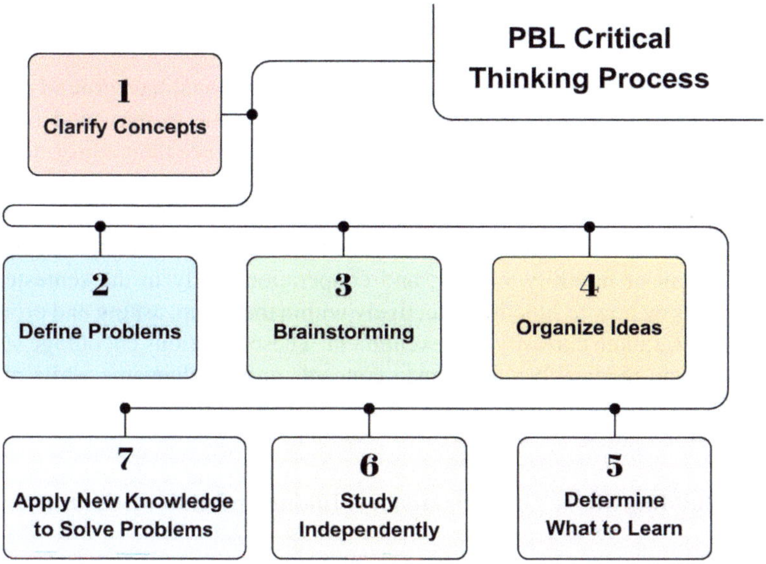

Fig. 5.3 The 7-step cognitive critical thinking process in PBL, ranging from concepts clarification to applying new knowledge to solve defined problems

5.4.2 Fostering Student-Led Inquiry

In a PBL curriculum, the cornerstone of learning is the student inquiry process. An effective facilitator poses thoughtful questions, but over time, students are expected to take ownership of the inquiry, asking most, if not all, of the critical questions. This approach nurtures their ability to acquire, comprehend, apply, analyze, synthesize, and evaluate information, fostering independent and critical thinking.

5.4.2.1 Collaborative Inquiry as a Driver of Learning

Unlike traditional didactics, where the lecturer poses questions to students and expects a response, PBL emphasizes inquiry as a collaborative effort among group members. Students initiate questions, and peers respond by seeking evidence-based solutions. These dynamic fosters active learning, as students identify knowledge gaps, authenticate responses, and build complex explanations through verbal discussions or presentations, such as PowerPoint slides. For instance, a group might collaboratively analyze acid-base imbalances and the body's compensatory mechanisms in a clinical scenario. Such discussions require students to integrate knowledge from basic and clinical sciences while working in subgroups to present their findings. Over time, students develop the confidence to initiate and answer questions independently, making inquiry a routine and integral part of their learning process.

5.4.2.2 Addressing Variability Among Learners

Students enter PBL with diverse educational and professional backgrounds, ranging from clinical experience as scribes or nurses to expertise in unrelated fields like engineering or education. These varied experiences influence their adjustment to the PBL process. According to Tai and Yuen (2007), transitions into PBL are unique, and facilitators must be mindful of these differences.

Facilitators play a crucial role in setting the tone for group dynamics by fostering an environment of humility, civility, and cooperation. Early in the semester, they guide students on how to function effectively within the group, asking and prompting questions to stimulate curiosity and excitement. These questions encourage students to explore basic medical/health science concepts and mechanisms while aligning with the facilitator guide's objectives.

5.4.2.3 Building Skills Through History-Taking and Role Assignments

A key aspect of the PBL process is the introduction of history-taking. Students learn to perform a complete patient history by participating in interactive interviews, often role-playing as physicians while the facilitator acts as the patient. Each student practices this skill, which is then expanded to include physical examination discussions, lab tests, and imaging related to the case. Over time, students adapt to this process, beginning to ask questions and lead discussions without facilitator input.

Facilitators ensure that all students experience various roles, such as reader, scribe, and physician/case presenter, to stimulate richer, broader discussions. By questioning themselves and one another, students critically evaluate their hypotheses and adjust their approaches. This inquiry process ultimately enhances their understanding of basic medical/health science concepts and clinical applications within the context of the case.

5.4.2.4 Inquiry's Role in Collaborative Knowledge Building

As students navigate the complexities of clinical cases, they encounter moments of doubt or puzzlement that drive deeper discussions. For example, a case involving respiratory acidosis might prompt students to analyze lab results, historical data, and physical findings to determine the underlying mechanisms. Through this co-construction of knowledge, students integrate evidence from multiple basic medical/health science disciplines, aligning their understanding with the clinical scenario. This dynamic aligns with the cognitive schema and affective domain approach discussed by Krathwohl et al. (1973). Students actively exchange ideas, build consensus, and scaffold knowledge collaboratively. Facilitators observe and listen, ensuring the group stays on track while allowing students to direct the discussion.

5.4.2.5 The Evolution of Independent Inquiry

With repeated practice, students develop the skills to independently seek and synthesize information. They analyze, evaluate, and organize data while internalizing individual and group values. Emotional responses within the group influence both personal growth and collective effectiveness, enabling students to arrive at well-reasoned diagnoses and solutions. By the end of a PBL case, students demonstrate their ability to comprehend, apply, and synthesize information. This process mirrors the professional ethical practices they will encounter in clinical settings, laying a foundation for their development as competent, reflective practitioners.

5.4.2.6 Integrating Professional and Ethical Growth

The inquiry-driven approach in PBL not only builds cognitive and technical skills but also fosters professional and ethical development. As students internalize values and validate or challenge their assumptions, they prepare for the collaborative and reflective demands of the clinical workforce. This dual focus on individual and group growth ensures that PBL equips students with both the intellectual and interpersonal skills needed for success.

5.4.3 Adapting to Group Dynamics

The PBL process requires time and practice for students to become proficient. Facilitators play a vital role in guiding groups through this progression, using the facilitator guide to ensure that discussions remain focused on the necessary concepts and mechanisms. This structured approach prevents tangential conversations and optimizes the group's time to meet the learning objectives.

5.4.3.1 Establishing Effective Group Dynamics

A healthy group dynamic is essential for PBL success. Facilitators oversee the group's interactions, promoting clinical reasoning in a collaborative atmosphere. They observe both individual and collective engagement, ensuring that each student contributes meaningfully to the group's progress. When necessary, facilitators intervene to maintain a productive flow of discussion. For example, if multiple students speak simultaneously, making information inaccessible to others, the facilitator steps in to restore order.

According to Tai and Yuen (2007), authentic activity lies at the heart of PBL, enabling students to analyze complex scenarios and explore conflicting explanations of basic medical/health science concepts or mechanisms relevant to the case. Through this process, facilitators ensure that the group maintains a constructive and inclusive environment conducive to critical thinking and problem-solving.

5.4.3.2 Adapting to Group Variations

No two PBL groups function identically, even with the same case materials. The dynamics of each group and session can vary significantly. For instance, early in the semester, groups may progress more slowly as students familiarize themselves with the PBL process. This slower pace is expected and necessary for building a strong foundation. Conversely, experienced groups often move at a faster pace, requiring facilitators to adjust to ensure that they do not overlook critical details or nuances in the case.

As noted by Preeti et al. (2013), PBL fosters an environment where students build upon their existing knowledge. Cross-functional feedback from peers and facilitators sharpens students' critical thinking and enhances accountability to themselves and the group. This dual focus on individual and group growth underscores PBL's role in knowledge acquisition and application.

5.4.3.3 The Unique Personality of Each Group

Each PBL group develops its own "personality," shaped by the unique combination of participants and their interactions. Facilitators are tasked with encouraging the group to develop a systematic, dynamic, and consultative approach to achieve learning outcomes with minimal intervention. Group maturity, which is defined by the ability to consult, research, and apply evidence to illustrate concepts or mechanisms, largely determines the outcomes of the PBL process.

Facilitators bring their own experiences and personalities to the PBL session, enriching the group's learning process. Typically, students work with two facilitators per semester, providing diverse perspectives and guidance. Additionally, new PBL groups are formed at the beginning of each semester, challenging students to adapt to new peers and facilitators. By the end of their PBL curriculum, students have honed their ability to collaborate, analyze, and solve problems effectively, demonstrating proficiency in the PBL process.

5.4.3.4 Facilitator's Role in Group Progression

Facilitators are instrumental in fostering a balance between group autonomy and guidance. They stimulate discussion, monitor group function, and ensure alignment with learning objectives. This iterative process allows groups to evolve, becoming more independent and confident in their ability to navigate complex clinical cases. Through consistent adaptation to group and session variations, PBL cultivates a rich learning environment that prepares students for the collaborative demands of clinical practice.

5.5 Facilitator-Led Scaffolding: Enhancing Engagement and Cognitive Growth in PBL

Effective student engagement in the PBL process is often facilitated through scaffolding, a teaching strategy that bridges gaps in knowledge and supports progressive learning. In PBL, each student brings prior knowledge, some of which may be relevant to the case at hand. The facilitator plays a crucial role as an active listener, observing the group's discussions and stepping in at opportune moments to ask questions or stimulate deeper exploration.

Scaffolding provides a structured framework for students to build upon their existing knowledge during PBL sessions. This process helps students navigate the complexities of clinical cases while developing critical thinking and problem-solving skills. Facilitators use scaffolding techniques to guide discussions, helping students connect concepts and mechanisms within the case context.

Healthcare profession students, individually and collectively, employ scaffolding during the metacognitive phases of PBL. They assess their understanding, identify gaps in knowledge, and seek additional information to enhance their learning process. As shown in Fig. 5.4, scaffolding facilitates a step-by-step approach to deeper learning, fostering a collaborative and dynamic learning environment.

Facilitators maintain an active and alert mindset throughout the PBL process, responding to content requests in sequence or out of sequence to ensure a productive learning environment. They avoid dictating what students should do, instead encouraging autonomy and collaboration. At the end of each session, facilitators guide the group through a wrap-up process, which serves two purposes:

1. **Individual Assessment**: Evaluating each student's performance and contributions.
2. **Group Assessment**: Reflecting on the group's overall dynamics and progress.

The wrap-up phase is integral to the learning process, allowing facilitators and students to consolidate their understanding of the case. This phase provides an opportunity to clarify any unresolved issues, reinforce key learning objectives, and evaluate the group's overall performance. Facilitators use this time to encourage reflection, helping students internalize what they have learned and prepare for the next session.

Facilitators are also responsible for monitoring essential tasks, such as the completion of SOAP note presentations and the development of comprehensive differential diagnoses. By creating space for participants to tackle complex concepts and mechanisms, facilitators ensure that the group fully engages with the material.

By employing scaffolding techniques and fostering a supportive yet challenging environment, facilitators enable students to engage effectively in the PBL process.

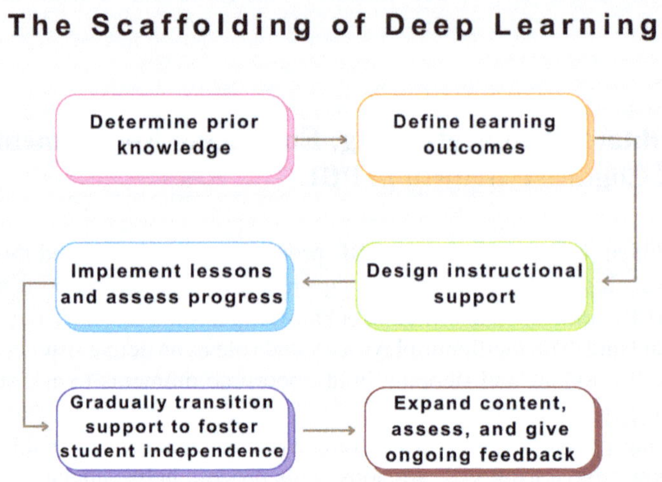

Fig. 5.4 The scaffolding thinking process in PBL for deep learning, a step-by-step approach that begins with identifying prior knowledge and progresses to expanding new content

This dynamic interaction not only enhances individual learning but also strengthens the collective cognitive growth of the group.

5.5.1 *Mastering the Art of Questioning in PBL: Cultivating Inquiry, Critical Thinking, and Collaborative Learning*

The ability to ask thoughtful and meaningful questions is fundamental to the PBL process, fostering critical thinking and deep engagement with clinical cases. Facilitators play a pivotal role in nurturing this skill among students by modeling and encouraging effective questioning techniques.

During PBL sessions, facilitators guide discussions by asking open-ended questions that prompt students to explore basic medical/health science concepts presented in a clinical case. Instead of answering student queries directly, facilitators respond with questions that encourage independent investigation (Hmelo-Silver & Barrows, 2006). This strategy not only reinforces the students' inquiry skills but also highlights the interconnected nature of independent learning and group dynamics in PBL.

Facilitators remain attentive to the facilitator guide, which outlines key topics and concepts to address in each case. They may interject with content-related questions to steer discussions productively but must remain mindful of session timing. Maintaining adherence to the overall schedule ensures that all cases are completed on time and that students are prepared to submit their test topics before examinations.

5.5.1.1 Students' Role in Asking Questions

In PBL, students progressively learn the art of questioning, which is essential for critical thinking and lifelong learning. The process is self-directed, and facilitators encourage students to ask their own questions, particularly as they become familiar with PBL dynamics. Over time, students' questioning skills evolve, leading to more frequent and sophisticated inquiries during sessions.

Effective questioning stimulates discussion, reinforces learning, and promotes critical thinking. When students express thoughts through questions and answers, they retain information more effectively (Kedrick et al., 2023). Additionally, questioning nurtures curiosity and fosters the spirit of scientific inquiry, integral to the PBL experience.

Productive questions in PBL are characterized by their ability to drive discussion, highlight key concepts, and deepen understanding. Higher-order questions, which require complex reasoning and synthesis of information, are particularly valuable. These questions build upon foundational knowledge, requiring students to:

- Read and understand broadly from assigned health science textbooks.
- Cite references appropriately from their readings.
- Engage the group in deeper learning by connecting concepts and mechanisms.

When students question each other, it signals active engagement and a healthy group dynamic. This collaborative inquiry allows the group to arrive at a consensus and demonstrates mastery of concepts.

Following a constructivist approach (Wood, 2003), facilitators listen for students to activate prior knowledge and build upon it, guiding them to validate new understanding through cross-referencing basic medical/health science texts. By doing so, facilitators support students in retaining knowledge effectively and creating a challenging yet stimulating PBL environment.

A PBL session driven by student questions fosters a culture of curiosity and collaborative learning. Students who actively engage in questioning are better equipped to synthesize information, develop critical thinking skills, and retain knowledge for future application. Facilitators, by fostering this questioning culture, ensure that the PBL process remains dynamic and impactful, ultimately preparing students for lifelong learning in the healthcare field.

5.5.2 Facilitator Strategies for Overcoming PBL Challenges

PBL presents several challenges for health professions students, primarily due to its self-directed nature, the complexity of integrating knowledge from diverse disciplines, and the large volume of reading required. Despite these challenges, there are effective strategies that both students and facilitators can adopt to enhance the learning process and ensure students' success in PBL.

One of the primary challenges students face in PBL is the overwhelming volume of reading. For many first-year students, especially those who are not accustomed to scientific reading or who lack a background in basic medical/health sciences, the amount of material can be intimidating. In the early stages, students often supplement their learning with audiovisual resources found online, but these resources are not always comprehensive and may lack the depth required for health professions education. To address this, facilitators should emphasize the importance of using foundational textbooks for in-depth learning. For example, textbooks like *Guyton and Hall's Textbook of Medical Physiology* offer detailed explanations of physiological mechanisms that are essential for understanding complex case studies. While audiovisual resources can serve as helpful supplements, they should not replace comprehensive textbook reading. Over time, as students become more familiar with the material, their reading efficiency and understanding of complex concepts improve.

Another challenge students encounter is grappling with complex mechanisms and conflicting information from different sources. When students struggle to understand certain concepts or encounter conflicting explanations, it is crucial that these issues are brought into the PBL discussions for collaborative problem-solving. Facilitators can guide the group by asking open-ended questions and prompting discussions to help clarify misunderstandings. For instance, if a group is struggling to understand the pathophysiology of a disease, the facilitator might encourage students to compare and contrast different theories presented in their textbooks. By discussing the conflicting explanations, students not only solidify their understanding but also develop the critical thinking skills necessary to navigate complex healthcare science knowledge.

First-year students are often anxious about missing important information during their self-directed learning. This anxiety can be particularly intense when they are unfamiliar with the PBL process. Facilitators play an essential role in alleviating this anxiety by creating a supportive environment where students feel comfortable sharing their concerns. Facilitators should respect students' emotions, listen to their concerns, and encourage active participation in the PBL sessions. One effective strategy is to assign students roles, such as presenter, scribe, or reader, which helps distribute the responsibility for learning and ensures that each student is engaged in the process. For example, the student who is assigned as the presenter might lead the group through the case study, while the scribe documents key points, and the reader summarizes additional relevant information. This approach not only helps students feel more confident but also reinforces the collaborative nature of PBL, where each participant contributes to the group's overall learning.

Facilitators also guide students in clinical reasoning by helping them create structured tasks and lists, such as the differential diagnosis list. This list is a tool for students to organize their thoughts and consider a range of possible conditions based on the patient's history and physical examination. One way to assist students in developing this list is by introducing the VINDICATE-P mnemonic, which covers a broad range of diagnostic categories: vascular, infection, neoplasm, drugs, inflammation/idiopathic, congenital, autoimmune, trauma, endocrine, and psychological conditions. By using this mnemonic, students are encouraged to think broadly and integrate knowledge across various healthcare science disciplines. For example, if a student is working on a case involving a patient with chest pain, they might use VINDICATE-P to consider not only cardiovascular issues like myocardial infarction (vascular) but also non-cardiac causes such as esophageal reflux (endocrine) or anxiety (psychological). This approach helps students develop a comprehensive understanding of the many factors that contribute to a patient's condition.

Throughout the PBL process, facilitators continuously promote inquiry and scaffolding by guiding students through the complexities of the case while encouraging them to ask more questions. As previously mentioned, scaffolding is a teaching strategy where facilitators support students' learning by gradually transferring responsibility to the students as they develop their skills. For instance, when students first encounter a complex concept, the facilitator might provide guiding questions or suggest resources, but over time, as students become more proficient, the facilitator steps back and allows them to direct their own learning. This approach helps students build confidence and independence in their clinical reasoning.

Facilitators can also contribute to the PBL examination process by submitting case-based multiple-choice questions (MCQs) to the PBL Director after each case. These questions are designed to assess the students' understanding of the concepts covered during the PBL sessions. Case-based questions are particularly valuable because they reflect real-world clinical scenarios, requiring students to apply their knowledge in a practical context. For example, after a case on diabetes management, the facilitator might submit a question that asks students to identify the most appropriate diagnostic test for a patient with suspected type 2 diabetes. This type of assessment encourages students to integrate basic medical/health science knowledge with clinical practice and reinforces key learning outcomes.

While PBL presents challenges, it also offers numerous opportunities for students to develop critical thinking, clinical reasoning, and self-directed learning skills. By employing strategies such as emphasizing textbook learning, encouraging collaborative problem-solving, assigning roles to students, and using structured tools like VINDICATE-P, both students and facilitators can overcome these challenges. Facilitators, by creating a supportive and structured learning environment, help students develop the skills they need to succeed in their healthcare science education and future clinical practice.

5.5.3 Facilitator Role in PBL Assessments

Facilitators play a vital role in evaluating student learning within the PBL framework by contributing to the pool of multiple-choice case-based questions (MCQs) used in assessments. These questions, submitted to the PBL Director, are typically created after a series of cases has been completed or once an individual case has been thoroughly explored by the group. The timeline and expectations for submitting these questions are established during facilitator group meetings at the beginning of each PBL session and are reiterated after the sessions conclude.

Case-based MCQs are carefully crafted to focus on the specific learning objectives and content covered during the PBL sessions. These questions are designed not just to test students' recall of information but to evaluate their understanding of basic medical/health science concepts and mechanisms in the context of clinical scenarios. For example, after a case involving the pathophysiology of congestive heart failure, a case-based MCQ might ask: *Which of the following compensatory mechanisms is most likely to occur in response to reduced cardiac output?* The answer choices could include reduced heart rate, peripheral vasodilation, activation of the renin-angiotensin-aldosterone system, or decreased myocardial oxygen demand. Students must apply their understanding of physiology and pathophysiology to choose the correct response, demonstrating integration of knowledge across disciplines.

Similarly, if a group has worked on a case involving diabetic ketoacidosis (DKA), a facilitator might construct a question such as: *Which laboratory finding is most consistent with a diagnosis of DKA?* The answer options could include elevated blood glucose, metabolic acidosis with an increased anion gap, hypokalemia, or low serum osmolality. These questions require students to analyze clinical data and correlate it with the pathophysiological processes underlying the condition.

The content of these questions can vary based on the dynamics and pace of each PBL group. Facilitators are encouraged to align their questions with the unique discussions and discoveries of their groups while adhering to the overall curriculum objectives. For instance, if one group dives deeply into the pharmacological management of asthma during their case discussions, an appropriate MCQ could ask: *Which of the following medications is most appropriate for the acute management of an asthma exacerbation?* The choices might include inhaled corticosteroids, long-acting beta-agonists, short-acting beta-agonists, or leukotriene receptor antagonists. This type of question evaluates the group's understanding of pharmacotherapy and its clinical application.

Azer (2003) highlights the benefits of using case-based scenarios in health professions education, particularly in solidifying students' grasp of basic medical/health science concepts and their clinical applications (Fig. 5.5). These scenarios bridge the gap between theoretical learning and clinical practice, ensuring that students not only understand the material but can also apply it effectively. Facilitators, by contributing thoughtfully constructed questions, play a crucial role in reinforcing this connection and supporting students in achieving a deeper, more integrated understanding of healthcare science knowledge.

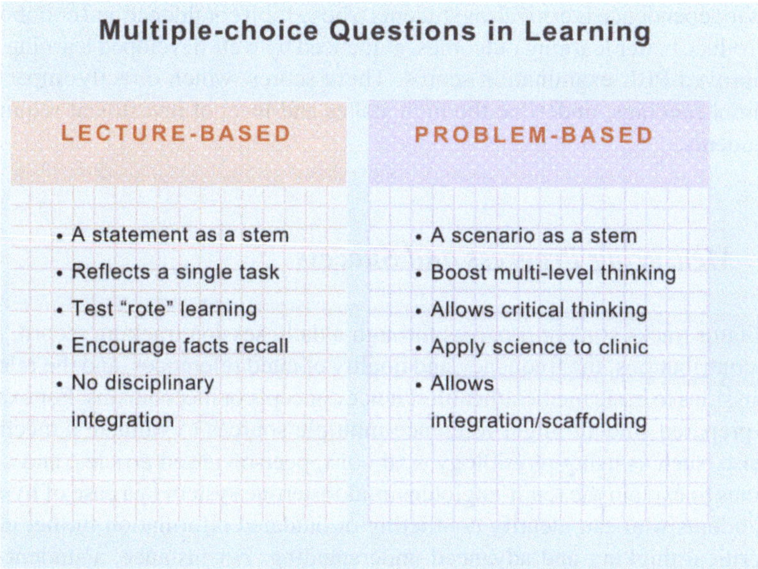

Fig. 5.5 Advantages to writing case-based multiple-choice questions for PBL examination, which differ significantly from questions used in lecture-based learning

5.6 Measuring the Impact of Facilitation in PBL

5.6.1 Defining Success: Goals for Effective PBL Facilitations

Facilitators must adopt a purposeful mindset and demonstrate a keen awareness of group dynamics, pacing, and content delivery to ensure effective PBL sessions. Managing a group of eight to nine students requires forethought, preparation, oversight, and practice. A successful facilitator skillfully sets the pace for the group while ensuring discussions remain focused and productive. This involves setting clear expectations, encouraging inquiry, and emphasizing the importance of identifying learning issues through diverse health science textbooks without overtly interceding or redirecting the group's focus. For example, a facilitator might encourage students to reference their assigned physiology textbook when discussing the Frank-Starling mechanism in a case involving heart failure.

The facilitator's attitude significantly influences the learning environment, setting the stage for students to be engaged, motivated, and empowered to explore health science concepts or mechanisms, whether familiar or unfamiliar. When students begin to direct their learning by asking their own questions and challenging their understanding, the facilitator has achieved a core goal of PBL: fostering self-directed learning. For instance, if a student asks, "*How does insulin resistance affect the progression of non-alcoholic fatty liver disease?*" and the group collaborates to answer, it demonstrates self-directed inquiry and teamwork.

This independence is critical, as students who exhibit confidence and collaboration often produce better learning outcomes, evidenced by well-developed learning topics and improved PBL examination scores. These scores, which directly impact GPA and school rankings, underline the high stakes and level of investment required by PBL students.

5.6.2 *Measuring Progress and Success*

A facilitator tracks student progress through a daily session tracking record, noting verbal contributions, the frequency and quality of cited references, and the relevance of discussions to basic medical/health science concepts or mechanisms. For example, a well-prepared student might reference multiple sources to validate a mechanism of disease, such as using physiology textbooks, peer-reviewed articles, and clinical guidelines to explain the renin-angiotensin-aldosterone system in a case of hypertension. Students who can identify conflicting or outdated information further demonstrate critical thinking and advanced understanding. For instance, a student might point out an older resource's lack of alignment with current clinical guidelines for anticoagulation therapy.

Non-verbal participation is also a critical measure of engagement, as attentive listening and thoughtful note-taking contributes to a group's dynamics. For instance, a facilitator may notice that a student who doesn't speak often is still engaged by taking detailed notes or nodding during discussions. Low or no participation negatively affects the group's learning outcomes, making accountability essential. Facilitators must address issues like tardiness and absenteeism promptly, as preparation and punctuality are vital for optimal learning.

To evaluate and improve facilitation, facilitators meet individually with students to discuss their performance and gather feedback on the facilitator's role. These meetings are an opportunity to use the tracking record and to ask specific questions about healthcare science knowledge, communication skills, professionalism, and interpersonal dynamics. For example, a facilitator might ask a student, "*How comfortable are you with synthesizing information from multiple sources? What additional support would help you improve your contributions during sessions?*" Such discussions allow facilitators to provide constructive feedback while gaining insights into their own effectiveness.

5.6.3 *Fostering Engagement, Equity, and Growth Through Facilitator Oversight*

Facilitators play a foundational role in shaping the learning environment of PBL groups by actively promoting accountability, equitable engagement, and intellectual growth among all students. Their influence goes far beyond moderating sessions. They serve as mentors, motivators, and strategic guides who create the conditions in which deep learning and meaningful collaboration can flourish.

One of the most effective ways facilitators support student growth is by encouraging group members to volunteer for challenging presentations or to explain complex biomedical mechanisms. For example, a student might be asked to walk the group through the physiological basis of acid-base disturbances within the context of a case involving metabolic acidosis. This task not only reinforces that student's understanding but also elevates the overall learning experience for the group by introducing peer teaching as a dynamic and collaborative element of PBL. This process empowers students to become active contributors rather than passive recipients of knowledge.

Facilitators must also be highly attuned to group dynamics, especially concerning participation equity. While some students may readily dominate discussions, others may hesitate to share ideas or ask questions without prompting. Skilled facilitators monitor these dynamics closely and respond with subtle interventions designed to encourage engagement without creating discomfort or embarrassment. For instance, if a student appears withdrawn or less active during discussions, the facilitator might gently pose a question such as, "What are your thoughts on how this mechanism could explain the patient's clinical presentation?" This strategy invites participation while validating the student's perspective and reinforcing that every contribution is valued.

Beyond facilitating dialogue, effective oversight requires facilitators to maintain a structured approach to assessing progress and guiding development. Facilitators set clear expectations early in the PBL cycle and regularly revisit them to ensure alignment with session objectives. They track individual and group performance through consistent observation, structured rubrics, and electronic tools such as eValue software, which allows facilitators to document student behaviors, learning outcomes, and professional attributes in real time. This data serves multiple purposes, including formative feedback, student self-assessment, referral to academic support services, and end-of-term evaluations. The availability of this documentation also ensures accountability and transparency in student assessment processes.

Over the course of several weeks, facilitators strategically use open-ended questioning to foster a culture of intellectual curiosity and inquiry. Students respond by becoming more adept at articulating complex thoughts, reassessing their interpretations, and asking targeted questions that deepen their understanding. For instance, in a case involving unexplained weight loss, students might pose questions such as, "How does the patient's thyroid panel correlate with these symptoms?" or "Could gastrointestinal malabsorption be contributing to the clinical picture?" These inquiries reflect students' growing competence in integrating clinical data with biomedical principles.

Using the clinical case as an organizing framework, students systematically analyze key elements such as chief complaint, patient history, physical examination findings, laboratory results, and additional diagnostic data. As emphasized by Hmelo-Silver (2004), this process allows students to deconstruct complex health problems into manageable components and identify underlying pathophysiological mechanisms. During group sessions, students are encouraged to question one another to clarify understanding and extend the discussion. For example, a student might ask a peer, "Can you explain how the renin angiotensin aldosterone system is contributing to this patient's hypertension?" or "What findings help rule out an autoimmune cause in this case?" Such peer-to-peer questioning promotes collaborative learning, strengthens conceptual understanding, and encourages critical reflection.

Importantly, the skills cultivated through the PBL process extend far beyond the classroom. Students develop the ability to think analytically, ask precise questions, communicate ideas clearly, and revise their thinking based on new evidence. These competencies are essential in clinical practice, where healthcare professionals must evaluate complex situations, formulate differential diagnoses, justify treatment decisions, and communicate effectively with colleagues, patients, and interdisciplinary teams. As Thomassen and Stentoft noted (2020), the iterative process of inquiry and discussion that defines PBL fosters habits of mind that support lifelong learning, a defining characteristic of competent and reflective health professionals.

By setting high expectations, modeling inquisitive thinking, and creating a supportive space for academic risk-taking, facilitators not only guide students through the content of the curriculum but also help shape their professional identities. The lessons students internalize about accountability, engagement, and teamwork during PBL sessions become enduring assets in their academic journey and future careers in healthcare.

5.6.4 Advancing Facilitator Excellence Through Student Feedback and Reflection

Student evaluations play a crucial role in enhancing facilitator effectiveness and improving the overall quality of the PBL experience. These evaluations are typically conducted at the end of each session or academic term, providing students with the opportunity to offer structured, constructive feedback on their facilitator's performance. Students complete a standardized evaluation form, which includes 14 questions assessing various facilitation skills and behaviors, with each item rated on a scale from 1 to 5, where 1 represents the lowest score and 5 the highest.

The evaluation focuses on key aspects of facilitation that significantly impact student engagement and learning. These include the timing and quality of the facilitator's questions, attentiveness during group discussions, the appropriateness of information shared, encouragement of balanced participation, and openness to receiving feedback. For instance, students are asked to evaluate whether the facilitator's questions promote critical thinking and meaningful group dialogue, whether the facilitator appropriately paces the session, and whether they create an environment where all students feel encouraged to participate.

The Facilitator Evaluation Form (Appendix) is a comprehensive tool designed to gather feedback on various dimensions of facilitation. It includes categories such as attentiveness, fostering equitable participation, and encouraging collaboration. Questions like "Does the facilitator allow enough time for the group to explore a problem before intervening?" and "Does the facilitator promote the development of differential diagnoses?" are used to assess the balance between guidance and student independence. By analyzing responses, facilitators gain valuable insights into their strengths and areas for growth, as well as specific suggestions for improvement.

Reviewing the evaluation results help facilitators better understand how their teaching style influences group dynamics and student performance. For example, if multiple students note that the facilitator's questions lack depth or fail to stimulate critical discussion, the facilitator may choose to refine their questioning techniques, focusing on more open-ended or integrative questions. Conversely, if feedback suggests that students feel over-guided or micromanaged, facilitators may need to step back, providing more opportunities for students to engage in self-directed learning.

In cases where feedback highlights issues with uneven group participation, facilitators can implement strategies to promote greater equity and involvement. These may include rotating leadership roles in discussions, actively inviting quieter students to share their perspectives, or designing activities that ensure all members contribute. Such approaches help create a more inclusive environment where every student feels empowered to participate and learn.

Additionally, student feedback can shed light on how effectively facilitators support higher-order thinking. By evaluating how well the facilitator promotes SOAP note presentations, the development of differential diagnoses, and the use of content-based questioning, facilitators gain insight into their ability to encourage critical thinking and clinical reasoning. Positive evaluations in these areas signal that the facilitator is successfully fostering intellectual rigor and cross-disciplinary integration.

The true value of student feedback lies in its ability to identify both strengths and areas for improvement, guiding facilitators toward continuous professional growth. This process of reflection and adaptation aligns with the core principles of PBL, where both students and facilitators engage in ongoing self-assessment and development. Facilitators who view student evaluations as constructive feedback, rather than as punitive measures, are better equipped to evolve and meet the diverse needs of their learners.

Incorporating student evaluations into facilitator development strengthens the PBL process by ensuring that facilitators remain responsive to the evolving dynamics of group learning while maintaining a commitment to excellence. When facilitators embrace feedback with openness and purpose, they model the values of lifelong learning, adaptability, and reflective practice that they seek to instill in their students.

5.6.5 *Enhancing PBL Sessions Through Reflective Wrap-Ups and Feedback*

Facilitators play a vital role throughout the PBL process, ensuring that sessions are thorough and productive while guiding students in analyzing relevant content. As the PBL process becomes consistent, broad learning topics across basic medical/health science disciplines emerge by the end of each clinical case. Many of these learning topics evolve into exam questions, reflecting students' identification of pertinent areas for assessment. To maintain consistency and foster growth, both facilitators and students should regularly evaluate each PBL session.

A critical facilitator's responsibility is to lead a reflective wrap-up after each session. A constructive wrap-up involves open discussion among students and the facilitator, assessing the quality of the session and the contributions of each participant. During this time, the group evaluates various parameters, including the depth of questions asked, the mechanisms discussed, and the roles played by participants. Additionally, teamwork, problem-solving skills, basic medical/health science knowledge, communication (such as clear presentations or eloquent explanations), patient care insights, preparation, appropriate citation of literature, and professionalism, such as attendance, punctuality, and respectful communication, are reviewed.

Wrap-ups offer students a valuable opportunity for reflection. They can voice concerns, seek clarification on challenging concepts, and identify areas for improvement for future sessions. For instance, if students struggle with citing appropriate references, the facilitator might suggest specific textbooks or resources for more effective research. Similarly, if communication challenges arise, the facilitator might propose structured presentation methods to enhance clarity and confidence.

Facilitators also use the wrap-up to provide targeted feedback. For example, they might comment on how well the group achieved the learning objectives for a clinical case or highlight areas where the discussion fell short. Facilitators can further encourage students by showing how collaborative efforts during the session enhance the group's understanding of complex concepts, surpassing what individual learning might achieve.

In addition to reflecting on group dynamics, facilitators may highlight specific examples from the session to reinforce key learning points. For instance, they might reference a student's analysis of a challenging mechanism or a particularly effective differential diagnosis discussion as exemplary. Ultimately, the wrap-up is not just a summary but an essential tool for continuous improvement. It helps both students and facilitators recognize the value of teamwork, refine their approaches to problem-solving, and ensure alignment with PBL objectives. Through reflective discussions and actionable feedback, wrap-ups pave the way for more effective and engaging PBL sessions.

5.6.6 Troubleshooting and Strategies for Effective Facilitation

PBL teams may face a variety of challenges that impact their effectiveness, including issues such as a lack of trust, dominance by certain individuals, insufficient preparation, or interpersonal conflicts. When these obstacles arise, facilitators must first assess the underlying causes by engaging in one-on-one discussions with students to gain insights from within the group. These conversations should be approached with empathy and an open mind, ensuring that students feel supported and understood. Once the root causes are identified, facilitators can work with the group to develop an action plan, which should be followed by ongoing feedback and progress monitoring. For example, if a few students dominate discussions, the facilitator could implement structured speaking turns or actively encourage quieter members to contribute. Acknowledging and praising improvements during wrap-ups can also reinforce positive changes and promote group unity.

When the group veers off course during a session, facilitators can use open-ended questions to help refocus the discussion without taking control. For instance, if the conversation moves into unrelated topics, a facilitator might ask, "How does this relate to the patient's chief complaint?" This approach encourages the group to stay on track while maintaining the collaborative, student-driven nature of PBL.

5.6.6.1 Addressing Engagement Challenges

Student engagement in PBL can vary significantly due to differences in preparation, personality, and learning preferences. Some students excel in verbal contributions, while others may demonstrate strength in listening, asking insightful questions, or researching resources. Facilitators must create an inclusive environment that values these differences while fostering active participation. For example, a student who excels in research might take on the role of the group's resource expert, while a more vocal student could lead discussions.

However, disengagement, such as lack of speaking, presenting, or contributing to tasks, is a clear sign of participation issues. In these cases, a private conversation with the student can help identify the root cause. For instance, if a student is struggling with time management, they may benefit from advice on task prioritization. Alternatively, a student feeling overwhelmed by the material might need guidance in finding more accessible resources. By offering personalized support, facilitators can help each student feel empowered to engage and contribute meaningfully to the group.

5.6.6.2 Managing Group Dynamics and the Affective Domain

The emotional dynamics within a PBL group play a crucial role in shaping both individual and collective learning. The affective domain, which directly influences

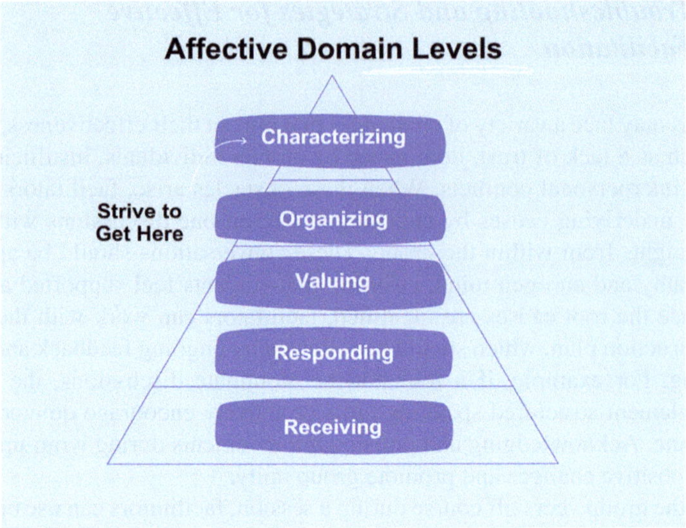

Fig. 5.6 The affective domain levels in PBL session, ranging from receiving information passively (receiving), actively participating (responding), appreciating teamwork (valuing), integrating new values (organizing), and demonstrating integrity and responsibility regularly (characterizing)

students' emotional engagement with the material and the group, follows a hierarchical structure (Fig. 5.6). This progression begins with the passive reception of information, moves through active responses, and culminates in the valuing, organizing, and integrating of critical details. For example, a group may begin by passively listing symptoms but later transition into actively debating differential diagnoses, ultimately synthesizing their findings into a cohesive understanding.

Utilizing tools like shared documents (e.g., Google Docs), often monitored by an e-scribe, can significantly enhance organizational skills and foster collaboration. This digital approach allows all group members to contribute in real time and track progress, creating a sense of collective responsibility. As students recognize the significance of their contributions, their emotional investment increases, fostering stronger group cohesion and motivating them to engage more deeply in the learning process.

5.6.6.3 Transitioning from Lecture to Facilitation

For facilitators accustomed to traditional lecturing, shifting to the PBL model requires a significant change in approach. Unlike lectures, where the instructor controls the flow of information, PBL facilitation empowers students to take charge of their learning. Facilitators guide the process, prompting students to engage in discussions, research evidence-based information, and uncover new concepts themselves.

This transition promotes intellectual humility, as students are challenged to navigate the dynamic and evolving landscape of healthcare science. For example, a facilitator might prompt the group to reconsider how a recent finding reshapes the understanding of a well-established mechanism. These discussions highlight the importance of adaptability and lifelong learning.

Successful facilitation ultimately fosters a collaborative environment where students develop essential problem-solving and decision-making skills. By creating a space that values inquiry, reflection, and mutual respect, facilitators help prepare students for the complexities of healthcare practice, while nurturing a culture of intellectual curiosity and professional growth.

Appendix: Lake Erie College of Osteopathic Medicine—Bradenton

Problem-Based Learning: Facilitator Evaluation Form

Facilitator Name: ______________________________

Date: ____________________

PBL Course (Circle One): PBL-I PBL-II PBL-III PBL-IV

Group Number: ______________

Please evaluate your facilitator by responding truthfully and objectively to the statements below. All responses will remain confidential. Use the following scale:

Scale:

5 = 100 | 4 = 90 | 3 = 80 | 2 = 70 | 1 = 60

---

1. The facilitator asks questions at appropriate times.

☐ 5 ☐ 4 ☐ 3 ☐ 2 ☐ 1

Comments:

---

2. The facilitator asks thought-provoking questions.

☐ 5 ☐ 4 ☐ 3 ☐ 2 ☐ 1

Comments:

---

3. The facilitator is attentive during group discussions.

☐ 5 ☐ 4 ☐ 3 ☐ 2 ☐ 1

Comments:

---

4. The facilitator shares relevant information at appropriate times.

☐ 5 ☐ 4 ☐ 3 ☐ 2 ☐ 1

Comments:

____

5. The facilitator encourages equal participation among group members.

☐ 5 ☐ 4 ☐ 3 ☐ 2 ☐ 1

Comments:

____

6. The facilitator is open to receiving feedback from the group.

☐ 5 ☐ 4 ☐ 3 ☐ 2 ☐ 1

Comments:

____

7. When asked for content help, the facilitator guides the group through questions rather than direct answers.

☐ 5 ☐ 4 ☐ 3 ☐ 2 ☐ 1

Comments:

____

8. The facilitator fosters a productive and collaborative learning environment.

☐ 5 ☐ 4 ☐ 3 ☐ 2 ☐ 1

Comments:

____

9. The facilitator guides without dominating group discussion.

☐ 5 ☐ 4 ☐ 3 ☐ 2 ☐ 1

Comments:

____

10. The facilitator promotes group reflection and evaluation at the end of meetings.

☐ 5 ☐ 4 ☐ 3 ☐ 2 ☐ 1

Comments:

____

11. The facilitator fosters strong learning relationships among group members.

☐ 5 ☐ 4 ☐ 3 ☐ 2 ☐ 1

Comments:

____

12. The facilitator encourages presentation of case progress reports (e.g., SOAP notes) at the beginning of meetings.

☐ 5 ☐ 4 ☐ 3 ☐ 2 ☐ 1

Comments:

____

13. The facilitator allows the group sufficient time to work through issues before intervening.

☐ 5 ☐ 4 ☐ 3 ☐ 2 ☐ 1

Comments:

____

14. The facilitator encourages systematic development of potential systems involved and differential diagnoses after each case history.

☐ 5 ☐ 4 ☐ 3 ☐ 2 ☐ 1

Comments:

____

____

Additional Comments:

____

____

____

References

Azer, S. A. (2003). Problem-based learning. Assessment in a problem-based learning course. *Biochemistry and Molecular Biology Education, 31*(6), 428–434.

Azer, S. A. (2011). Introducing a problem-based learning program: 12 tips for success. *Medical Teacher, 33*(10), 808–813. https://doi.org/10.3109/0142159X.2011.558137

Barrows, H. S. (1998). The essentials of problem-based learning. *Journal of Dental Education, 62*(9), 630–633.

Fonteijn, H. T. H., & Dolmans, D. H. J. M. (2019). Group work and group dynamics in PBL. In *The Wiley handbook of problem-based learning* (pp. 199–220). https://doi.org/10.1002/9781119173243.ch9

Gallardo, K., Valle, A., & Saldana, A. (2021). Strengthening the comprehension process in medical students: Applying problem-based learning accompanied by the reasoning procedural map. *Interdisciplinary Journal of Problem-Based Learning, 15*(2). https://doi.org/10.14434/ijpbl.v15i2.28726

Gibbon, C., & Marcangelo, C. (2012). A PBL evaluation toolkit: Building the evidence-based to understand effective practices. *Procedia-Social and Behavioral Sciences, 47*(2021), 1686–1691. https://doi.org/10.1016/j.sbspro.2012.06.833

Hmelo-Silver, C. E. (2004). Problem-based learning: What and how do students learn? *Educational Psychology Review, 16*(3), 235–266. https://doi.org/10.1023/B:EDPR.0000034022.16470.f3

Hmelo-Silver, C. E., & Barrows, H. S. (2006). Goals and strategies of a problem-based learning facilitator. *Interdisciplinary Journal of Problem-Based Learning, 1*(1), 4.

Hung, W., Jonassen, D. H., & Liu, R. (2008). Problem-based learning. In *Handbook of research on educational communications and technology* (pp. 485–506). Routledge.

Kedrick, K., Schrater, P., & Koutstaal, W. (2023). The multifaceted role of self-generated question asking in curiosity-driven learning. *Cognitive Science, 47*(4), e13253. https://doi.org/10.1111/cogs.13253

L'Ecuyer, K. M., Pole, D., & Leander, S. A. (2015). The use of PBL in an interprofessional education course for health care professional students. *Interdisciplinary Journal of Problem-Based Learning, 9*(1). https://doi.org/10.7771/1541-5015.1497

Preeti, B., Ashish, A., & Shriram, G. (2013). Problem-based learning(PBL)-an effective approach to improving learning outcomes in medical teaching. *Journal of Clinical and Diagnostic Research, 7*(12), 2896–2897.

Salinitri, F. D., Wilhelm, S. M., & Crabtree, B. L. (2015). Facilitating facilitators: Enhancing PBL through a structured facilitator development program. *Interdisciplinary Journal of Problem-Based Learning, 9*(1). https://doi.org/10.7771/1541-5015.1509

Spahic, H., Goplerud, D., Blatt, C., Murphy, M., Golden, W. C., & Pahwa, A. (2023). Promoting clinical reasoning with meta-memory techniques to teach broad differential diagnosis generation in a pediatric core clerkship. *Diagnosis (Berlin), 10*, 242. https://doi.org/10.1515/dx-2023-0038

Tai, G. X. L., & Yuen, M. C. (2007). Authentic assessment strategies in problem-based learning. In *Proceedings Ascilite Singapore 2007* (pp. 983–993).

Thomassen, A. O., & Stentoft, D. (2020). Being explicit about critical thinking and reflective practice as competencies in PBL: A review of existing research and theory. In *Abstracts, Congress Problem-Based Learning 2016, June 16–17, 2016, Zürich, Switzerland* (pp. 41–42).

Wood, D. F. (2003). ABC of learning and teaching in medicine: Problem based learning. *British Medical Journal, 326*, 328–330.

Chapter 6
The Problem-Based Learning Examination

Santiago Lorenzo

6.1 The Role of Examinations in Problem-Based Learning

Assessments may be formative or summative. In the realm of PBL, examinations are summative, typically occurring at the end of each block, right after a series of PBL cases. Examinations are a vital component in the education of healthcare professionals (Ricci et al., 2018). PBL is most effective when examinations focus on understanding principles that link concepts, rather than just understanding individual concepts or their applications (Dochy et al., 2003; Gijbels et al., 2005). Effective PBL examinations can integrate factual knowledge with problem-solving principles, using multiple-choice questions, patient management problems, and objective-structured practical examinations (Chakravarty et al., 2005). Properly used, an examination will aid in accomplishing key curricular goals, such as providing direction and motivation for further learning (Boud, 2000; Gipps, 2008; Shepard, 2000) identifying areas of improvement (Boud, 2000; Schuwirth & Van der Vleuten, 2011) and supporting future learning (Boud, 2000; Eva et al., 2016; Martinez & Lipson, 1989; Rushton, 2005; Schuwirth & Van der Vleuten, 2011; Shepard, 2000). This outcome is particularly important in PBL, where educational experiences and previous strategies vary from student to student. Because of such a powerful influence on student learning (Ricci et al., 2018), examinations must be designed with high-quality questions that will further identify educational goals and reflect professionalism. Student mastery of material, rather than memorization, is the major overriding intent of a well-developed examination in the PBL curriculum (van der Vleuten & Schuwirth, 2019). It has been reported that performance-based testing in PBL measures not only factual knowledge but also the application of knowledge in clinical settings, often resulting in better clinical reasoning skills compared to traditional methods (Schwartz et al., 1997).

S. Lorenzo (✉)
Lake Erie College of Osteopathic Medicine, Bradenton, FL, USA
e-mail: slorenzo@lecom.edu

S. Lorenzo and B. Zhang (eds.), *Mastering Problem-Based Learning in Health Profession Programs*, https://doi.org/10.1007/978-3-032-05405-0_6

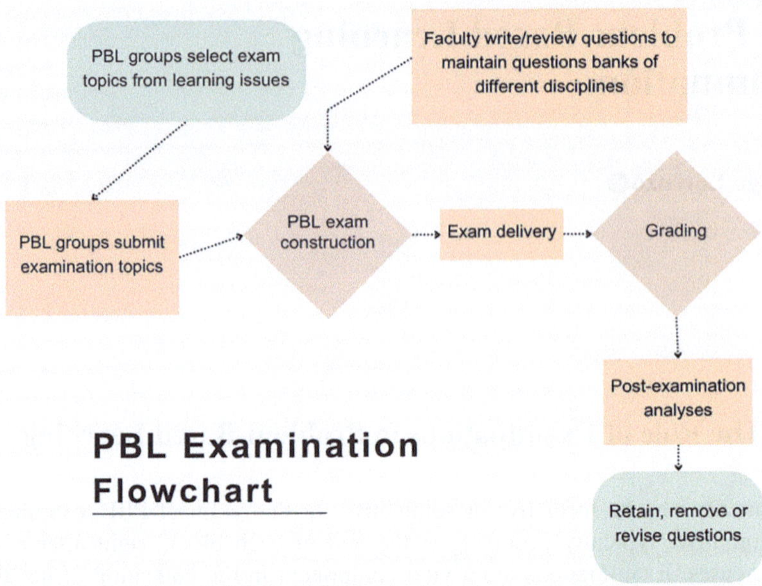

Fig. 6.1 The steps and procedures in PBL examination include exam construction, delivery, grading and post-examination analysis

The following section describes the details for custom-designed discrete PBL examinations. Additional details are also provided concerning topic collection and administration, data collection and analysis, item writing and banking, and scoring of each of these examinations. The steps and procedures (Fig. 6.1) in this chapter have been refined over several years of trial and error at the author's institution. These procedures, however, should be flexible and adapt to the specific needs of each healthcare program and student body involved.

6.2 Student Selection of Examination Topics and Submission Process

One of the foundational principles of PBL is that it places students at the center of their own learning process, encouraging a high level of autonomy and responsibility in identifying, researching, and mastering learning issues. This self-directed approach empowers students to engage actively with case materials and fosters a deeper understanding of health-related concepts (van der Vleuten & Schuwirth, 2019; Zaveri et al., 2019). Rather than passively absorbing information, students in a PBL curriculum are expected to independently identify gaps in their knowledge, explore relevant health-related literature, and integrate this information into their understanding of the case. The ability to independently navigate health-related literature and synthesize relevant information is a crucial skill for future healthcare professionals (Dolmans et al., 2016; Schmidt et al., 2011).

The selection of learning issues and examination topics is a multi-step process that begins within the initial PBL sessions (Fig. 6.2). As the group collaboratively reviews the case and identifies key clinical signs, symptoms, and pathophysiological mechanisms, each student is encouraged to select specific learning issues aligned with their interests and knowledge gaps. These learning issues must be clinically relevant and rooted in the objectives of the health professions program. The choice of topics is not arbitrary but should be guided by the case presentation, program competencies, and alignment with the core knowledge domains covered in national licensing examinations such as COMLEX-USA and USMLE.

This process of selecting learning issues not only promotes accountability and intellectual curiosity but also mirrors the real-world clinical reasoning that physicians must perform daily. In clinical settings, healthcare professionals must rapidly identify pertinent information, prioritize learning needs, and apply evidence-based knowledge to solve patient problems (Schmidt et al., 2015). PBL fosters these

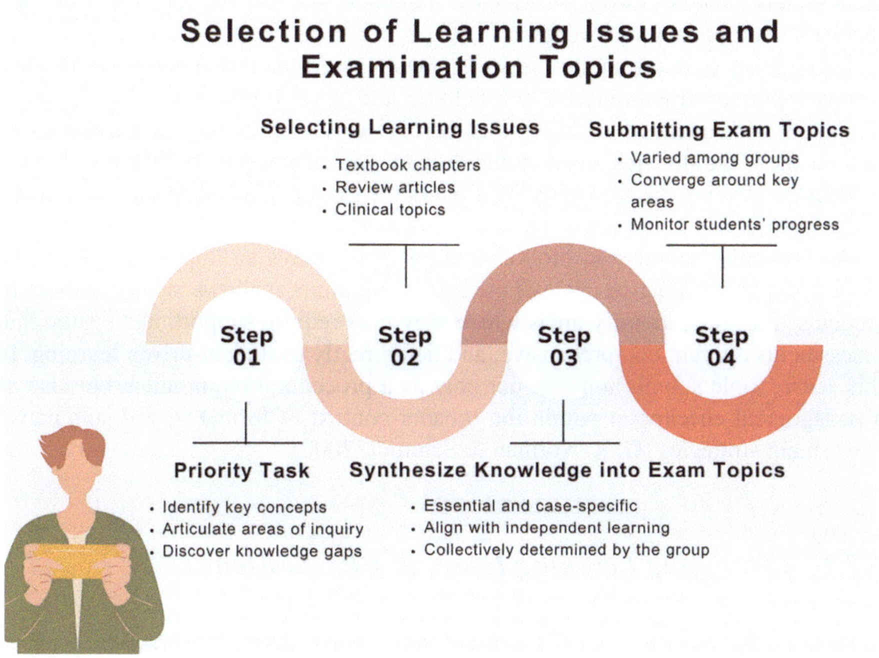

Fig. 6.2 The selection of learning issues and examination topics is a multi-step process, including identifying knowledge gaps, selecting learning issues, extracting exam topics and submitting them

same metacognitive skills, making students better prepared for lifelong learning in medicine.

Effective selection of learning issues requires students to identify and articulate key concepts and areas of inquiry that emerge from the clinical case. These issues should be broad enough to encourage exploration and integration of multiple disciplines, yet focused enough to guide meaningful research and discussion. For example, a case on chronic kidney disease might prompt learning issues such as "*Mechanisms underlying glomerular filtration*," "*Electrolyte imbalances in renal dysfunction*," or "*Role of the renin-angiotensin-aldosterone system in blood pressure and fluid regulation*." These learning issues allow students to investigate complex physiological, biochemical, and clinical relationships in depth. Well-formulated learning issues serve as the foundation for independent study, foster collaboration during PBL sessions, and ensure alignment with curricular goals and the development of essential clinical reasoning skills.

Once a case is completed, typically after the second or third session, students are expected to synthesize the knowledge they have gained into formal examination topics, which will be discussed later in this chapter. Briefly, these examination topics form the foundation of their assessments and must be submitted by a designated deadline. In many programs, including our own, students are required to submit these topics via email to the Course Director or through an online learning management system such as Canvas, where faculty members review and approve or provide feedback on topic appropriateness.

To support students in this process, faculty facilitators may provide rubrics, sample topics, or structured feedback, helping students refine their choices and ensure alignment with intended learning outcomes. However, facilitators are careful not to "spoon-feed" the students, maintaining the pedagogical integrity of PBL by allowing students to develop the autonomy required in their future clinical practice (Dolmans et al., 2016).

Additionally, submission of examination topics plays an important role in the assessment and evaluation cycle of the PBL curriculum. It allows faculty to monitor students' progress, identify areas where they may require support, and ensure that assessments are fair, comprehensive, and tied directly to student-driven learning. In this sense, topic submission acts not only as a procedural requirement but also as a pedagogical checkpoint within the broader context of formative and summative assessment strategies (G. R. Norman & Schmidt, 2000).

6.2.1 Identifying Learning Issues in PBL Sessions

In Problem-Based Learning (PBL), one of the central tasks students face during each session is identifying appropriate and meaningful learning issues. These learning issues serve as focal points for independent study, group discussion, and the integration of foundational science with clinical reasoning. This identification process occurs collaboratively within the group and is informed by critical engagement with the clinical case. It involves dissecting the scenario through iterative questioning, dialogue, and reflection.

Following the progressive disclosure model foundational to PBL, facilitators present case information in incremental segments, releasing new data only after the current content has been thoroughly discussed and relevant learning issues have been identified (Barrows, 2000). This stepwise disclosure encourages analytical thinking and hypothesis generation while fostering the development of self-directed learning skills. The role of the facilitator is not to provide answers but to stimulate student inquiry by prompting metacognitive reflection and curiosity. Facilitators may encourage students to consider the following types of questions:

- What are the potential underlying pathophysiological mechanisms of the presenting condition?
- Which diagnostic tools or laboratory tests are needed, and what are their clinical indications?
- What pharmacological agents are relevant, and what are their mechanisms of action?
- How do clinical features connect to foundational concepts in physiology, pathology, microbiology, and pharmacology?

These kinds of guiding questions help anchor learning issues in the clinical scenario while broadening them to encompass related foundational knowledge. For example, in a case involving a patient with suspected congestive heart failure, appropriate learning issues might include "The pathophysiology of left and right heart failure," "Mechanisms of compensatory responses in reduced cardiac output," and "Pharmacologic management of chronic heart failure." These learning issues are intentionally broader than narrowly focused questions, which ensures that students engage with larger conceptual frameworks rather than isolated facts (Van Der Vleuten & Schuwirth, 2005). By engaging in this process, students develop skills in prioritization, synthesis of health-related knowledge, and evidence-based reasoning (Dolmans et al., 2016). Furthermore, this self-directed selection of topics ensures that students learn contextually relevant material, reinforcing the integration of basic and clinical sciences (Schmidt et al., 2011).

Most learning issues are best conceptualized as larger academic units, such as textbook chapters, review articles, or comprehensive clinical topics, rather than discrete, testable questions. This broad framing allows students to explore the depth and breadth of complex systems and conditions, thereby fostering the integration of basic and clinical sciences (Dolmans et al., 2016). Some learning issues arise directly from uncertainties or knowledge gaps that students identify in real-time during the discussion. Others may be introduced toward the end of the case to ensure comprehensive coverage of associated conditions, differential diagnoses, or long-term management considerations (Barrows, 1996; Dolmans et al., 1994).

Importantly, learning issues should be framed at an appropriate level of generality. A topic that is too narrow may result in rote memorization rather than conceptual understanding. For instance, a proposed learning issue such as "What does the first heart sound represent?" is overly specific and would be better reframed as "Heart sounds" or even "The cardiac cycle." This broader topic would allow students to engage with the physiology of heart sounds, their relation to valve function, timing in the cardiac cycle, and their diagnostic significance, leading to a more integrated and clinically relevant understanding (Hmelo-Silver, 2004).

Moreover, the collaborative nature of this process fosters important skills such as teamwork, respectful dialogue, and the capacity to articulate and defend reasoning in front of peers. These are not only critical for academic development but also mirror the competencies expected of practicing healthcare professionals. Over time, consistent practice in identifying and exploring learning issues enhances students' abilities to prioritize health science knowledge, differentiate essential information from peripheral detail, and navigate the health science literature with increasing independence (Hmelo-Silver, 2004; Norman & Schmidt, 1992).

In summary, the process of identifying learning issues is central to the success of the PBL approach. By engaging students in active, reflective, and collaborative exploration of clinically relevant concepts, it cultivates the habits of lifelong learning, critical appraisal, and integrative thinking that are essential for professional practice in healthcare.

6.2.2 Difference Between "Learning Issues" and "Examination Topics"

A core objective of the group meeting in PBL is to collectively identify basic biomedical science topics that all group members do not yet understand. These unknowns are surfaced through an iterative process of inquiry and reflection as students analyze the case. As they engage with a progressively disclosed clinical scenario, such as that of a 55-year-old male presenting with chest pain, they are prompted to generate a series of probing questions aimed at uncovering the underlying pathophysiological mechanisms. For instance, initial questions may include:

- *Why* does the patient experience chest pain?
- *How* does myocardial ischemia develop at the physiological level?
- *What* are the possible differential diagnoses based on his symptoms and risk factors?

As the case unfolds with additional clinical information (e.g., elevated troponin levels or ST-segment elevation on ECG), students refine their inquiries to address more targeted concepts:

- *Why* does an ST-segment elevation indicate myocardial infarction rather than unstable angina?
- *How* does atherosclerosis contribute to coronary artery occlusion?
- *What* treatment options exist, and how do they work physiologically?

By engaging in this ongoing questioning process, students ensure a deeper understanding of the case, integrating foundational sciences with clinical reasoning.

This process of constant questioning fosters deeper cognitive engagement and reinforces the integration of foundational science with clinical reasoning (Hmelo-Silver, 2004). Every page of the case, regardless of whether it presents novel findings or normal laboratory values, serves as a springboard for identifying underlying biomedical science concepts. Even normal lab results are worth discussing, as they provide opportunities to explore why certain abnormalities are absent and what that implies at the pathophysiological level. Through this lens, students identify knowledge gaps and record them as "learning issues." These are intended to be explored through self-directed learning before the next group session.

Because students typically do not know the case diagnosis during the initial phase, their learning issues tend to be broad and exploratory. This ambiguity is pedagogically intentional, as it compels students to consider multiple possibilities and learn how to evaluate and prioritize clinical data. Literature has shown that such ambiguity-driven exploration helps students develop stronger clinical reasoning skills and promotes deeper learning (Dolmans et al., 2005; Schmidt et al., 2009).

Upon completion of the case and full disclosure of the diagnosis, students collaboratively generate a list of "examination topics." These are distilled from the more numerous and diverse learning issues explored throughout the case. Unlike learning issues, which are broad and not tied to specific diagnoses, examination topics are focused and centered around particular diagnoses. They are carefully selected to represent the most central biomedical science concepts essential to understanding the case's pathophysiology, clinical presentation, diagnostic findings, and treatment rationale. For example, in a case concerning acute myocardial infarction, early learning issues might include general topics such as "mechanisms of chest pain" or "ECG interpretation." By the end of the case, once the diagnosis is known, students refine their focus to examination topics such as "ST-elevation myocardial infarction (STEMI) pathophysiology" or "pharmacological action of beta-blockers in acute coronary syndrome." This targeted approach aligns with the concept of "constructive alignment," where learning activities and assessments are tightly linked to desired learning outcomes (Biggs, 1996).

It is also important to recognize that examination topics differ among groups due to the inherently self-directed and collaborative nature of PBL. Each group's path of inquiry can vary based on the questions they prioritize, their unique knowledge gaps, and the specific discussions that unfold during group meetings. This variation is not a flaw but a strength of the PBL model: it supports personalized learning and fosters diverse approaches to complex clinical problems (Barrows, 1986). Consequently, each group submits its own list of examination topics, and each group's exam is uniquely tailored based on those topics (see Tables 6.1 and 6.2). However, given that all groups are working from the same cases, some commonalities naturally emerge, especially around core concepts required to explain the patient's key clinical findings (Schmidt et al., 2011). To illustrate, in a case focused on cystic fibrosis, universally relevant examination topics might include the CFTR gene mutation, chloride ion transport in epithelial cells, and mucociliary clearance dysfunction in the lungs. These align closely with standard educational objectives found in healthcare professions curricula. However, some groups may choose to explore deeper into psychosocial dimensions, such as the impact of chronic illness on quality of life or the role of genetic counseling in family planning, which are topics that, while not central to the pathophysiology, enrich the holistic understanding of the disease and reflect students' individual learning interests.

Table 6.1 Learning issues vs. examination topics

Learning issues	Examination topics
Hemoglobin structure and function	Physiology Ch. 33: Red Blood Cells, Anemia, and Polycythemia
Mechanism of red blood cell synthesis	Biochemistry Ch. 42: The Biochemistry of Erythrocytes and Other Blood Cells
White blood cell components	Physiology Ch. 34: Resistance of the Body to Infection: Leukocytes, Granulocytes, the Monocyte-Macrophage System, and Inflammation
Why did the patient have edema? Fluid/electrolyte balance	Pathology Ch. 3: Inflammation and Repair
Mechanism of dyspnea: What causes shortness of breath?	Physiology Ch. 40: Principles of Gas Exchange; Diffusion of Oxygen and Carbon Dioxide Through the Respiratory Membrane
What is a PFT? What does it measure?	Physiology Ch. 38: Pulmonary Ventilation
Cholesterol synthesis and metabolism	Biochemistry Ch. 32: Cholesterol Absorption, Synthesis, Metabolism, and Fate
What is rheumatoid arthritis	Immunology Ch. 19: Hypersensitivity Disorders
What are gram-positive bacteria?	Microbiology Ch. 19: Streptococcus and Enterococcus
How do statins work?	Pharmacology Ch. 35: Agents Used in Dyslipidemia

Table 6.2 Exam topics clarified

Appropriate exam topics	Inappropriate exam topics
Derived from the case's learning issues and thoroughly explored during group discussions.	Selected solely because they appear straightforward or less challenging.
Essential for understanding the fundamental biomedical mechanisms presented in the case.	Peripheral topics not directly related to the case's core health science concepts.
Chosen collaboratively by the group, ensuring consensus among all members.	Based on individual assumptions about what might be tested, without group agreement.
Reflective of topics the group has actively studied and discussed in depth.	Subjects that the group has not yet reviewed or lacks sufficient understanding of.
Focused on diagnosis-specific content that aligns with the case's clinical scenarios.	Overly broad or general topics that do not pertain to specific diagnoses within the case.

In summary, while learning issues are student-identified questions that guide initial exploration, examination topics represent a post-hoc synthesis of essential, diagnosis-centered content. This structured yet flexible approach to learning supports both standardization of core competencies and the cultivation of learner autonomy, a balance supported by evidence from multiple PBL studies (Albanese & Mitchell, 1993; Neville, 2009).

Because all PBL groups work through the same clinical cases, there is a shared foundational framework that guides the learning process. As a result, there is a significant degree of overlap in the core concepts and fundamental basic science mechanisms addressed across all groups. This shared foundation ensures that the PBL examination focuses on the essential health science content embedded within each case. Consequently, examination topics selected by different groups should converge around key areas of relevance, even though the learning journeys may differ. The focus of these examinations is on assessing students' understanding of core physiological, pathological, and biochemical principles that explain the signs and symptoms presented in the case (Schmidt et al., 2011).For example, after completing a case involving a pediatric patient diagnosed with cystic fibrosis, students from various groups will likely identify a consistent set of essential learning objectives, despite having explored different paths during the case. These essential objectives include the ability to:

- Identify the etiology and pathophysiological mechanisms underlying cystic fibrosis, particularly focusing on the dysfunction of the CFTR gene and how this affects chloride ion transport and mucus viscosity.
- Recognize the autosomal recessive inheritance pattern of cystic fibrosis and understand the genetic mutations most commonly involved, such as ΔF508.
- Describe the characteristic clinical manifestations and symptomatology associated with the disease, including chronic pulmonary infections, pancreatic insufficiency, and growth delays.
- Explain the diagnostic criteria for cystic fibrosis, including sweat chloride testing, newborn screening, and genetic analysis
- Discuss how cystic fibrosis affects multiple organ systems, particularly the respiratory, digestive, and reproductive systems, and explore how these complications interrelate.
- Explain treatment options, including pharmacologic therapies such as CFTR modulators (e.g., ivacaftor and lumacaftor), airway clearance techniques, nutritional interventions, and, in severe cases, lung transplantation.

While these core objectives are generally shared across all groups and form the basis of the assessment, the self-directed nature of PBL encourages students to explore tangential topics based on their own interests and perceived knowledge gaps. As a result, some groups may extend their inquiry into additional learning areas. For example, certain groups may:

- Investigate the role of multidisciplinary teams in managing chronic illnesses like cystic fibrosis, emphasizing collaboration among pulmonologists, dietitians, physical therapists, and social workers to optimize patient outcomes.
- Explore the psychosocial dimensions of living with a chronic disease, including the impact on mental health, adherence to treatment regimens, and quality of life for patients and their families.
- Study potential complications and comorbidities, such as diabetes mellitus, liver disease, and infertility, and how these are managed within a long-term care framework.
- Examine the latest research and emerging therapies in cystic fibrosis care, such as gene therapy, mRNA-based treatments, or novel CFTR modulators currently in clinical trials.

This individualized approach means that while all students master a core set of knowledge, their learning experiences and examination topics may differ based on the depth and direction of their inquiry. Such flexibility in topic selection aligns with adult learning theory, which emphasizes autonomy, relevance, and self-motivation as central to effective education (Knowles, 1984). This structure allows each group to tailor their learning experience to their own interests and academic needs, thus enriching the learning environment and promoting intellectual curiosity and engagement.

By fostering varied, yet rigorous, learning pathways, PBL accommodates different learning styles while ensuring alignment with curriculum goals and assessment standards. Although examination content is group-specific, the shared clinical cases and foundational objectives ensure sufficient commonality for a fair and comprehensive evaluation across all PBL groups. This dual structure of individualized exploration within a shared framework reflects the strength of PBL in promoting both standardized core knowledge acquisition and personalized academic development (Dolmans et al., 2005).

6.2.3 Poor Exam Topic Choice Strategies

As students progress through PBL, their ability to identify and formulate appropriate examination topics improves. However, depending on their stage of development, they may require additional guidance. Facilitators play a crucial role in ensuring that students select examination topics that align with the case's learning objectives, reinforce essential health-related knowledge, and prepare them for future assessments, including board licensing examinations.

Below are common poor examination topic selection strategies and how facilitators can intervene to promote better decision-making:

- **Avoiding examination topics because they are too difficult (even if they are highly relevant to the case)**: Some students may shy away from complex topics, fearing that they require too much effort to understand. However, difficult topics often represent core health science concepts that are essential for clinical reasoning (Dolmans et al., 2016). Facilitators should encourage students to embrace challenging topics, emphasizing that grappling with complexity fosters deeper learning and prepares them for real-world clinical problem-solving (Schmidt et al., 2011).

- **Selecting examination topics based solely on brevity**: Students sometimes opt for topics that require minimal reading rather than those that are most relevant to the case. While efficiency is important, this strategy can lead to gaps in knowledge. Facilitators should remind students that examination topics should be chosen based on their educational value and relevance to the case rather than the number of pages covered in a textbook (Hmelo-Silver, 2004).
- **Avoiding examination topics based on unverified claims that they are not covered on board licensing exams**: Some students might dismiss crucial topics due to hearsay about their relevance to licensing exams. However, high-stakes exams such as the USMLE and COMLEX evolve, and clinically significant topics remain integral to health science education (van der Vleuten & Schuwirth, 2019). Facilitators should stress that mastering foundational knowledge is crucial for both assessments and future clinical practice, regardless of perceived exam emphasis.
- **Excluding topics due to group dynamics, such as dominant voices overshadowing others**: In some groups, more vocal students may steer the discussion away from certain topics, even if they are pertinent to the case. Facilitators should ensure that all members have an equal opportunity to contribute and that topic selection is based on academic merit rather than social dynamics (Zaveri et al., 2019). A structured approach, such as voting or requiring justification for topic choices, can help maintain objectivity.
- **Choosing topics unrelated to the case**: Some students may select topics that have not been studied in previous courses simply to diversify their learning, even if those topics do not apply to the case. While broad learning is valuable, examination topics should directly reinforce the understanding of the current case and its associated pathophysiology, diagnostics, and treatment (Barrows, 1996). Facilitators should help students distinguish between curiosity-driven learning and case-relevant learning.
- **Reading and learning a highly relevant topic but failing to submit it as an examination topic**: Occasionally, students study crucial concepts but do not list them as examination topics, leading to gaps in assessment coverage. This may occur due to oversight or a lack of confidence in selecting core topics. Facilitators should encourage students to align their independent learning with examination topic submissions to ensure that all critical aspects of the case are properly evaluated (Schmidt et al., 2011).
- **Avoiding topics because students have previously taken a course in the subject**: Some students may dismiss topics they perceive as redundant, assuming prior coursework has already covered them sufficiently. However, health science knowledge builds on reinforcement and integration across disciplines (Dolmans et al., 2016). Even if a topic has been previously studied, its relevance within

a new clinical context may deepen understanding. Facilitators should encourage students to revisit and integrate foundational concepts within the case framework.

By addressing these poor selection strategies, facilitators can guide students toward making well-informed decisions about their examination topics. Encouraging students to select topics that are comprehensive, clinically relevant, and aligned with the case ensures that their PBL experience translates into meaningful learning that prepares them for future healthcare challenges.

6.2.4 *Identifying and Formulating Learning Issues for Examination*

When students evaluate their performance in identifying learning issues, the most frequent self-criticism is that the learning issues are too broad or poorly defined. These problems may be avoided if the students remember to organize their learning issues in two ways: by basic medical/health science disciplines and by levels of organization. There are seven basic medical/health science disciplines, and within each of these disciplines, there are seven levels of organization.

The basic medical/health science disciplines:

- Anatomy (including Histology, Embryology, and Neuroanatomy)
- Biochemistry (including Medical Genetics and Nutrition)
- Behavioral Science
- Microbiology (including Immunology)
- Pathology
- Pharmacology
- Physiology

The seven levels of organization:

- The Molecular Level
- The Cellular Level
- The Tissue Level
- The Organ Level
- The Organ System Level
- The Whole Patient Level
- The Family and Community Level

If these are kept in mind when formulating learning issues, and even more important when studying, the student can feel confident that a given issue is being approached with the appropriate breadth and depth. Not all disciplines and levels apply to every learning issue, but if each topic is analyzed from this perspective, then oversight can be minimized. One of the basic principles in healthcare professions is the treatment of the entire patient instead of a limited focus on the disease. By treating each learning

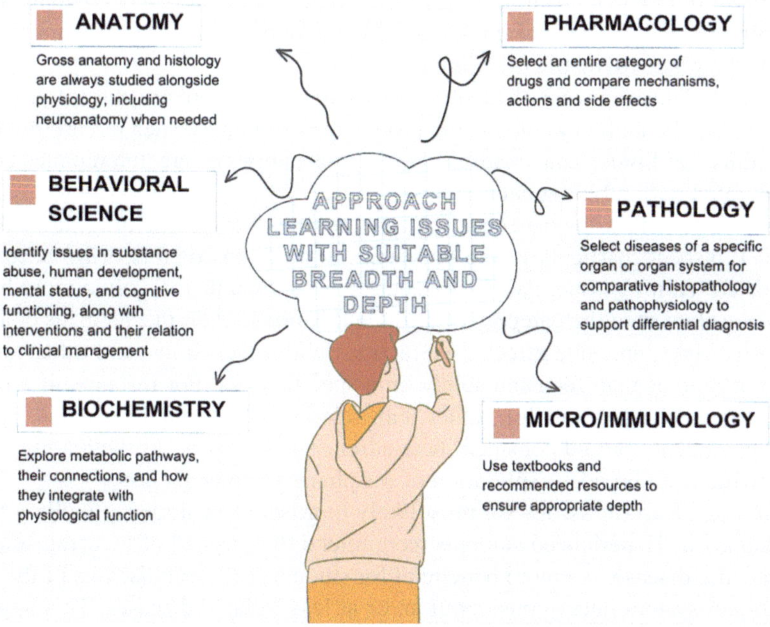

Fig. 6.3 Guidance or advice given to students when selecting learning issues is tailored to be specific to different subjects

issue at the seven levels of organization, students will develop a mindset consistent with the appropriate practice of quality medical care.

The following thoughts should help students make decisions when choosing learning issues. It is important to note that novice learners often need some guidance or advice from the facilitator when identifying potential learning issues (Fig. 6.3).

- When selecting learning issues, those that deal with the *physiology* of organs and organ systems will come most easily. However, remember that whenever an organ or organ system is brought up, students must also keep gross *anatomy* and *histology* in mind and study that as well. Also, when appropriate, any *neuroanatomy* involved in the control of the organ or system should be included.
- Learning issues involving *behavioral science, including substance use, human development, mental status, cognitive functioning, and mental health*, are occasionally relegated to a secondary position in comparison to medical or healthcare-related problems. There's a misconception that these issues are merely ancillary matters, not necessitating direct attention from healthcare professionals, or are deemed the exclusive domain of psychiatrists. However, the relationship between the mind and body is strong and research repeatedly indicates that behavior and health are highly correlated (Umberson & Montez, 2010). When confronted with such matters, students often explore into determining how to effectively identify

problems in these areas and discern when these factors warrant pharmacological and non-pharmacological interventions. Additionally, they may contemplate the ramifications these factors could have on a patient's diagnoses, treatment plans, and adherence to treatment regimens.

- When students engage with learning issues about biochemistry, they often explore the metabolic pathways of specific groups of compounds, such as carbohydrates, proteins, or lipids, and examine how these pathways are interconnected and integrated within biological systems.
- When a patient in the case receives treatment with a specific drug, the *pharmacology* aspect, particularly the properties and actions of that drug, becomes a selected learning issue. Past experiences have shown that it's often more beneficial to select an entire category of drugs and compare their mechanisms of action, relative risks, and side effects, interactions with other drugs, and other relevant factors, rather than focusing solely on a specific drug. For instance, if a patient is treated with propranolol, rather than selecting "propranolol" as the learning issue, students should consider "beta-adrenergic blockers" as the learning issue, allowing for a broader exploration of the pharmacological class.
- *Pathology* learning issues are most likely to arise when students finally arrive at a diagnosis. Experienced students recommend that instead of focusing solely on a specific disease, it's more beneficial for students to select diseases of the organ or organ system under consideration, or at least related diseases. This approach enables students to dive into comparative histopathology and pathophysiology concerning the differential diagnosis of the organ or organ system. By exploring a broader range of diseases of the same organ or system, students can better understand the underlying mechanisms and variations in presentation, aiding in more accurate diagnosis and management. For example, let's say the case involves a patient presenting with respiratory symptoms. Instead of selecting a single disease like pneumonia as the learning issue, students might broaden their focus to diseases of the respiratory system or related conditions. They could explore diseases such as asthma, chronic obstructive pulmonary disease (COPD), pulmonary embolism, lung cancer, or tuberculosis.
- *Microbiology and Immunology* learning issues will present themselves at obvious times. There might be a tendency to deal with these more superficially than is desirable. Students should use the textbooks and other recommended resources as topic guides.

6.3 Structure of a PBL Examination

PBL examinations are structured in a way that enhances student learning and assessment of basic medical/health sciences knowledge applied to a clinical scenario. Although the PBL examination is composed exclusively of multiple-choice questions, there are three different categories of questions included, all of which are knowledge-based: case-based questions, pre-assigned readings (see below), and group-specific topics. All three categories of questions are well represented in a PBL examination, so students must study and prepare for all of them. Depending on the stage in the PBL development and the degree of overlap of topics between groups, the proportion of the number of questions may vary. For example, early in the PBL curriculum, students might receive more pre-assigned readings to familiarize them with the PBL process and foundational concepts. On the other hand, as students progress and become more adept at self-directed learning, the curriculum might reduce (or eliminate) pre-assigned readings, instead increasing the overlap of examination topics across all groups. In any case, the proportion of questions related to a specific topic will depend on the chapter's length and its relevance to the case. Longer chapters typically contain more content and will have more questions, and chapters closely related to the case's central issues will have more questions as well.

6.3.1 Case-Based Questions

Case-based questions are an important component of the PBL examination. This section will highlight the process of identifying important concepts from a particular case and the subsequent development of questions to test those concepts.

Case-based questions are questions directly related to the case, and all PBL groups should have discussed them during the PBL sessions. Very simply, these are questions that are derived from the underlying basic medical/health science mechanisms that are so central to the case that ALL groups must have learned and discussed them during the case. It has been shown that case-based questions are highly relevant for learning and are well-received by students, as they encourage the application of clinical knowledge and problem-solving skills, making them an effective tool in PBL environments (Durak et al., 2007).

Case-based questions are designed to encourage students to pay attention to the cases and explore deeply into the basic medical/health science mechanisms causing the PBL patient's conditions. To achieve such a goal, a condensed version of each completed PBL case is given during the examination, plus all the pertinent tests and lab results. The case presentation should take one page or less, followed by a series of basic medical/health science mechanism questions about the case. These questions are always "big picture" questions that the students would ask of themselves *during* the case. For example, the patient may present with anemia. The students would ask themselves, "What is anemia, and what may cause it?" One of the case-based questions that could be asked is the mechanism of erythropoiesis.

Students are instructed and constantly reminded to ask the *why's, what's, and how's* of every case and the related laboratory tests. For example, if the patient in the case has pitting edema, students should be asked about the specific basic medical/health science mechanisms that are responsible for the accumulation of fluid in the tissues and the reason for pitting, which is different from non-pitting, and a possible case-based question would test students about these mechanisms. Another example, during a hepatitis case, the liver function test may show elevations of ALT and AST.

Students should ask what these enzymes are, what they do, and how they are out of the normal range. Therefore, an appropriate case-based question could ask students to identify the function of one of these liver enzymes. Every group receives the same case-based questions. The case-based questions aim to encourage the group to explore all the basic medical/health science mechanisms from the case "during" the PBL session. For example, if during the PBL case the patient was prescribed a specific drug, a feasible case-based question would be to ask what the mechanism of action of that drug is. Students typically score high on these questions. Although case-based questions are typically multiple-choice, other formats such as short answer or fill-in-the-blank questions could be utilized.

Once the final case of a block or semester concludes, a 7–10-day period known as "review week" begins. During this time, the PBL Director undertakes the critical task of constructing individualized examinations for each PBL group. The construction of these examinations is a meticulous and time-intensive process. Each exam is tailored to align with the specific exam topics selected by the group, ensuring that the questions reflect the depth and scope of their discussions throughout the block. This customization requires the Director to carefully review each group's chosen topics and design questions that are diagnosis-specific and mechanism-driven.

The exam development process involves creating a variety of question formats, including single-best-answer multiple-choice questions, fill-in-the-blank items, and matching questions. Each format serves distinct assessment purposes: multiple-choice questions assess a broad range of content efficiently and objectively; fill-in-the-blank questions test recall and understanding without cues; and matching questions evaluate recognition and understanding of relationships between concepts. Healthcare professional programs have the flexibility to design examinations using these formats (or any other format) in a manner that best aligns with their curricular goals and assessment strategies. This adaptability ensures that assessments are tailored to measure the intended competencies effectively. Each question is meticulously vetted to ensure scientific accuracy, appropriate complexity, and integration across disciplines. Given the individualized nature of these assessments, the Director's role during review week is pivotal in ensuring that each exam accurately reflects the group's academic journey and learning objectives. Although facilitators do not meet with students during this period, review week serves as a bridge between the collaborative learning experience and the rigorous assessment that follows, emphasizing the importance of tailored evaluation in the PBL curriculum.

6.3.2 Pre-Assigned Readings

These questions come from any pre-assigned readings given to the students before the start of an examination block. Although typically the pre-assigned readings are from specific textbook chapters, they can also be in any other format, such as PowerPoint presentations, video lectures, journal articles, etc. Pre-assigned readings may or may not be on a particular examination. Due to several factors, pre-assigned readings are often deemed more essential in the early stages of the PBL curriculum. While PBL emphasizes student-driven learning, learners typically gravitate towards topics directly relevant to the cases they encounter. Consequently, they may overlook foundational concepts crucial for comprehending later chapters in textbooks. To address this gap, foundational topics are sometimes pre-assigned to students with readings carefully selected to align with the system or topic of the PBL cases in the examination block. For example, to better understand Chapter 8: Cholinoreceptor-Blocking Drugs in Pharmacology, it may be best to pre-assign introductory chapters such as Chapter 2: Drug Receptors and Pharmacodynamics and Chapter 5: Pharmacogenomics. While the primary aim of PBL is to foster self-directed learning, pre-assigned reading remains vital, particularly in the initial stages of the PBL curriculum when students are still acclimating to the PBL process and philosophy, making structured guidance essential for laying a strong educational foundation.

6.3.3 Group-Specific Examination Topics

These are the questions from the specific chapters chosen by each PBL group. Selected examination topics by students make up the bulk of the examination and are different for every PBL group. However, every group completes the same cases for a given PBL examination block. Thus, the topics selected across groups will have some degree of commonality. The number of questions from each examination topic is related to the scope and complexity of the subject. If the topic requires most of the students' time to master, they will receive more questions on that topic in the exam. If the topic is very small, either in content or page numbers (or both), they will receive fewer questions. This is necessary because there are only a few "big picture" and clinically relevant topics to ask from a topic small in scope with fewer pages.

As an example, following the completion of a case on sickle cell disease, a PBL group opted to focus on the chapter about erythropoiesis in the physiology textbook (Chapter 33: Red Blood Cells, Anemia, and Polycythemia). They deemed this topic crucial for comprehending the pathogenesis of sickle cell disease. Consequently, an examination question stemming from this chapter might inquire about the impact of erythropoietin on the production of new red blood cells.

6.4 Examination Construction

Faculty members review the question bank of a specific discipline by their area of expertise to ensure that only high-quality questions are included in the examination. They edit questions that can be improved (due to poor wording, ambiguity, or poor statistical data), and they write new questions regularly. Creating a high-quality examination is no easy task, particularly when several different high-quality examinations must be created simultaneously. It requires motivation, excellent time management skills, and effective communication among the examination PBL director, faculty members, and students.

As previously described, PBL examinations are comprised of the following categories of questions (Fig. 6.4):

- Case-based questions
- Pre-assigned readings (if any)
- Group-specific examination topics

All groups receive the same number of questions, regardless of how many topics were chosen by the group. Conserving the equality of each question's weight on the examination is essential. In doing so, different numbers of questions are given to different groups in each topic category. For example, one group may have chosen a total of 30 examination topics, while another may have chosen a total of 27 topics. The group choosing 27 topics will necessarily receive more questions in each topic category to have the same overall number of questions as the group choosing 30 topics.

The total number of topics selected for each group can be tracked using a spreadsheet. The spreadsheet of topics serves many purposes and is the backbone of the organization needed to accomplish the task of building several discrete exams. As topics are submitted, they are entered into the spreadsheet using the number 1 in the

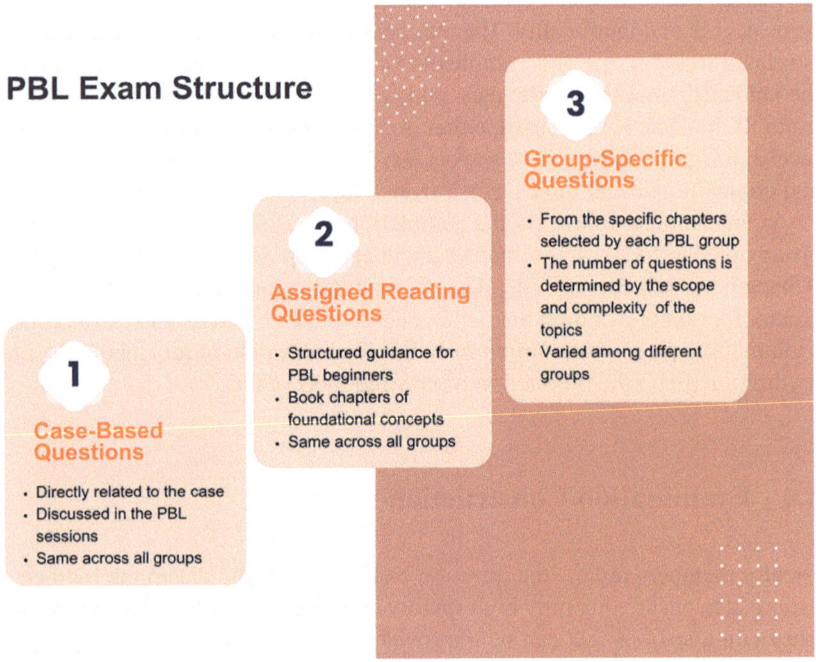

Fig. 6.4 PBL examinations consist of the three categories of questions: case-based questions, pre-assigned reading questions, and group-specific questions

cell corresponding to the specific group and the topic chosen (Fig. 6.5). The total number of examination topics is summed at the bottom of the spreadsheet for each group. While compiling the examination, the number 1 can be changed to the number of items in that topic area so that the sum for a group will total the number of questions on the examination (Fig. 6.5). This process is done for each group individually until the sums for all groups are the same. This is an essential part of examination construction. Students often express concerns about the fairness of examination questions, particularly when groups select different chapters for study. However, it's crucial to emphasize that questions are meticulously crafted, edited, and reviewed by faculty experts with appropriate training backgrounds. As a result, every question employed is deemed fair and appropriate for assessment.

When groups choose different chapters, the content covered will naturally vary, leading to questions on diverse topics with varying levels of difficulty. While some questions may indeed be more challenging than others, it's important to note that the distribution of question difficulty balances out across groups. Consequently, no

	Topic Selection					Numbner of Questions				
Group #	1	2	3	4	5	1	2	3	4	5
Biochemistry (5th ed)										
29 Digestion and Transport of Dietary Lipids	1	1			1	5	5			5
31 Synthesis of Fatty Acids, Triacylglycerols, and the Major Membrane Lipids			1					6		
32 Cholesterol Absorption, Synthesis, Metabolism, and Fate		1			1		6			5
33 Metabolism of Ethanol	1				1	5				5
42 The Biochemistry of Erythrocytes and Other Blood Cells		1	1	1			6	6	6	
43 Blood Plasma Proteins, Coagulation, and Fibrinolysis	1	1			1	5	5			5
44 Liver Metabolism				1	1				5	5
Microbiology (9th ed)										
18 staphylococcus and related gram-positive cocci	1		1			5		5		
19 streptococcus and enterococcus	1	1	1	1	1	5	5	6	5	5
21 listeria and related Gram-positive bacteria	1		1			5		5		
22 Mycobacterium and related acid-fast bacteria	1	1	1	1	1	5	5	6	6	5
23 Neisseria and related genera	1		1	1		5		6	6	
24 Haemophilus and related bacteria		1		1	1		5		6	5
25 Enterobacteriaceae	1		1	1		5		6	6	
35 Chlamydia	1					5				
43 Human Herpesviruses	1	1	1	1	1	5	5	6	6	5
Pathology (10th Ed)										
3 Inflammation and Repair	1	1	1	1	1	5	5	6	6	5
4 Hemodynamic Disorders, Thromboembolic Disease, and Shock	1	1	1	1	1	5	5	6	6	5
Pharmacology (15th ed)										
10 Adrenoceptor Antagonist Drugs	1			1	1	5			6	5
11 Antihypertensive Agents		1	1	1	1		6	6	6	5
12 Vasodilators & the Treatment of Angina Pectoris					1					5
13 Drugs Used in Heart Failure			1					6		
14 Agents Used in Cardiac Arrhythmias	1	1		1	1	5	6		6	6
15 Diuretic Agents	1	1			1	5	6			6
Physiology (14th ed)										
9 Cardiac Muscle; The Heart as a Pump and Function of the Heart Valves	1	1	1	1	1	5	6	6	6	6
10 Rhythmical Excitation of the Heart	1	1	1	1	1	5	6	6	6	6
11 The Normal Electrocardiogram	1	1				5	6			
35 Resistance of the Body to Infection: II. Immunity and Allergy		1	1	1			6	6	6	
36 Blood Types; Transfusion; Tissue and Organ Transplantation	1		1	1		5		6	6	
37 Hemostasis and Blood Coagulation		1			1		6			6
Total	20	18	17	17	19	100	100	100	100	100

Topic Selection: Mark with a "1" each topic the groups select

Number of Questions: Add questions to each chosen topic to achieve desired total number of questions for exam (this example has 100 questions)

Fig. 6.5 A sample spreadsheet to track topic selection and the number of questions, which can be effectively organized using Excel

single group is disproportionately burdened with difficult questions compared to others.

In practice, the examination score averages across groups typically exhibit minimal variance, typically within a range of 3–4% between the highest and lowest group averages. Additionally, when questions from past examinations are utilized, historical statistics are leveraged to ensure a comparable degree of difficulty. Indeed, with new questions lacking historical statistics, variations in difficulty are to be expected, with some questions posing greater challenges than others. Despite differences in question difficulty, the overall examination results tend to cluster around the average range. This suggests that while individual questions may vary in difficulty, the collective impact of the assessment process tends to yield consistent outcomes across PBL groups. Thus, while the challenge level of individual questions may vary, the overall assessment remains robust and reflective of students' understanding and performance within the PBL curriculum.

6.5 PBL Examination Construction Guidelines

The following guidelines are utilized by faculty members responsible for constructing PBL examinations, as well as by those involved in item writing and examination administration. These procedures ensure the reliability, validity, and educational appropriateness of assessments used throughout the curriculum. The focus is on creating examinations that fairly and accurately assess student progress while fostering the critical thinking and clinical reasoning skills essential for healthcare practice (Fig. 6.6).

6.5.1 General Guidelines for Examination Construction

- Examinations must accurately gauge the appropriate difficulty level relative to the student's stage of training within their respective healthcare professional program. This principle is essential to support progressive skill development and ensure the readiness of students for future clinical responsibilities (Case & Swanson, 2002). The appropriate level of complexity should reflect not only the professional program, such as medicine, physician assistant studies, nursing, dentistry, or pharmacy, but also whether the student is in the early preclinical stages or approaching their clinical rotations.
- Exam questions should challenge students to demonstrate mastery of basic medical/health science knowledge at a healthcare professional in training level rather than at a graduate research or PhD student level. The distinction ensures alignment with national competency expectations and board examination standards, emphasizing the application of knowledge in clinical contexts over purely theoretical exploration (Downing & Haladyna, 2004).

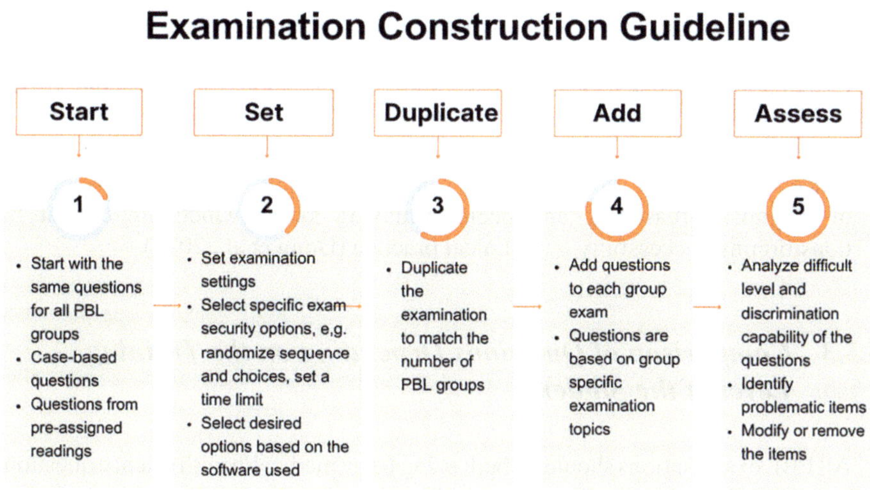

Fig. 6.6 Construct a PBL examination step by step is an organized process that can be carried out efficiently

- Examinations must be constructed on an ongoing basis as new PBL case topics are released. This rolling approach ensures that assessment materials stay current and aligned with recently discussed cases, reinforcing active learning principles and minimizing content gaps (Schuwirth & Van der Vleuten, 2011).
- All faculty members are expected to contribute examination items within their area of expertise. Collaboration across disciplines enhances the quality and breadth of assessments, promotes content integration, and models interdisciplinary teamwork for students, which is a critical skill in modern healthcare environments (Hrynchak et al., 2014).

6.5.2 *Guidelines for Examination Items*

- Item authors must be thoroughly familiar with established multiple-choice question writing guidelines, such as those outlined in the *National Board of Medical Examiners' Constructing Written Test Questions for the Basic and Clinical Sciences* (NBME, 2021) and the *NBOME Item Writing Guide* (NBOME, 2006). Adherence to these standards improves question quality by reducing ambiguity, minimizing cueing, and enhancing item validity.
- Every examination question must be verifiable by references within required textbooks or approved supplemental resources. This practice ensures that assessments remain fair and objective, supporting both student learning and due process in the event of grade challenges (Case & Swanson, 2002).
- Questions should be based on "big picture" objectives typically found at the beginning of each textbook chapter. Additionally, examination items should be

constructed using the specific learning objectives from each of the PBL cases discussed during the curriculum. This dual anchoring to general and case-specific goals enhances content validity and promotes integration of knowledge across different health science domains (Schuwirth & Van der Vleuten, 2011).

- Questions must have clinical relevance or emphasize important foundational concepts. Clinically contextualized questions support students' development of diagnostic reasoning and decision-making skills, which are crucial for transitioning successfully into clinical practice (Dong et al., 2014).

6.5.3 Comparison of Questions Depending on the Training Level of the Student

- All PBL examinations should be built using basic medical/health science questions presented within a clinical context, reflecting the realities of healthcare practice where foundational science underpins patient care decisions. This approach aligns with contemporary evidence supporting contextual learning as superior to isolated rote memorization (Norman, 2005).
- Clinical scenarios should be written following item writing guidelines provided by licensing bodies such as the NBME and NBOME. Properly written clinical vignettes simulate real world cases and encourage students to engage in higher order thinking processes such as analysis, synthesis, and evaluation (Case & Swanson, 2002).
- In the early phases of the PBL curriculum, such as during the first semester, PBL examinations may include a small proportion of direct recall questions, generally comprising about 10–20% of the overall examination. These questions assess foundational knowledge necessary for more complex cognitive applications later. However, the majority of questions, even early on, should present clinical scenarios requiring the application of basic medical/health science principles to patient-centered problems (Schuwirth & Van der Vleuten, 2011).
- For students in the latter stages of their training, PBL examinations should increasingly consist of basic medical/health science questions embedded in comprehensive clinical cases. At this stage, examinations should be dominated by case-based questions, each testing understanding of several critical concepts from the PBL cases covered. Group-specific examination topics should also be incorporated to assess collaboration and group learning outcomes. By the end of the PBL curriculum, the expectation is that students can interpret complex clinical scenarios independently and apply their foundational knowledge toward diagnosis and management (Dong et al., 2014).

6.6 Post-Examination Analyses

The scoring of PBL examinations is performed automatically through examination delivery software platforms such as ExamSoft or equivalent programs. These platforms facilitate efficient grading and offer immediate feedback to both faculty and students. However, because the PBL format often necessitates discrete examinations for each group, the subsequent statistical analyses are highly dependent on the specific analytical capabilities of the examination software used. In the case of small group assessments, where the number of test takers is relatively low (for example, $n = 8$ if there are eight students in a group), the statistical measures produced must be interpreted with caution. In such instances, the validity and reliability of certain metrics, including difficulty indices and discrimination indices, may be compromised due to the small sample size (Downing & Haladyna, 2004).

Ideally, for robust post-examination analysis, all examination items used across different PBL groups should be aggregated into a larger item bank, and their statistical properties assessed collectively. Pooling data from multiple groups enhances the sample size and improves the reliability of item analysis outcomes (Tavakol & Dennick, 2011). However, whether this aggregation is feasible depends on the functionalities available within the examination software platform. Some platforms offer flexible data merging and comparative reporting tools, while others may not support cross-examination item aggregation.

Despite these challenges, several best practices in post-examination analysis can be implemented, even with small samples, to enhance the quality of examinations and inform future item development. These best practices, adapted from recommendations by Rudolph et al. (2019), are outlined below:

- Questions that exhibit a difficulty factor of less than 0.40 are flagged for further scrutiny. A low difficulty factor, such as 0.40, suggests that only 40% of students answered the item correctly, indicating that the item may be excessively difficult or possibly flawed.
- The upper and lower quartile method is employed to assess the discrimination capability of each question. This involves comparing the performance of the top 25% of students to the bottom 25%. A well-discriminating item is one where high-performing students answer correctly more frequently than low-performing students (Ebel & Frisbie, 1991).
- Analysis of the frequency of selection of specific answer choices can reveal questions with two plausible correct answers. If an alternative distractor is chosen nearly as frequently as the keyed correct answer, it may indicate ambiguity in the item or multiple correct interpretations.
- Once problematic items are identified, they are reviewed by a content expert. The expert evaluates whether the item was simply a very difficult but valid question, whether multiple correct answers exist, or whether the item lacks a clearly correct answer altogether. Content expertise is critical in making fair and educationally sound judgments (Downing & Haladyna, 2004).

- Based on the content expert's evaluation, a recommendation is made regarding whether the item should be modified, removed from scoring, or retained without changes. These decisions should align with established institutional policies for examination integrity and fairness.

To illustrate how these practices are applied, consider the following example from a post-examination analysis:

- **Question A**: Difficulty factor = 0.49, Discrimination index = 0.41
- **Question B**: Difficulty factor = 0.51, Discrimination index = 0.06

Although both questions are moderately difficult, given that only about half of the students answered each correctly, their discrimination indices tell different stories. Question A has a strong discrimination index of 0.41, suggesting that it effectively differentiates between students who have mastered the material and those who have not. Conversely, Question B, with a low discrimination index of 0.06, appears unable to distinguish high performers from low performers, indicating potential issues such as poor question construction, ambiguity, or content misalignment.

Based on these results, it would be educationally appropriate to retain Question A for future use while considering the removal or revision of Question B. However, such decisions should not be made in isolation. The PBL director should establish formalized criteria for post-examination item evaluation and decision-making. These criteria may include specific cutoff values for difficulty and discrimination indices, contextual factors related to examination goals, and standards specific to the healthcare profession program (Downing & Haladyna, 2004). Below is a post-examination analysis checklist designed for Problem-Based Learning (PBL) directors. This tool can be adapted and customized to align with the specific needs of healthcare professional programs.

Faculty Post Examination Analyses Checklist
Purpose: To guide faculty through the review and evaluation of PBL examination items after each administration.
1. Exam Scoring and Initial Review • Confirm exam scoring completed automatically via examination platform (e.g., ExamSoft). • Retrieve statistical reports from examination software for each examination group.
2. Validity of Statistical Data • Acknowledge small sample size if group size is low (e.g., n = 8); interpret statistics cautiously. • If possible, pool data from multiple groups for more robust statistical analysis.
3. Item Difficulty Evaluation • Identify items with a difficulty factor <0.40. • Flag these items for further review.
4. Item Discrimination Analysis • Use upper and lower quartile comparisons to evaluate item discrimination. • Identify items with a discrimination index <0.20 for closer scrutiny. • Recognize strong items with discrimination indices >0.30–0.40.

(continued)

(continued)

Faculty Post Examination Analyses Checklist
5. Distractor Analysis • Examine frequency of each answer choice selection. • Identify potential issues: – Multiple correct answers – Poorly constructed distractors – Ambiguous or confusing item wording
6. Expert Content Review • Content expert reviews each flagged item. • Determine if issues are due to: – Excessive difficulty – Multiple plausible correct answers – Lack of a correct answer • Make a formal recommendation: – Retain item – Revise item – Remove item
7. Final Decision and Documentation • Apply formalized cutoff criteria (as set by PBL director or program). • Record decisions for each flagged item with justifications. • Update item bank accordingly for future use.
8. Handling Failures • Identify students scoring below institutional passing threshold (typically <70%). • Design remediation opportunities focused on specific missed learning objectives. • Offer targeted remediation exams if necessary.
Notes: • Statistical measures must be interpreted carefully when sample size is small. • Aggregating items across groups strengthens reliability of post examination analysis. • Content expertise is essential for valid post examination review.

As we focus primarily on the summative assessment aspects of PBL examinations in this chapter, it is important to recognize the possibility of student failure. Generally, a performance below 70% is considered failing, although the passing threshold may differ based on the policies of individual healthcare education programs. In the event of examination failure, students should be offered remediation opportunities. Remediation examinations should be carefully designed to focus on the specific learning objectives or major concepts that the student did not master, promoting targeted learning and eventual competency achievement. Formative assessment strategies, which differ in purpose and approach from summative assessments, will be discussed separately in Chap. 7.

6.7 Conclusions

As discussed in this chapter, examinations in PBL play a pivotal role in driving student learning and remain a cornerstone of the educational process. Well-constructed PBL examinations not only evaluate student knowledge but also encourage integration and application of foundational concepts within clinical contexts, thus fostering deeper understanding and critical thinking skills essential for healthcare professionals (Hmelo-Silver, 2004). According to Zaveri et al. (2019), the implementation of PBL assessments consistently correlated with students performing above the national average on first-level licensing board examinations, highlighting the effectiveness of this approach in preparing students for high-stakes professional certification.

PBL examinations serve multiple valuable functions beyond simple assessment. They identify knowledge gaps, which can then be addressed through targeted remediation and further learning opportunities, thereby promoting mastery and reducing future clinical errors (Schmidt et al., 2011). These assessments also motivate students to engage actively with course material, knowing that evaluation is closely tied to clinical relevance and practical application (Dolmans et al., 2005). Furthermore, systematic examination construction and post-examination analysis provide essential quality assurance, ensuring that assessments remain fair, valid, and aligned with evolving curricular goals and professional competencies (Cook & Artino, 2016).

The influence of adept examination design extends beyond measurement. It can reinforce key elements of the PBL process itself, such as collaborative learning, problem-solving, and clinical reasoning, by aligning examination items with the cases discussed and the learning objectives emphasized throughout the curriculum (Norman & Schmidt, 1992). This alignment ensures that assessments are not isolated hurdles but integrated components of a cohesive educational strategy, thereby enhancing the overall learning experience.

In conclusion, carefully designed and executed PBL examinations not only assess and enhance students' mastery of basic medical/health science concepts in clinical contexts but also support continuous curricular improvement and student motivation. These outcomes ultimately contribute to the development of competent, reflective healthcare professionals ready to deliver high-quality patient care. Future chapters will further explore formative assessments and their role in complementing summative evaluations to create a comprehensive and effective assessment framework within PBL curricula.

References

Albanese, M. A., & Mitchell, S. (1993). Problem-based learning: A review of literature on its outcomes and implementation issues. *Academic Medicine: Journal of the Association of American Medical Colleges, 68*(1), 1. https://doi.org/10.1097/00001888-199301000-00012

Barrows, H. S. (1986). A taxonomy of problem-based learning methods. *Medical Education, 20*(6), 481–486. https://doi.org/10.1111/j.1365-2923.1986.tb01386.x

Barrows, H. S. (1996). Problem-based learning in medicine and beyond: A brief overview. *New Directions for Teaching and Learning, 1996*(68), 3–12. https://doi.org/10.1002/tl.37219966804
Barrows, H. S. (2000). *Problem-based learning applied to medical education* (Revised ed.). Southern Illinois University, School of Medicine.
Biggs, J. (1996). Enhancing teaching through constructive alignment. *Higher Education, 32*(3), 347–364. https://doi.org/10.1007/BF00138871
Boud, D. (2000). Sustainable assessment: Rethinking assessment for the learning society. *Studies in Continuing Education, 22*(2), 151–167. https://doi.org/10.1080/713695728
Case, S. M., & Swanson, D. B. (2002). *Constructing written test questions for the basic and clinical sciences* (3rd ed.). National Board of Medical Examiners. Retrieved from https://www.researchgate.net/publication/242759434_Constructing_Written_Test_Questions_For_the_Basic_and_Clinical_Sciences
Chakravarty, M., Latif, N. A., Abu-Hijleh, M. F., Osman, M., Dharap, A. S., & Ganguly, P. K. (2005). Assessment of anatomy in a problem-based medical curriculum. *Clinical Anatomy, 18*(2), 131–136. https://doi.org/10.1002/ca.20038
Cook, D. A., & Artino, A. R. (2016). Motivation to learn: An overview of contemporary theories. *Medical Education, 50*(10), 997–1014. https://doi.org/10.1111/medu.13074
Dochy, F., Segers, M., Van den Bossche, P., & Gijbels, D. (2003). Effects of problem-based learning: A meta-analysis. *Learning and Instruction, 13*(5), 5. https://doi.org/10.1016/S0959-4752(02)00025-7
Dolmans, D. H. J. M., Schmidt, H. G., & Gijselaers, W. H. (1994). The relationship between student-generated learning issues and self-study in problem-based learning. *Instructional Science, 22*(4), 251–267. https://doi.org/10.1007/BF00891779
Dolmans, D. H. J. M., De Grave, W., Wolfhagen, I. H. A. P., & van der Vleuten, C. P. M. (2005). Problem-based learning: Future challenges for educational practice and research. *Medical Education, 39*(7), 7. https://doi.org/10.1111/j.1365-2929.2005.02205.x
Dolmans, D. H. J. M., Loyens, S. M. M., Marcq, H., & Gijbels, D. (2016). Deep and surface learning in problem-based learning: A review of the literature. *Advances in Health Sciences Education: Theory and Practice, 21*(5), 1087–1112. https://doi.org/10.1007/s10459-015-9645-6
Dong, T., Swygert, K. A., Durning, S. J., Saguil, A., Gilliland, W. R., Cruess, D., DeZee, K. J., LaRochelle, J., & Artino, A. R. (2014). Validity evidence for medical school OSCEs: Associations with USMLE® step assessments. *Teaching and Learning in Medicine, 26*(4), 379–386. https://doi.org/10.1080/10401334.2014.960294
Downing, S. M., & Haladyna, T. M. (2004). *Validity threats: Overcoming interference with proposed interpretations of assessment data., 25*(1), 33–41.
Durak, H. I., Caliskan, S. A., Bor, S., & Van Der Vleuten, C. (2007). Use of case-based exams as an instructional teaching tool to teach clinical reasoning. *Medical Teacher, 29*(6), e170–e174. https://doi.org/10.1080/01421590701506866
Ebel, R. L., & Frisbie, D. A. (1991). *Essentials of educational measurement*. Prentice Hall.
Eva, K. W., Bordage, G., Campbell, C., Galbraith, R., Ginsburg, S., Holmboe, E., & Regehr, G. (2016). Towards a program of assessment for health professionals: From training into practice. *Advances in Health Sciences Education: Theory and Practice, 21*(4), 897–913. https://doi.org/10.1007/s10459-015-9653-6
Gijbels, D., Dochy, F., Van den Bossche, P., & Segers, M. (2005). Effects of problem-based learning: A meta-analysis from the angle of assessment. *Review of Educational Research, 75*(1), 27–61. https://doi.org/10.3102/00346543075001027
Gipps, C. (2008). *Beyond testing: Towards a theory of educational assessment*. Routledge. https://doi.org/10.4324/9780203486009
Hmelo-Silver, C. E. (2004). Problem-based learning: What and how do students learn? *Educational Psychology Review, 16*(3), 3. https://doi.org/10.1023/B:EDPR.0000034022.16470.f3
Hrynchak, P., Takahashi, S. G., & Nayer, M. (2014). Key-feature questions for assessment of clinical reasoning: A literature review. *Medical Education, 48*(9), 870–883. https://doi.org/10.1111/medu.12509

Knowles, M. S. (1984). *The adult learner: A neglected species*. Gulf Pub. Co., Book Division. Retrieved from http://archive.org/details/adultlearnernegl0000know

Martinez, M. E., & Lipson, J. I. (1989). Assessment for learning. *Educational Leadership, 46*(7), 73–75.

NBME. (2021). *NBME item-writing guide*. Retrieved from https://www.nbme.org/item-writing-guide

NBOME. (2006). *NBOME item-writing guide*. Retrieved from https://pdfcoffee.com/comlex-iw-guide-2006-pdf-free.html

Neville, A. J. (2009). Problem-based learning and medical education forty years on. *Medical Principles and Practice, 18*(1), 1–9. https://doi.org/10.1159/000163038

Norman, G. (2005). Research in clinical reasoning: Past history and current trends. *Medical Education, 39*(4), 418–427. https://doi.org/10.1111/j.1365-2929.2005.02127.x

Norman, G. R., & Schmidt, H. G. (1992). The psychological basis of problem-based learning: A review of the evidence. *Academic Medicine: Journal of the Association of American Medical Colleges, 67*(9), 9. https://doi.org/10.1097/00001888-199209000-00002

Norman, G. R., & Schmidt, H. G. (2000). Effectiveness of problem-based learning curricula: Theory, practice and paper darts. *Medical Education, 34*(9), 721–728. https://doi.org/10.1046/j.1365-2923.2000.00749.x

Ricci, M., St-Onge, C., Xiao, J., & Young, M. (2018). Students as stakeholders in assessment: How students perceive the value of an assessment. *Perspectives on Medical Education, 7*(6), 352–361. https://doi.org/10.1007/s40037-018-0480-3

Rudolph, M. J., Daugherty, K. K., Ray, M. E., Shuford, V. P., Lebovitz, L., & DiVall, M. V. (2019). Best practices related to examination item construction and post-hoc review. *American Journal of Pharmaceutical Education, 83*(7), Article 7. https://doi.org/10.5688/ajpe7204

Rushton, A. (2005). Formative assessment: A key to deep learning? *Medical Teacher, 27*(6), 509–513. https://doi.org/10.1080/01421590500129159

Schmidt, H. G., van der Molen, H. T., te Winkel, W. W. R., & Wijnen, W. H. F. W. (2009). Constructivist, problem-based learning does work: A meta-analysis of curricular comparisons involving a single medical school. *Educational Psychologist, 44*(4), 227–249. https://doi.org/10.1080/00461520903213592

Schmidt, H. G., Rotgans, J. I., & Yew, E. H. J. (2011). The process of problem-based learning: What works and why. *Medical Education, 45*(8), 8. https://doi.org/10.1111/j.1365-2923.2011.04035.x

Schmidt, H. G., Wagener, S. L., Smeets, G. A. C. M., Keemink, L. M., & van der Molen, H. T. (2015). On the use and misuse of lectures in higher education. *Health Professions Education, 1*(1), 12–18. https://doi.org/10.1016/j.hpe.2015.11.010

Schuwirth, L. W. T., & Van der Vleuten, C. P. M. (2011). Programmatic assessment: From assessment of learning to assessment for learning. *Medical Teacher, 33*(6), 478–485. https://doi.org/10.3109/0142159X.2011.565828

Schwartz, R. W., Burgett, J. E., Blue, A. V., Donnelly, M. B., & Sloan, D. A. (1997). Problem-based learning and performance-based testing: Effective alternatives for undergraduate surgical education and assessment of student performance. *Medical Teacher, 19*(1), 19–23. https://doi.org/10.3109/01421599709019341

Shepard, L. A. (2000). The role of assessment in a learning culture. *Educational Researcher, 29*(7), 4–14. https://doi.org/10.3102/0013189X029007004

Tavakol, M., & Dennick, R. (2011). Making sense of Cronbach's alpha. *International Journal of Medical Education, 2*, 53–55. https://doi.org/10.5116/ijme.4dfb.8dfd

Umberson, D., & Montez, J. K. (2010). Social relationships and health: A flashpoint for health policy. *Journal of Health and Social Behavior, 51*(Suppl), S54–S66. https://doi.org/10.1177/0022146510383501

Van Der Vleuten, C. P. M., & Schuwirth, L. W. T. (2005). Assessing professional competence: From methods to programmes. *Medical Education, 39*(3), 309–317. https://doi.org/10.1111/j.1365-2929.2005.02094.x

van der Vleuten, C. P. M., & Schuwirth, L. W. T. (2019). Assessment in the context of problem-based learning. *Advances in Health Sciences Education, 24*(5), 903–914. https://doi.org/10.1007/s10459-019-09909-1

Zaveri, N., Coty, M., McCarver, V., Vidic, C., Nolan, T., Nath, S., & Vanier, C. (2019). Changes to an active learning curriculum in osteopathic medical education: Effects on exam outcomes and board scores. *Medical Science Educator, 29*(1), 1. https://doi.org/10.1007/s40670-018-00674-1

Chapter 7
Formative Feedback for Students in Problem-Based Learning

Santiago Lorenzo

7.1 Feedback in PBL

In the context of PBL, feedback to health profession students can be formative or summative (Fig. 7.1). Summative feedback, in the form of PBL examinations, has been extensively discussed in Chap. 6.

Formative feedback, on the other hand, plays a pivotal role in supporting student growth and enhancing learning outcomes. Formative feedback can be defined as information communicated to students intended to modify their thinking or behavior to improve learning (Shute, 2008). It is an interactive process designed to identify areas of strength and opportunities for improvement, allowing students to refine their knowledge and skills iteratively. Studies have consistently shown that formative feedback is a crucial factor for learning and performance purposes (Bandura & Cervone, 2000; Fletcher & Perry, 2002; Ilgen et al., 1979). Formative feedback should be provided regularly throughout the PBL block and after each PBL session. Such feedback can take various forms, including oral comments during debriefing sessions, written evaluations, or structured rubrics that assess specific competencies. Facilitators should aim to deliver feedback in a timely, constructive, and actionable manner. Providing specific examples and suggestions help students understand how to bridge gaps in their learning and build upon their existing strengths. Moreover, the feedback process in PBL should be a two-way interaction. Students should be encouraged to reflect on the feedback they receive and engage in dialogue with their facilitators to clarify expectations and address misunderstandings. Incorporating self-assessment and peer feedback can further enrich the learning experience by promoting metacognition and fostering collaborative skills among students.

S. Lorenzo (✉)
Lake Erie College of Osteopathic Medicine, Bradenton, FL, USA
e-mail: slorenzo@lecom.edu

S. Lorenzo and B. Zhang (eds.), *Mastering Problem-Based Learning in Health Profession Programs*, https://doi.org/10.1007/978-3-032-05405-0_7

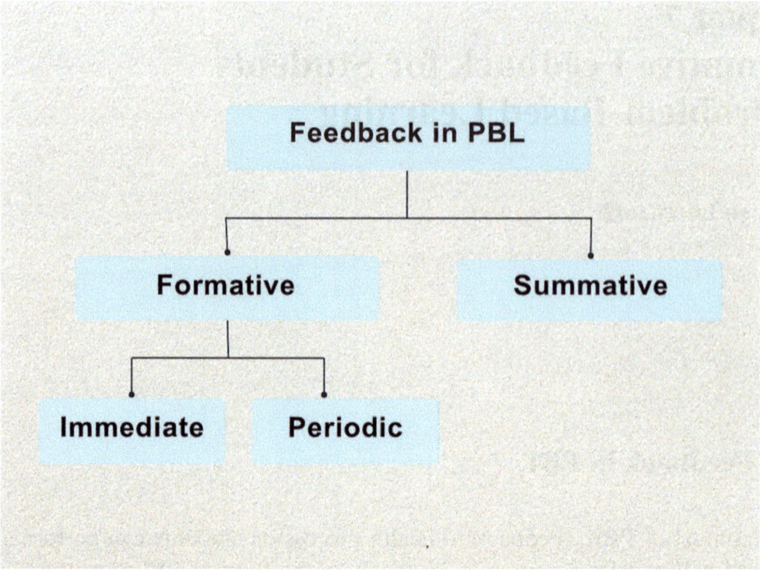

Fig. 7.1 Different types of feedback in PBL include formative and summative feedback

7.1.1 Formative Feedback: Purpose and Mechanisms of Delivery

The feedback to students in PBL aims to provide them with information about their progress toward a desired goal (Shute, 2008). Studies have shown that students can remain motivated if there is a close alignment between the student's goals and their expectations that these goals can be achieved (Fisher & Ford, 1998). There must be an appropriate balance when setting the goals, which is critical for the development of knowledge and skills of students in PBL. If the goals are not realistic and set too high, the student will experience failure and become discouraged. Conversely, if the goals are set too low, the success of the student attaining the goal will lose its power to motivate them to keep growing and learning (Shute, 2008). Facilitators must consider the students' development stage in their academic career to ensure that the goals are challenging but attainable. For example, a novice PBL student will not have the same goal expectations as a more seasoned PBL student when it comes to finding information in textbooks or other reliable resources and relating the information from multiple resources on a particular concept.

Several cognitive mechanisms underlie the effective use of formative feedback in PBL, including scaffolding, metacognition, cognitive load management, self-explanation, and retrieval practice (Fig. 7.2). These mechanisms help students process complex information, integrate new knowledge, and improve long-term retention. It can identify gaps between a student's current level of performance and their desired level of achievement, serving as a key motivational factor in learning (Song &

Keller, 2001). Additionally, it can reduce cognitive load, particularly for students who struggle with self-directed learning (Paas et al., 2003). Novice learners in PBL may find the process overwhelming, as they are required to engage deeply with clinical problems without prior structured instruction. Providing targeted formative feedback can alleviate cognitive strain, making it easier for students to process and retain information. Moreover, formative feedback is instrumental in correcting procedural errors, inappropriate task approaches, and misconceptions, ensuring that students develop accurate and effective problem-solving skills (Ilgen et al., 1979).

Scaffolding is one way formative feedback supports student learning. By providing structured guidance early in the learning process, tutors help students navigate complex problems, gradually reducing support as they gain confidence and competence (Wood et al., 1976). For instance, a tutor may begin by offering prompts and guiding questions to help students identify relevant learning issues in a clinical case. Over time, as students become more proficient, the tutor withdraws this support, allowing them to direct their own learning (Hmelo-Silver, 2004). Another critical cognitive mechanism is metacognition, which enables students to monitor and regulate their own thinking. Through self-reflection and peer review, students can assess their understanding, identify knowledge gaps, and adjust their study strategies

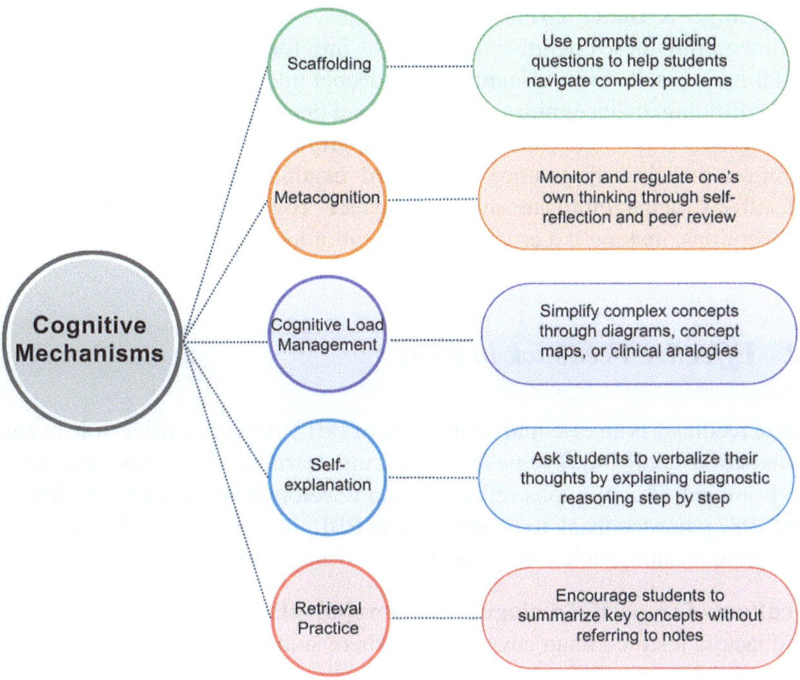

Fig. 7.2 The cognitive mechanisms underlying effective formative feedback in PBL include: scaffolding, metacognition, cognitive load management, self-explanation, and retrieval practice

accordingly. Tutors can facilitate this process by encouraging students to articulate their reasoning aloud, helping them recognize areas that need further development (Kostons et al., 2010; Schraw & Dennison, 1994).

Cognitive load management is another essential function of formative feedback, as it helps students process and retain information more efficiently. By simplifying complex health science concepts through diagrams, concept maps, or clinical analogies, tutors can structure discussions to minimize extraneous cognitive load, improving comprehension and problem-solving abilities (Sweller, 1988; van Merriënboer & Sweller, 2005). Additionally, self-explanation, the process of verbalizing one's thought process, reinforces learning by integrating new information with prior knowledge (Chi et al., 1989). In a PBL setting, tutors may ask students to explain their diagnostic reasoning step by step, prompting them to engage in deeper cognitive processing and strengthening their understanding of key concepts (Berthold et al., 2008).

Retrieval practice, the process of actively recalling information, is another powerful tool for improving long-term retention and knowledge application. At the end of a PBL session, students can be encouraged to summarize key concepts without referring to their notes. Revisiting previous cases in later discussions also reinforces knowledge retention and transferability, ensuring that learning is not only momentarily acquired but deeply ingrained for future clinical application (Karpicke & Blunt, 2011; Roediger & Butler, 2011).

By integrating these cognitive mechanisms into formative feedback, PBL fosters critical thinking, self-directed learning, and deeper understanding of medical knowledge. Scaffolding, metacognition, cognitive load management, self-explanation, and retrieval practice all contribute to enhanced problem-solving abilities and better preparation for clinical practice and board examinations. Additionally, formative feedback helps motivate students, reduce cognitive overload, and correct misconceptions, making it a crucial component of an effective PBL curriculum.

7.1.2 Effective Feedback in PBL

Effective feedback is an essential component of PBL, playing a critical role in guiding students toward self-improvement, reinforcing learning objectives, and fostering an environment of continuous reflection and development (Boud & Molloy, 2013; Schön, 1987). For feedback to be effective in PBL, it must align with key principles that promote meaningful learning experiences (Ende, 1983; Walsh, 2005) (Fig. 7.3).

- **A culture of respectful dialogue between students and the facilitator**: Effective feedback is fostered in an environment where students and facilitators engage in respectful dialogue. Creating a safe, constructive space allows students to express their thoughts, clarify uncertainties, and actively engage with the material. A facilitator can initiate this dialogue by acknowledging the student's efforts before offering constructive criticism. For instance, starting with, "*I appreciate how you*

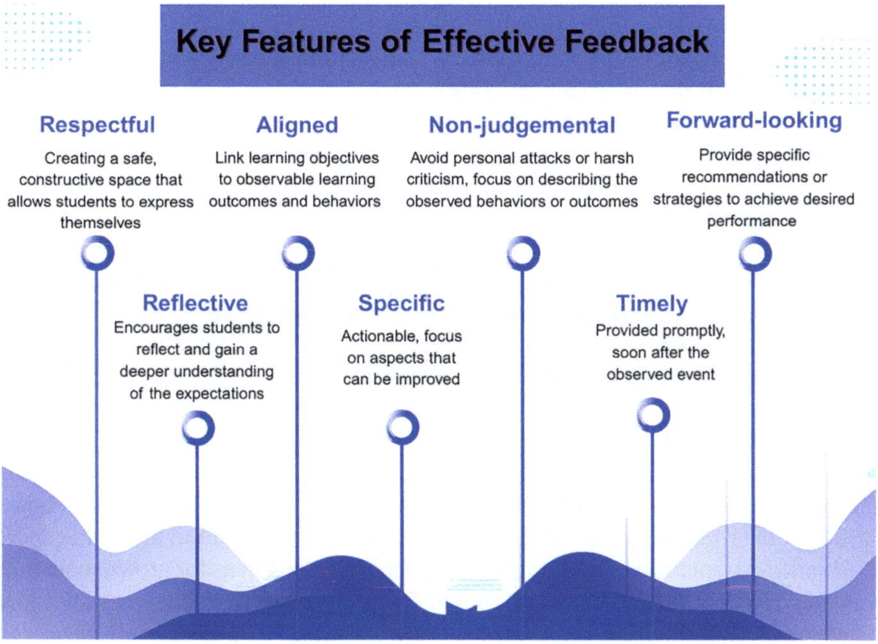

Fig. 7.3 Key features of effective feedback include being respectful, reflective, aligned with learning objectives and outcomes, specific, non-judgmental, timely and forward-looking

approached today's case. Let's discuss what worked well and explore areas for improvement," encourages open discussion and receptivity to feedback (Sargeant et al., 2009).

- **Encouraging student self-assessment of performance and understanding of expectations**: Effective feedback in PBL encourages students to reflect on their performance and gain a deeper understanding of the expectations set for them. By guiding students to evaluate their own performance and understand expectations, they develop metacognitive skills essential for lifelong learning (Eva & Regehr, 2008). Facilitators might prompt self-reflection by asking, "*How do you think you performed in identifying key learning issues today? What strategies could help you improve next time?*" This practice reinforces active learning and accountability (Sadler, 1989).
- **Link learning objectives to observable learning outcomes and behaviors**: To enhance the impact of feedback, it is essential to link learning objectives to observable learning outcomes and behaviors (Hattie & Timperley, 2007). Feedback should be directly connected to students' actions and demonstrate how these align with expected competencies. For example, if a student is working on differential diagnosis, a facilitator might say, "*You identified several potential diagnoses. Let's*

examine how each aligns with the patient's symptoms and consider which diagnostic tests would be most appropriate." This ensures clarity and applicability in future clinical scenarios (Shute, 2008).

- **Specific, focused on what is changeable**: PBL feedback should be specific and focused on aspects that can be improved or changed. Vague or general feedback is less helpful in guiding students toward desired improvements. By pinpointing specific areas for development, students can take actionable steps to enhance their performance (Kluger & DeNisi, 1996). Instead of saying, "*Your explanation was unclear*," a facilitator should provide actionable guidance such as, "*When presenting a patient case, try structuring your response chronologically. This will improve clarity and coherence.*" Targeted feedback allows students to make concrete improvements and develop competence in key areas (Nicol & Macfarlane-Dick, 2006).
- **Non-judgmental, descriptive, and framed as positively as possible**: Effective feedback should be non-judgmental and descriptive, avoiding personal attacks or harsh criticism. It should focus on describing the observed behaviors or outcomes, rather than making assumptions or judgments about the individual. Feedback should be framed positively, highlighting strengths and areas for growth constructively (Archer, 2010). Criticism should focus on observed behaviors rather than personal attributes. For instance, rather than stating, "*You completely misunderstood glycolysis*," a facilitator could say, "*Your interpretation of glycolysis was a good start. Let's revisit some key steps and see how they apply to the case.*" This approach promotes a growth mindset and resilience (Dweck, 2006).
- **Well-timed, close to the event**: Feedback is most effective when provided promptly, ideally soon after the observed event or performance, which allows students to connect the feedback with their recent experiences, making it more relevant and actionable. Immediate feedback helps students draw direct connections between their performance and the guidance given. After a group discussion, a facilitator might say, "*Your explanation of the pathophysiology of Alzheimer's Disease was thorough. Next time, consider summarizing key points to maintain engagement and clarity.*" Timely feedback supports retention and application of knowledge (Ericsson et al., 1993).
- **Specific recommendations for achieving desired performance**: Effective feedback goes beyond pointing out areas for improvement; it provides specific recommendations or strategies for achieving the desired performance (Henderson et al., 2019). Through actionable guidance, students can develop a more defined path to enhance their skills or understanding. For example, a facilitator might suggest, "*To strengthen your critical thinking skills, summarize each learning issue in your own words before consulting resources. This will help clarify your understanding and pinpoint knowledge gaps.*" Providing actionable steps empowers students to take ownership of their learning journey (Brookhart, 2017).

Incorporating these characteristics into the PBL feedback process cultivates a supportive and productive learning environment. By fostering respectful dialogue, encouraging self-assessment, linking feedback to objectives, providing specific and actionable recommendations, and ensuring a timely, non-judgmental approach, PBL facilitators can significantly enhance students' educational experiences. This structured feedback framework ultimately equips health profession students with the critical thinking and self-directed learning skills necessary for their future careers (Epstein, 2007).

7.2 Timing of Feedback

Students receive both immediate and periodic feedback in PBL (Fig. 7.4). Immediate feedback is provided to students during the "Wrap-up" segment during the last few minutes of the PBL session. Periodic feedback, delayed in nature, could occur during the halfway point of an examination block and consists of a one-on-one meeting between the facilitator and the student. In PBL, it is important to provide immediate and periodic feedback to support the student's learning process. Immediate feedback allows students to receive timely information about their performance and progress, while delayed periodic feedback provides an opportunity for deeper reflection and integration of learning. Research has suggested that low-achieving students may benefit more from immediate feedback, whereas high-achieving students may prefer or benefit from delayed feedback (Gaynor, 1981; Roper, 1977).

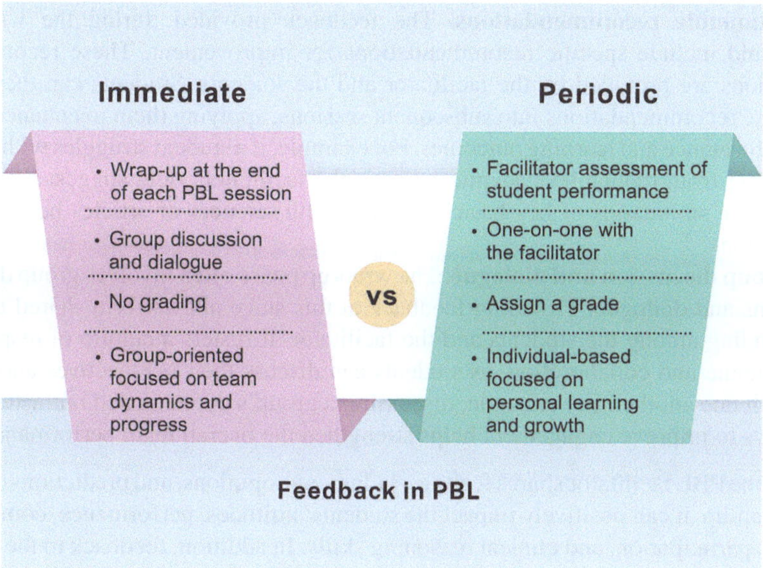

Fig. 7.4 Immediate and periodic feedback in PBL are two forms of formative feedback

7.2.1 Immediate Feedback

In PBL, immediate feedback is typically provided at the end of the session during the wrap-up phase. It consists of self, peer, and group assessments. This type of feedback can be used to assess and address group processes, student contributions, communication skills, and professional behavior. The sooner corrective information is provided (such as at the end of the PBL session), the more likely efficient retention will result (Phye & Andre, 1989). While the timing may vary depending on the PBL implementation according to the specific health professions program, providing feedback during the wrap-up serves several purposes:

- **Consolidation of learning**: The wrap-up phase presents an opportunity to consolidate what has been learned during the session. By providing immediate feedback at this point, students can reflect on their performance, connect it to the learning objectives, and solidify their understanding. For example, a facilitator might point out how effectively a student summarized the case objectives or referenced a specific basic medical/health science concept.
- **Reflective thinking**: Immediate feedback during the wrap-up encourages students to engage in reflective thinking, which prompts them to contemplate their approach, problem-solving strategies, and contributions to the group. This reflective process allows for profound learning and self-assessment. For instance, a facilitator might ask, "How could you have approached the differential diagnosis differently?" to stimulate deeper consideration.
- **Actionable recommendations**: The feedback provided during the wrap-up should include specific recommendations for improvement. These recommendations are provided by the facilitator and the students. Students can then take these recommendations into subsequent sessions, applying them to enhance their performance and learning outcomes. For example, if a student struggles with referencing from reputable academic sources, the facilitator could suggest preparing concise summaries of key basic medical/health sciences or articles before PBL sessions.
- **Group discussion and dialogue**: The wrap-up phase often involves group discussions and dialogue. Providing feedback at this stage allows for a shared understanding among the students and the facilitator. It fosters a culture of respectful dialogue and collaboration, as students can discuss their perspectives and learn from one another. For example, discussing a group's dynamic and brainstorming ways to improve engagement helps strengthen the overall team performance.

When the PBL facilitator shares feelings, judgments, opinions, and predictions during the wrap-up, it can positively impact the students' attitudes, performance, communication, participation, and clinical reasoning skills. In addition, feedback to the group can help improve cohesive group performance. While immediate feedback during the wrap-up phase is valuable, facilitators should also understand that it is essential to provide ongoing feedback throughout the PBL session. Encouraging students to present a concise summary mid-discussion or asking them to clarify a concept in real time allows for immediate adjustments and learning. Combining both immediate and ongoing feedback contributes to a comprehensive feedback loop that supports continuous learning and growth in PBL.

7.2.2 *Periodic Feedback*

An integral facet of the PBL process involves the Facilitator Assessment of Student Performance (FASP). A sample FASP form is shown below and can be modified as needed (Table 7.1):

This assessment requires facilitators to assign a grade to each student in the group based on the student's performance during the PBL sessions, which typically include the integration of medical knowledge, research-like skills, clinical reasoning, and professionalism (Neve et al., 2018).

The rationale behind FASP grades and their feedback is to encourage students to prepare before the PBL session, engage in discussions, and collaborate as a team during the discussion sessions. Depending on the healthcare profession program, the FASP grade may be composed of different categories, including medical knowledge, interpersonal communication skills, and patient care. The FASP is an assessment of the student's current level of training. Typically, a passing grade for the FASP is set at 70% or above. However, individual health professions programs reserve the right to establish their own passing criteria. In instances where students do not meet the passing grade, they may receive counseling from either the facilitator or the PBL director. This guidance aims to help students refine their approach in subsequent PBL sessions, facilitating their improvement and overall success.

In addition to the final FASP grade, there should be a mid-FASP meeting between the facilitator and each student at the halfway point. A typical PBL block of cases might include 12–16 2-h sessions with an examination at the end of that block. Halfway through that block, the facilitator completes the FASP form and then meets one-on-one with each of the students for about 15 min. This evaluation is private between the student and the facilitator. The facilitator can also solicit feedback from the student regarding PBL sessions and the facilitator's contributions. These meetings are extremely important as students will get some insights and feedback on their performance in the PBL sessions and on the areas for potential improvement. For example, if a student consistently struggles with participation, the facilitator might suggest specific strategies such as preparing discussion points in advance or summarizing key concepts for the group. Facilitators are encouraged to share with the students an actual grade, which offers students a clearer understanding of their performance in PBL when they receive their final FASP grade. Students often demonstrate significant improvement in their performance during PBL sessions following the receipt of formative feedback through the mid-FASP meeting. They value the feedback provided and actively adjust their behavior and interaction with peers based on the facilitator's input. For instance, if a facilitator addresses a student's limited participation or contributions during PBL sessions, the student typically exhibits noticeable

Table 7.1 The Facilitator Assessment of Student Performance (FASP) form (Lake Erie College of Osteopathic Medicine—Bradenton, 2025)

Facilitator Assessment of Student Performance (FASP)

Much less than expected	0–3
Less than expected	4–6
Met expectations	7–8
Exceeded expectations	9
Greatly exceeded expectations	10

The final score is calculated as the percentage of 100 points, the maximum score.

Part 1

1. Medical Knowledge
   (a) Displays adequate preparation by citing appropriate references.
   (b) Displays adequate preparation by articulating ideas, concepts, and mechanisms.
   (c) Chooses relevant chapters as learning topics.
   (d) Demonstrates sound critical thinking skills.
2. Interpersonal and Communication Skills
   (a) Prepared to present case-specific progress reports.
   (b) Encourages discussions and teamwork among group members.
   (c) Offers constructive observations during sessions and in wrap-up.
3. Patient Care
   (a) Integrates preclinical sciences with mechanisms of homeostasis and disease.
4. Professionalism
   (a) Provides appropriate feedback to group members and facilitator.
   (b) Demonstrates respect for group members and facilitator.

Part 2

Attendance & Punctuality

Students have unexcused absences—minus 10 points for each.

Student is late for the start of a group session—minus 5 points for each occurrence.

Comments: What are the student's greatest strengths?

Comments: What can the student do to improve his/her performance?

Follow-up Actions Required?

If you suspect that this student is having difficulty in any of the following areas and would like to ensure that help is provided, please check the "YES" box in response to the statements below. If not, check the "NO" box.

YES/NO

I have concerns regarding this student's academic performance.

I have concerns regarding this student's professional behavior and/or demeanor.

I have concerns regarding this student's attendance and/or punctuality.

changes in subsequent sessions, aiming to enhance their FASP score and demonstrate improvement. Alternatively, a student who receives feedback about over-dominating discussions might consciously work to foster more balanced group interactions.

In summary, both immediate and periodic feedback are adopted in PBL to encourage students' learning. Delayed feedback holds significance for promoting the transfer of learning, especially concerning concept-formation tasks, whereas immediate feedback may be more efficient, particularly in the short term, and for honing procedural skills, such as the ability to reference specific sources during the PBL session (Corbett & Anderson, 2001; Schroth, 1992).

7.3 Strategies for Effective Feedback in PBL

Formative feedback in PBL is a powerful tool for improving learning outcomes and promoting the development of expertise in health professions students. By incorporating the principles of effective feedback, facilitators can create a supportive and productive learning environment that nurtures students' growth and success (Fig. 7.5).

7.3.1 Personalize Feedback to Motivate Students

Motivation plays a significant role in students' performance, and feedback can be a potent tool in influencing their efforts and achievements (Covington & Omelich, 1984). The concept of goal orientation is an important aspect to consider when designing instruction and providing feedback, as it can impact how students respond to the feedback and approach tasks within a PBL session (Dempsey et al., 1993). Goal orientation refers to the different ways in which students are motivated to pursue various types of goals. Two primary orientations are typically identified: learning orientation and performance orientation (Dweck, 1986). Facilitators should carefully observe each student during the PBL session so they can better determine if a student is learning-oriented or performance-oriented. Learning orientation is characterized by a focus on the process of learning itself. Students with a learning

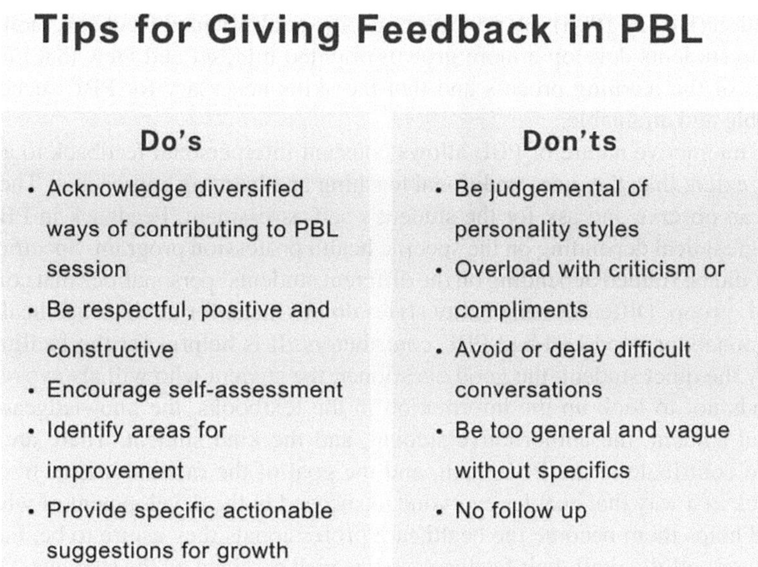

Fig. 7.5 Do's and don'ts when giving feedback in PBL

orientation are more interested in increasing their competence, developing new skills, and mastering new situations. They believe that intelligence and abilities can be developed and improved over time through effort and learning. Such students tend to view challenges as opportunities for growth and are less concerned about external evaluations. On the other hand, performance orientation is characterized by a focus on demonstrating competence to others and seeking positive evaluations from others. Students with a performance orientation are more concerned about showing their abilities and being judged favorably by others. They often believe that intelligence and abilities are fixed traits, leading them to seek validation and avoid situations where they might be judged negatively. Students who are learning-oriented will be more receptive to the facilitator's feedback and will tend to be more successful than performance-orientation students (Button et al., 1996; Fisher & Ford, 1998; VandeWalle et al., 1999).

Studies have found that the way feedback is delivered can have different effects on students with different goal orientations (Dweck & Leggett, 1988). For students with a learning orientation, feedback that emphasizes effort, improvement, and strategies for growth tends to be more effective and motivating. Such feedback reinforces their belief that they can improve and encourages them to persevere when facing challenges. Conversely, students with a performance orientation may be more motivated by feedback that highlights their accomplishments and compares them favorably to others. However, this type of feedback might also create a fear of failure and discourage students from taking risks or seeking out challenging tasks where they may not excel immediately (Farr et al., 1993). By providing meaningful formative feedback in PBL, facilitators can play a crucial role in influencing students' goal orientation and shifting their focus from a performance orientation to a learning orientation (Hoska, 1993). By providing specific goal-oriented feedback, facilitators can help students develop a more growth-oriented mindset and view that mistakes are part of the learning process and that the skills necessary for PBL success are malleable and attainable.

The interactive nature of PBL allows constant interpersonal feedback to a much greater extent than the more traditional teaching and learning approaches. The facilitator can observe and ask for the student's self-assessment. Feedback in PBL can vary a great deal depending on the specific health profession program. Specific feedback could be framed depending on the different students' personalities that compose the PBL group. Different personality styles do not make for good or bad healthcare professionals or good and bad PBL contributors. It is helpful for the facilitator to identify the quiet student, the good questioner, the student who will always respond but tends not to look up the information in the textbooks, the knowledgeable but doubtful student, the authoritative student, and the kind student. There are many ways to contribute to the PBL team, and the goal of the facilitator is to frame the feedback in a way that enables everyone to succeed in the development of who they are and helps them become the healthcare professionals they aspire to be. Facilitators must carefully craft their feedback so it is well received by the students. For that goal to be met, the facilitator needs to help each student own the learning. A group atmosphere of acceptance, openness, trust, sharing, mutual respect, and support is conducive to better feedback.

7.3.2 Comprehensive Feedback Approach

In PBL, feedback plays a crucial role in motivating students to achieve higher levels of performance. This feedback can take two forms: constructive feedback and positive feedback. Both types of feedback are indispensable in supporting student learning and motivation. By combining constructive feedback and positive feedback, PBL facilitators can devise a well-rounded approach to support and encourage students' development. Constructive feedback focuses on identifying areas for improvement and providing specific suggestions for growth. It aims to guide students in recognizing their weaknesses, rectifying misconceptions, and refining their problem-solving skills. Constructive feedback highlights areas where students can enhance their knowledge, critical thinking, and collaboration. When facilitators provide constructive feedback to students, they empower students to take actionable steps toward enhancing their performance in PBL. Positive feedback acknowledges and reinforces students' strengths, achievements, and effective strategies or behaviors during a PBL session. It recognizes their preparation, efforts, problem-solving skills, and contributions to group discussions. Positive feedback fosters a supportive and encouraging learning environment, boosting students' confidence, motivation, and self-esteem. It reinforces the idea that their efforts are valued and that they are on the right track, inspiring them to continue their progress and excel further. Research has shown that a combination of constructive and positive feedback is effective in promoting student engagement, self-regulation, and intrinsic motivation in PBL (Hmelo-Silver, 2004; Kusurkar et al., 2013). This comprehensive feedback approach recognizes students' progress, supports their ongoing development, and creates a positive feedback loop that fosters continuous learning and improvement.

Feedback in PBL should also be specific. Feedback specificity is defined as the depth of information presented to students (Goodman et al., 2004). There are opportunities for facilitators to provide specific feedback to students. For example, during the wrap-up portion of the PBL session, facilitators can address issues and offer meticulous suggestions for improvement. Another opportunity to provide specific feedback would be at the FASP meeting at the halfway point of the examination block. During the one-on-one meeting between the facilitator and student, specific and tailored feedback can be shared. Numerous studies have shown that specific feedback is significantly more effective as it provides the students with details on how to improve their performance, rather than just indicating whether the student's performance is adequate or not (Bangert-Drowns et al., 1991; Pridemore & Klein, 1991). For students, vague feedback is useless and frustrating (Williams, 1997), as they feel uncertain about how to act (Fletcher & Perry, 2002) and may need increased cognitive processing to understand the intended feedback message (Bangert-Drowns et al., 1991), which ultimately can lead to lower levels of learning and diminished motivation to respond to the feedback (Ashford, 1986; Kluger & DeNisi, 1998).

It is essential to balance constructive and positive feedback to prevent overwhelming students with excessive information or conflicting messages. Prioritizing key areas for improvement based on learning objectives, acknowledging strengths alongside areas for development, and providing specific, actionable feedback are essential strategies (Hattie & Timperley, 2007; Price et al., 2010; Sadler, 2010). Alternating between highlighting strengths and suggesting areas for improvement, breaking down feedback into manageable chunks, and encouraging self-reflection and goal setting also contribute to maintaining motivation and engagement (Garrison & Kanuka, 2004; Price et al., 2010). Fostering open dialogue between students and facilitators to clarify feedback and address concerns is crucial for effective feedback delivery (Garrison & Kanuka, 2004). By adopting these strategies, educators can ensure that students receive the guidance and support they need to thrive in PBL environments without feeling overwhelmed or discouraged.

7.3.3 Incorporating Technology to Enhance Formative Feedback

Advancements in digital tools and platforms offer valuable opportunities to enhance the delivery, tracking, and effectiveness of formative feedback in PBL. Technology facilitates timely, structured, and interactive feedback that aligns with student-centered learning principles. By integrating various digital tools, educators can optimize feedback processes, encourage self-directed learning, and improve engagement in PBL settings. One of the keyways technologies enhances formative feedback is through online feedback platforms. These platforms enable facilitators to provide structured, individualized, and immediate feedback to students, which is crucial in maintaining engagement and guiding improvement (Gikandi et al., 2011). Digital platforms such as Turnitin Feedback Studio, Peergrade, and Formative provide structured mechanisms for facilitators to annotate student work, offer inline comments, and track revisions over time. These tools support feedback loops where students can iterate on their work based on received input, promoting deeper learning (Nicol & Macfarlane-Dick, 2006).

Collaborative document editing tools like Google Docs and Microsoft Office 365 allow for real-time feedback and interactive collaboration between students and facilitators (Garrison & Kanuka, 2004; Lonn & Teasley, 2009). These tools facilitate seamless tracking of feedback history, version control, and simultaneous editing, thereby enabling an interactive and transparent feedback process. Real-time commenting features in these platforms allow facilitators to pinpoint areas needing improvement while also fostering peer-to-peer feedback, a crucial element in PBL that enhances critical thinking and communication skills (Van den Boom et al., 2007).

Learning Management Systems (LMS) such as Moodle, Canvas, and Blackboard offer built-in feedback functionalities that can be leveraged to streamline formative assessment and communication. These platforms provide centralized storage of feedback, progress tracking, and asynchronous communication, ensuring that feedback remains accessible and organized for both facilitators and students (Price et al., 2011). LMS tools also enable adaptive feedback features, such as automated quizzes with immediate response explanations, helping students identify gaps in their understanding and adjust their study strategies accordingly (Shute, 2008).

Video, audio, and mobile applications present additional avenues for enhancing formative feedback. Video feedback tools such as Flipgrid and Loom enable facilitators to provide personalized, nuanced feedback that may be more engaging and impactful than traditional text-based responses (Henderson & Phillips, 2015). Voice recording tools within LMS platforms or standalone applications like Kaizena allow facilitators to offer audio feedback, which research suggests can be more expressive and supportive compared to written feedback alone (Ice et al., 2007).

Technology also plays a crucial role in tracking and analyzing feedback patterns, student engagement, and learning progress over time. Data analytics embedded within LMS platforms and feedback tools can provide insights into how students interact with feedback, which feedback strategies are most effective, and which areas require further emphasis (Winstone et al., 2017). By leveraging artificial intelligence and machine learning, educators can even automate certain aspects of feedback, such as providing initial assessments on written responses or suggesting relevant resources based on student queries (Lee & Moore, 2024).

By integrating these digital tools and platforms into PBL environments, educators can optimize the delivery and tracking of formative feedback, promote active learning, and support student development more effectively. However, it is essential to ensure that the use of technology aligns with pedagogical best practices and does not replace meaningful human interaction in feedback processes. A balanced approach—where technology augments but does not overshadow personalized feedback—is crucial for maintaining the integrity of formative assessment in PBL.

7.4 Feedback Implementation Challenges

Implementing effective formative feedback in a PBL setting presents a complex set of challenges. These challenges span logistical, pedagogical, cultural, and institutional dimensions. Understanding and addressing these barriers is critical to maximizing the educational value of formative feedback. Below are common challenges and expanded strategies for overcoming them effectively in the context of health professions education (Fig. 7.6).

- **Time constraints**: PBL sessions are already intensive, often requiring significant preparation and facilitation. Adding structured feedback mechanisms can be perceived as burdensome, especially in programs with tight academic schedules

Feedback Implementation Challenges and Solutions

Challenges	Description	Solution
Time Constraints	PBL sessions require significant preparation and facilitation	Integrating brief but meaningful feedback moments into existing PBL structures
Lack of Formal Training	Facilitators lack familiarity with effective feedback strategies and don't see feedback as essential to learning	Invest in faculty development, recognition, and a reward system
Resistance to Critique	Open critiques are avoided in hierarchical or collectivist cultures	Facilitators model respectful feedback practices and emphasize professional growth
Limited Resources	Constrained budget limits time, personnel, and technological support	Prioritize feedback strategies that are scalable and efficient
Mis-alignment	Facilitators sometimes deliver vague or overly general comments that do not reflect specific PBL goals	Develop and distribute rubrics that clarify expectations and competencies
Inconsistency	Multiple facilitators of different groups may cause inconsistent student experiences due to feedback variability	Calibration exercises, training refreshers, shared templates, and guidelines can help align facilitator practices.
Feedback Overload	Unfocused or excessive feedback results in confusion and disengagement	Offer targeted, manageable feedback, encourage self-assessment and feedback response plans

Fig. 7.6 Challenges and solutions in feedback implementation are multi-faceted, including overcoming time constraints, lack of formal training, resistance to critique, limited resources, misalignment, inconsistency, and feedback overload

(Schönrock-Adema et al., 2012). However, feedback does not need to be a separate activity. Integrating brief but meaningful feedback moments into existing PBL structures can minimize additional time demands. For instance, during the wrap-up segment of each session, facilitators can engage students in reflective dialogue to highlight strengths and identify areas for improvement. Peer-to-peer feedback during group reflection can further distribute responsibility and deepen metacognitive awareness. Programs may also implement rotating roles where students offer structured peer feedback using simple rubrics (Hattie & Timperley, 2007).

- **Faculty training and buy-in**: Many facilitators in PBL are content experts without formal pedagogical training, and some may be unfamiliar with effective feedback delivery strategies(C. J. Watling & Ginsburg, 2019). Others may not view feedback as essential to student learning. Addressing this requires institutional investment in faculty development. Training should include hands-on workshops and video demonstrations. Sharing success stories where feedback significantly improved student outcomes can help promote engagement and support. Institutions should also consider recognizing and rewarding effective feedback practices to increase faculty motivation (Cantillon & Sargeant, 2008).

- **Cultural resistance to critique**: In some educational settings, particularly those influenced by hierarchical or collectivist cultures, students and faculty may avoid open critique. Feedback might be seen as confrontational or disrespectful (Carless & Boud, 2018). Facilitators must build psychological safety by modeling respectful feedback practices and emphasizing professional growth. Introducing group-level observations and anonymized examples can reduce discomfort. Over time, creating a feedback culture centered around learning rather than evaluation can normalize open dialogue and improve receptiveness.
- **Resource allocation**: Providing consistent formative feedback can require significant resources, including time, personnel, and technological support. These limitations can be particularly acute in institutions with constrained budgets (van de Ridder et al., 2008). Programs should prioritize feedback strategies that are scalable and efficient. For example, using existing platforms like Canvas or Zoom can support asynchronous or remote feedback. Feedback checklists, digital rubrics, or mobile apps may help reduce the administrative burden and improve standardization. Where feasible, trained peer tutors or academic coaches can assist in supporting students' learning through feedback.
- **Aligning feedback with learning objectives**: Feedback must be closely aligned with the intended learning outcomes to be meaningful and actionable. Facilitators sometimes deliver vague or overly general comments that do not reflect specific PBL goals (Ramani et al., 2017). Institutions should develop and distribute rubrics that clarify expectations and competencies. Tools such as the Facilitator Assessment of Student Participation (FASP) form can ensure alignment and improve the clarity of feedback. Facilitators should be encouraged to link feedback directly to learning objectives and provide specific guidance on how students can improve (Boud & Molloy, 2013).
- **Consistency across facilitators**: With multiple facilitators leading different groups, variability in feedback practices can lead to inconsistent student experiences. Some facilitators may provide detailed formative comments while others offer minimal input (Eva et al., 2012). Calibration exercises, where faculty discuss hypothetical scenarios and compare their feedback approaches, can promote consistency. Regular faculty meetings and training refreshers should reinforce institutional feedback standards. Shared digital feedback templates or institutional guidelines can also help align practices across facilitators and ensure that students receive equitable learning experiences.
- **Feedback overload**: Overloading students with feedback, especially when it is unfocused or excessive, can result in confusion and disengagement. Students may not know which comments to prioritize or how to act on them (Henderson et al., 2019). Facilitators should aim to offer targeted, manageable feedback. For example, focusing on one strength and one area for improvement in each session allows students to process feedback more effectively. Encouraging students to reflect on and set personal learning goals based on received feedback enhances their ability to use feedback constructively. Structured self-assessment tools and feedback response plans can also support this process.

Addressing feedback implementation challenges in PBL requires intentional planning, faculty engagement, and consistent evaluation. By embedding feedback into the PBL process, aligning it with learning goals, and building a supportive feedback culture, programs can transform feedback into a powerful educational tool. Proactive strategies that prioritize clarity, timeliness, and student engagement can significantly enhance the quality of student learning and promote long term development of professional competencies.

7.5 Feedback Training for Facilitators

Training facilitators to provide effective formative feedback in PBL is essential for promoting student development in critical thinking, communication, self-reflection, and professional identity. Given the complex and interactive nature of PBL, facilitators must not only guide content exploration but also help students grow through timely and meaningful feedback. A comprehensive training program should integrate theory, practical application, and ongoing support to help facilitators improve their feedback skills in ways that align with program goals and learner needs (Fig. 7.7).

- **Workshops and seminars**: Structured workshops and seminars provide foundational knowledge and skill development in feedback delivery. These events should focus on the unique characteristics of feedback in a PBL context, such

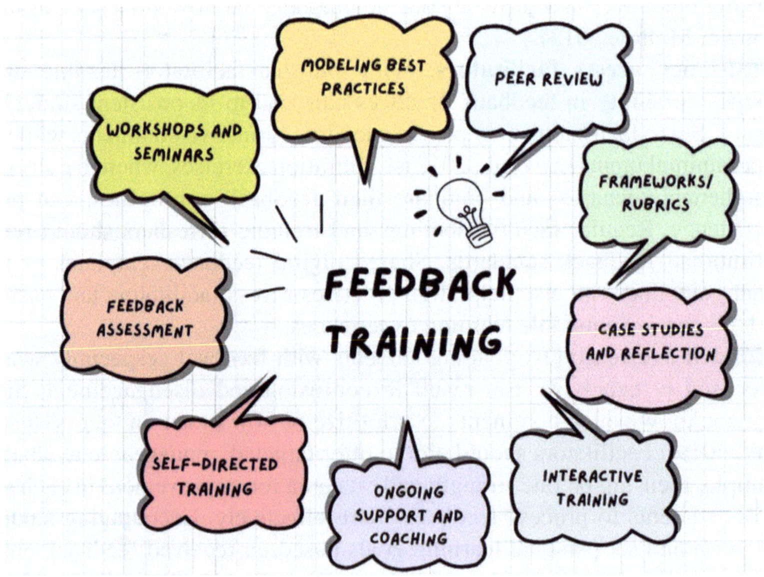

Fig. 7.7 A comprehensive feedback training program for PBL facilitators should integrate theory, practical application, and ongoing support improve skills in giving feedback

as facilitating self-directed learning, enhancing group dynamics, and supporting professional behaviors. Sessions should include simulated PBL scenarios to allow facilitators to practice giving and receiving feedback in real time. Evidence shows that facilitators benefit from structured training programs where they can rehearse skills and receive input in a supportive environment (Clynes & Raftery, 2008).

- **Modeling best practices**: Demonstrating effective feedback delivery helps facilitators visualize what high-quality feedback looks and sounds like. Trainers can use videos or role play to illustrate best practices. For example, feedback modeled using the "Ask Tell Ask" technique encourages learner reflection and active engagement (Cantillon & Sargeant, 2008). After demonstrations, structured discussion should follow to highlight elements such as clarity, specificity, tone, and alignment with learning objectives.
- **Peer observation and feedback**: Observing peers during PBL sessions and offering constructive feedback is another valuable strategy. Facilitators often learn best from watching others in similar roles, followed by guided reflection. Peer observation not only fosters a community of practice but also supports the standardization of feedback quality across facilitators. Feedback peer review systems have been found to increase both confidence and consistency in clinical and educational settings (Watling & Ginsburg, 2019).
- **Feedback frameworks and rubrics**: Training should include instruction on feedback frameworks that provide structure and alignment with program goals. Rubrics such as the Facilitator Assessment of Student Performance (FASP) form can be used to link facilitator observations with specific skills or competencies, such as reasoning, teamwork, and professionalism. Clear frameworks help facilitators generate feedback that is focused, actionable, and objective (Veloski et al., 2006). For instance, rather than offering vague comments such as "*participation needs work*," a rubric-informed comment would be, "*You shared relevant ideas during the early phase of the discussion, and I encourage you to build on peers' contributions more consistently to deepen group integration.*"
- **Case studies and reflection**: Realistic case studies based on feedback dilemmas provide rich opportunities for facilitator learning. These cases can involve challenging situations such as disengaged students, interpersonal tension in the group, or concerns about professionalism. Facilitators can analyze these cases using guided reflection frameworks, such as Gibbs' Reflective Cycle or the Kolb Experiential Learning Model, to identify strategies for handling similar scenarios (Mann et al., 2009).
- **Interactive training activities**: Active learning strategies such as brainstorming sessions, group problem solving, and feedback rewriting exercises can deepen understanding and reinforce learning. For example, facilitators can be given samples of poor or vague feedback and work in small groups to revise them into more targeted and constructive messages. Activities should encourage facilitators to share personal experiences and challenges, reinforcing the message that feedback is a complex, nuanced skill that develops over time (Sargeant et al., 2009).

- **Feedback training materials**: Self-directed learning resources should be developed to support continuous professional development. These can include handbooks, video tutorials, quick-reference guides, and curated readings from medical education literature. Making these resources available through an online learning platform ensures accessibility and allows facilitators to revisit content as needed. Studies have shown that structured online modules and blended learning models can be effective in improving feedback competence (C. Watling et al., 2013).
- **Ongoing support and coaching**: A one-time workshop is rarely sufficient to foster sustained change. Ongoing mentorship and coaching should be available for facilitators, especially during their first year. Experienced facilitators or education leaders can provide direct observation and personalized feedback to newer facilitators. Regular debrief sessions following PBL cycles can also provide a platform for collaborative problem solving and experience sharing (Archer, 2010).
- **Feedback evaluation and reflection**: Facilitators should also receive feedback on their feedback. Evaluation tools such as student satisfaction surveys, peer assessments, and facilitator self-evaluation forms can provide useful data for reflection. Encouraging facilitators to review their own written or verbal feedback allows them to assess whether their messages are consistent, specific, and constructive. Embedding self-reflection into facilitator development cultivates a growth mindset and supports long term excellence in teaching (Eva et al., 2012).

By implementing a comprehensive training approach that includes theory, skills practice, peer support, and continuous evaluation, PBL programs can significantly improve the quality of formative feedback. Well-trained facilitators are essential to creating learning environments where students feel supported, challenged, and empowered to grow professionally and academically.

References

Archer, J. C. (2010). State of the science in health professional education: Effective feedback. *Medical Education, 44*(1), 101–108. https://doi.org/10.1111/j.1365-2923.2009.03546.x

Ashford, S. J. (1986). Feedback-seeking in individual adaptation: A resource perspective. *Academy of Management Journal, 29*(3), 465–487. https://doi.org/10.2307/256219

Bandura, A., & Cervone, D. (2000). *Self-evaluative and self-efficacy mechanisms of governing the motivational effects of goal systems* (p. 214). Psychology Press.

Bangert-Drowns, R. L., Kulik, C.-L. C., Kulik, J. A., & Morgan, M. (1991). The instructional effect of feedback in test-like events. *Review of Educational Research, 61*(2), 213–238. https://doi.org/10.3102/00346543061002213

Berthold, K., Renkl, A., & Eysink, T. H. (2008). Assisting self-explanation prompts are more effective than open prompts when learning with multiple representations. *Instructional Science, 37*(4), 345–363. https://doi.org/10.1007/s11251-008-9051-z

Boud, D., & Molloy, E. (2013). *Feedback in higher and professional education: Understanding it and doing it well* (1st ed.). Routledge. Retrieved from https://www.routledge.com/Feedback-in-Higher-and-Professional-Education-Understanding-it-and-doing-it-well/Boud-Molloy/p/book/9780415692298

Brookhart, S. M. (2017). *How to give effective feedback to your students* (2nd ed.). ASCD. Retrieved from https://www.ascd.org/books/how-to-give-effective-feedback-to-your-students-2nd-edition?chapter=feedback-the-long-view-does-feedback-improve-learning

Button, S. B., Mathieu, J. E., & Zajac, D. M. (1996). Goal orientation in organizational research: A conceptual and empirical foundation. *Organizational Behavior and Human Decision Processes, 67*(1), 26–48. https://doi.org/10.1006/obhd.1996.0063

Cantillon, P., & Sargeant, J. (2008). Giving feedback in clinical settings. *British Medical Journal (Clinical Research Edition), 337*, a1961. https://doi.org/10.1136/bmj.a1961

Carless, D., & Boud, D. (2018). The development of student feedback literacy: Enabling uptake of feedback. *Assessment & Evaluation in Higher Education, 43*(8), 1315–1325. https://doi.org/10.1080/02602938.2018.1463354

Chi, M. T. H., Bassok, M., Lewis, M. W., Reimann, P., & Glaser, R. (1989). Self-explanations: How students study and use examples in learning to solve problems. *Cognitive Science, 13*(2), 145–182. https://doi.org/10.1207/s15516709cog1302_1

Clynes, M. P., & Raftery, S. E. C. (2008). Feedback: An essential element of student learning in clinical practice. *Nurse Education in Practice, 8*(6), 405–411. https://doi.org/10.1016/j.nepr.2008.02.003

Corbett, A. T., & Anderson, J. R. (2001). Locus of feedback control in computer-based tutoring: Impact on learning rate, achievement and attitudes. In *Proceedings of the SIGCHI Conference on Human Factors in Computing Systems* (pp. 245–252). https://doi.org/10.1145/365024.365111

Covington, M. V., & Omelich, C. L. (1984). Task-oriented versus competitive learning structures: Motivational and performance consequences. *Journal of Educational Psychology, 76*(6), 1038.

Dempsey, J. V., Driscoll, M. P., & Swindell, L. K. (1993). Text-based feedback. In *Interactive Instruction and Feedback* (pp. 21–54). Educational Technology Publications.

Dweck, C. S. (1986). Motivational processes affecting learning. *American Psychologist, 41*(10), 1040.

Dweck, C. S. (2006). *Mindset: The new psychology of success* (p. x, 276). Random House.

Dweck, C. S., & Leggett, E. L. (1988). A social-cognitive approach to motivation and personality. *Psychological Review, 95*(2), 256.

Ende, J. (1983). Feedback in clinical medical education. *Journal of the American Medical Association, 250*(6), 777–781.

Epstein, R. M. (2007). Assessment in medical education. *The New England Journal of Medicine, 356*(4), 387–396. https://doi.org/10.1056/NEJMra054784

Ericsson, K. A., Krampe, R. T., & Tesch-Römer, C. (1993). The role of deliberate practice in the acquisition of expert performance. *Psychological Review, 100*(3), 363–406. https://doi.org/10.1037/0033-295X.100.3.363

Eva, K. W., & Regehr, G. (2008). "I'll never play professional football" and other fallacies of self-assessment. *The Journal of Continuing Education in the Health Professions, 28*(1), 14–19. https://doi.org/10.1002/chp.150

Eva, K. W., Armson, H., Holmboe, E., Lockyer, J., Loney, E., Mann, K., & Sargeant, J. (2012). Factors influencing responsiveness to feedback: On the interplay between fear, confidence, and reasoning processes. *Advances in Health Sciences Education: Theory and Practice, 17*(1), 15–26. https://doi.org/10.1007/s10459-011-9290-7

Farr, J. L., Hofmann, D. A., & Ringenbach, K. L. (1993). Goal orientation and action control theory: Implications for industrial and organizational psychology. *International Review of Industrial and Organizational Psychology, 8*(2), 193–232.

Fisher, S. L., & Ford, J. K. (1998). Differential effects of learner effort and goal orientation on two learning outcomes. *Personnel Psychology, 51*(2), 397–420. https://doi.org/10.1111/j.1744-6570.1998.tb00731.x

Fletcher, C., & Perry, E. L. (2002). Performance appraisal and feedback: A consideration of national culture and a review of contemporary research and future trends. In *Handbook of industrial, work and organizational psychology* (Personnel psychology) (Vol. 1, pp. 127–144). Sage Publications Ltd.

Garrison, D. R., & Kanuka, H. (2004). Blended learning: Uncovering its transformative potential in higher education. *The Internet and Higher Education, 7*(2), 95–105. https://doi.org/10.1016/j.iheduc.2004.02.001

Gaynor, P. (1981). The effect of feedback delay on retention of computer-based mathematical material. *Journal of Computer-Based Instruction, 8*(2), 28–34.

Gikandi, J. W., Morrow, D., & Davis, N. E. (2011). Online formative assessment in higher education: A review of the literature. *Computers & Education, 57*(4), 2333–2351. https://doi.org/10.1016/j.compedu.2011.06.004

Goodman, J. S., Wood, R. E., & Hendrickx, M. (2004). Feedback specificity, exploration, and learning. *Journal of Applied Psychology, 89*(2), 248–262. https://doi.org/10.1037/0021-9010.89.2.248

Hattie, J., & Timperley, H. (2007). The power of feedback. *Review of Educational Research, 77*(1), 81–112. https://doi.org/10.1016/j.iheduc.2004.02.001

Henderson, M., & Phillips, M. (2015). Video-based feedback on student assessment: Scarily personal. *Australasian Journal of Educational Technology, 31*(1), 1. https://doi.org/10.14742/ajet.1878

Henderson, M., Ryan, T., & Phillips, M. (2019). The challenges of feedback in higher education. *Assessment & Evaluation in Higher Education, 44*(8), 1237–1252. https://doi.org/10.1080/02602938.2019.1599815

Hmelo-Silver, C. E. (2004). Problem-based learning: What and how do students learn? *Educational Psychology Review, 16*(3), 235–266. https://doi.org/10.1023/B:EDPR.0000034022.16470.f3

Hoska, D. M. (1993). Motivating learners through CBI feedback: Developing a positive learner perspective. In J. V. Dempsey & G. C. Sales (Eds.), *Interactive instruction and feedback*. Educational Technology Publications.

Ice, P., Curtis, R., Phillips, P., & Wells, J. (2007). Using asynchronous audio feedback to enhance teaching presence and students' sense of community. *Journal of Asynchronous Learning Networks, 11*(2), 3–25.

Ilgen, D. R., Fisher, C. D., & Taylor, M. S. (1979). Consequences of individual feedback on behavior in organizations. *Journal of Applied Psychology, 64*(4), 349–371. https://doi.org/10.1037/0021-9010.64.4.349

Karpicke, J. D., & Blunt, J. R. (2011). Retrieval practice produces more learning than elaborate studying with concept mapping. *Science, 331*(6018), 772–775. https://doi.org/10.1126/science.1199327

Kluger, A. N., & DeNisi, A. (1996). The effects of feedback interventions on performance: A historical review, a meta-analysis, and a preliminary feedback intervention theory. *Psychological Bulletin, 119*(2), 254–284. https://doi.org/10.1037/0033-2909.119.2.254

Kluger, A. N., & DeNisi, A. (1998). Feedback interventions: Toward the understanding of a double-edged sword. *Current Directions in Psychological Science, 7*(3), 67–72. https://doi.org/10.1111/1467-8721.ep10772989

Kostons, D., van Gog, T., & Paas, F. (2010). Self-assessment and task selection in learner-controlled instruction: Differences between effective and ineffective learners. *Computers & Education, 54*(4), 932–940. https://doi.org/10.1016/j.compedu.2009.09.025

Kusurkar, R. A., Croiset, G., Galindo-Garré, F., & Ten Cate, O. (2013). Motivational profiles of medical students: Association with study effort, academic performance and exhaustion. *BMC Medical Education, 13*, 87. https://doi.org/10.1186/1472-6920-13-87

Lake Erie College of Osteopathic Medicine—Bradenton. (2025). Facilitator Assessment of Student Performance (FASP) form. Internal institutional document.

Lee, S. S., & Moore, R. L. (2024). Harnessing Generative AI (GenAI) for automated feedback in higher education: A systematic review. *Online Learning*. https://doi.org/10.24059/olj.v28i3.4593

Lonn, S., & Teasley, S. D. (2009). Saving time or innovating practice: Investigating perceptions and uses of learning management systems. *Computers & Education, 53*(3), 686–694. https://doi.org/10.1016/j.compedu.2009.04.008

Mann, K., Gordon, J., & MacLeod, A. (2009). Reflection and reflective practice in health professions education: A systematic review. *Advances in Health Sciences Education, 14*(4), 595–621. https://doi.org/10.1007/s10459-007-9090-2

Neve, H., Bull, S., Lloyd, H., Gilbert, K., & Mattick, K. (2018). Evaluation of an innovative, evidence-guided, PBL approach. *The Clinical Teacher, 15*(2), 156–162. https://doi.org/10.1111/tct.12656

Nicol, D. J., & Macfarlane-Dick, D. (2006). Formative assessment and self-regulated learning: A model and seven principles of good feedback practice. *Studies in Higher Education, 31*(2), 199–218. https://doi.org/10.1080/03075070600572090

Paas, F., Renkl, A., & Sweller, J. (2003). Cognitive load theory and instructional design: Recent developments. *Educational Psychologist, 38*(1), 1–4. https://doi.org/10.1207/S15326985EP3801_1

Phye, G. D., & Andre, T. (1989). Delayed retention effect: Attention, perseveration, or both? *Contemporary Educational Psychology, 14*(2), 173–185. https://doi.org/10.1016/0361-476X(89)90035-0

Price, M., Handley, K., Millar, J., & O'Donovan, B. (2010). Feedback: All that effort, but what is the effect? *Assessment & Evaluation in Higher Education, 35*, 277–289. https://doi.org/10.1080/02602930903541007

Price, M., Handley, K., & Millar, J. (2011). Feedback: Focusing attention on engagement. *Studies in Higher Education, 36*(8), 879–896. https://doi.org/10.1080/03075079.2010.483513

Pridemore, D. R., & Klein, J. D. (1991). Control of feedback in computer-assisted instruction. *Educational Technology Research and Development, 39*(4), 27–32. https://doi.org/10.1007/BF02296569

Ramani, S., Könings, K., Mann, K. V., & van der Vleuten, C. (2017). Uncovering the unknown: A grounded theory study exploring the impact of self-awareness on the culture of feedback in residency education. *Medical Teacher, 39*(10), 1065–1073. https://doi.org/10.1080/0142159X.2017.1353071

Roediger, H. L., & Butler, A. C. (2011). The critical role of retrieval practice in long-term retention. *Trends in Cognitive Sciences, 15*(1), 20–27. https://doi.org/10.1016/j.tics.2010.09.003

Roper, W. J. (1977). *Feedback in computer assisted instruction*. Programmed Learning and Educational Technology.

Sadler, D. R. (1989). Formative assessment and the design of instructional systems. *Instructional Science, 18*(2), 119–144. https://doi.org/10.1007/BF00117714

Sadler, D. R. (2010). Beyond feedback: Developing student capability in complex appraisal. *Assessment & Evaluation in Higher Education, 35*, 535–550. https://doi.org/10.1080/02602930903541015

Sargeant, J. M., Mann, K. V., van der Vleuten, C. P., & Metsemakers, J. F. (2009). Reflection: A link between receiving and using assessment feedback. *Advances in Health Sciences Education: Theory and Practice, 14*(3), 399–410. https://doi.org/10.1007/s10459-008-9124-4

Schön, D. A. (1987). *Educating the reflective practitioner: Toward a new design for teaching and learning in the professions* (p. xvii, 355). Jossey-Bass.

Schönrock-Adema, J., Bouwkamp-Timmer, T., van Hell, E. A., & Cohen-Schotanus, J. (2012). Key elements in assessing the educational environment: Where is the theory? *Advances in Health Sciences Education: Theory and Practice, 17*(5), 727–742. https://doi.org/10.1007/s10459-011-9346-8

Schraw, G., & Dennison, R. S. (1994). Assessing metacognitive awareness. *Contemporary Educational Psychology, 19*(4), 460–475. https://doi.org/10.1006/ceps.1994.1033

Schroth, M. L. (1992). The effects of delay of feedback on a delayed concept formation transfer task. *Contemporary Educational Psychology, 17*(1), 78–82. https://doi.org/10.1016/0361-476X(92)90048-4

Shute, V. J. (2008). Focus on formative feedback. *Review of Educational Research, 78*(1), 153–189. https://doi.org/10.3102/0034654307313795

Song, S. H., & Keller, J. M. (2001). Effectiveness of motivationally adaptive computer-assisted instruction on the dynamic aspects of motivation. *Educational Technology Research and Development, 49*(2), 5–22. https://doi.org/10.1007/BF02504925

Sweller, J. (1988). Cognitive load during problem solving: Effects on learning. *Cognitive Science, 12*(2), 257–285. https://doi.org/10.1207/s15516709cog1202_4

van de Ridder, J. M. M., Stokking, K. M., McGaghie, W. C., & ten Cate, O. T. J. (2008). What is feedback in clinical education? *Medical Education, 42*(2), 189–197. https://doi.org/10.1111/j.1365-2923.2007.02973.x

Van den Boom, G., Paas, F., & van Merriënboer, J. J. G. (2007). Effects of elicited reflections combined with tutor or peer feedback on self-regulated and learning outcomes. *Learning and Instruction, 17*(5), 532–548. https://doi.org/10.1016/j.learninstruc.2007.09.003

van Merriënboer, J. J. G., & Sweller, J. (2005). Cognitive load theory and complex learning: Recent developments and future directions. *Educational Psychology Review, 17*(2), 147–177. https://doi.org/10.1007/s10648-005-3951-0

VandeWalle, D., Brown, S. P., Cron, W. L., & Slocum, J. W., Jr. (1999). The influence of goal orientation and self-regulation tactics on sales performance: A longitudinal field test. *Journal of Applied Psychology, 84*(2), 249.

Veloski, J., Boex, J. R., Grasberger, M. J., Evans, A., & Wolfson, D. B. (2006). Systematic review of the literature on assessment, feedback and physicians' clinical performance: BEME Guide No. 7. *Medical Teacher, 28*(2), 117–128. https://doi.org/10.1080/01421590600622665

Walsh, A. (2005). The tutor in PBL: A novice's guide.

Watling, C. J., & Ginsburg, S. (2019). Assessment, feedback and the alchemy of learning. *Medical Education, 53*(1), 76–85. https://doi.org/10.1111/medu.13645

Watling, C., Driessen, E., van der Vleuten, C. P. M., Vanstone, M., & Lingard, L. (2013). Beyond individualism: Professional culture and its influence on feedback. *Medical Education, 47*(6), 585–594. https://doi.org/10.1111/medu.12150

Williams, S. E. (1997). Teachers' written comments and students' responses: A socially constructed interaction. Retrieved from https://eric.ed.gov/?id=ED408589

Winstone, N. E., Nash, R. A., Rowntree, J., & Parker, M. (2017). 'It'd be useful, but I wouldn't use it': Barriers to university students' feedback seeking and recipience. *Studies in Higher Education, 42*(11), 2026–2041. https://doi.org/10.1080/03075079.2015.1130032

Wood, D., Bruner, J. S., & Ross, G. (1976). The role of tutoring in problem solving. *Child Psychology & Psychiatry & Allied Disciplines, 17*(2), 89–100. https://doi.org/10.1111/j.1469-7610.1976.tb00381.x

Chapter 8
Technology in Problem-Based Learning

Sarmad Ghazi, Serene Shaham, and Voicu S. Ciobanu

Information and communication technologies (ICT) play a pivotal role in today's PBL by facilitating and enhancing the learning process (Pearson, 2006). It features the technological tools used to support or enhance the learning experience in areas of knowledge acquisition, interpersonal interactions, assessment, and reflection (OCED, 2016). Besides online PBL, this chapter delves into the efficacy of multiple strategies for leveraging technology in the PBL classroom. It examines five ways in which technology can improve problem-based learning: (1) E-learning; (2) technology facilitated health professions education simulations, (3) technology-facilitated collaboration, (4) real-time response systems for enhanced engagement, and (5) technology facilitated assessment.

8.1 Online PBL

Online PBL is not brand new though it has never gained its momentum since the pandemic when all schools and classes had to migrate swiftly due to the lockdown. The traditional PBL is tightly structured, as described in previous chapters. Yet we all understand that the online version cannot be the exact copy of its in-person original.

S. Ghazi (✉)
College of Osteopathic Medicine, California Health Sciences University (CHSU), Clovis, CA, USA
e-mail: sghazi@chsu.edu

S. Shaham
Houston Methodist Research Institute, Houston, TX, USA
e-mail: sashaham@houstonmethodist.org

V. S. Ciobanu
College of Medicine, Roseman University of Health Sciences, Las Vegas, NV, USA
e-mail: vciobanu@roseman.edu

S. Lorenzo and B. Zhang (eds.), *Mastering Problem-Based Learning in Health Profession Programs*, https://doi.org/10.1007/978-3-032-05405-0_8

The role of technology is not to replace the human interaction (even if it was used like that during the pandemic restrictions) but to be a tool used to enhance, leverage, stimulate the act of learning, especially active learning, and increase the student's engagement.

8.1.1 Running an Online PBL

It is crucial to retain the characteristic natures of PBL when migrating it online, and they are: (a) the use of problems to initiate the learning process; (b) collaborative learning activities in small groups; (c) student-centered learning; (d) the guiding role of the facilitator; and (e) sufficient time for self-study (Hung et al., 2019).

Some essential elements are kept the same when running PBL online, such as the size of the small group. A facilitator designs learning and reasoning strategies and facilitates student learning through modeling and coaching, mainly using questioning techniques. As students gain experience with PBL, facilitators can gradually reduce scaffolding in the hope that collaborative learning groups will assume a substantial portion of facilitation duties. Students in each small groups rotate the following roles: "leader" or "moderator," "case presenter," "web searcher," "scribe," and "participants."

Some PBL curricula also include the role of "assistant leader." The moderator is instrumental in guiding the team through the learning process, organizing the discussion, ensuring that everyone has an opportunity to contribute, ensuring that no one dominates the discussion, keeping time, and keeping the group's focus. The assistant leader will work with the leader to assign the roles of the case presenter, web searcher, and scribe. The scribe is responsible for tracking team members' contributions, as well as their assigned tasks and utilized resources, whereas the web searcher is accountable for locating high-quality resources. Everyone else actively engages and performs designated tasks to enable the group to solve the case. Owing to the lack of the students' prior knowledge to explain the problem, learning issues are formulated to guide the self-study activities. Students acquire new information by studying resources (e.g., books, articles, and websites) or consulting their facilitator. After a period of independent study, students return to their groups to discuss their findings and apply their newly acquired knowledge to the problem at hand (Hung et al., 2019).

The well-structured online PBL includes three stages: pre-stage (pre-class preparation), in-stage (in-class challenge), and post-stage (feedback and reflection) (Fig. 8.1). During the pre-stage, the facilitator may conduct a pre-class orientation or workshop that emphasizes the online PBL activity's principles, roles, and process. Students review the pre-stage workflow manual and the principles of online etiquette, complete the assigned readings and pre-recorded lectures, and choose their team leader and assistant leader. A crucial aspect of this stage is identifying the introverted students and encouraging them to participate more in online PBL, as they may find it easier to do that than in the traditional classroom. Recognizing camera-shy students is also necessary, as they may require additional help. Furthermore, it is essential to identify students who are not tech-savvy, provide them with a technology instructional manual, and set up a meeting with the information technology department to address any potential problems. One of the key paths to success is the proper selection of the participants in the group. Students should be different enough from each other to provide different perspectives to enhance the act of learning but also similar enough so they can work well together as a team engaged in active learning.

During the in-class phase, the facilitator will remind the team to adhere to online etiquette to limit disruptive behavior. In addition, the facilitator will encourage students to contribute both verbal and written explanations. The facilitator then assesses the students' readiness to analyze the problem and integrate their knowledge during the PBL discussion. This can be accomplished through a brief series of multiple-choice questions (MCQs) reflective of the PBL assignment's level of knowledge. Such online real-time quiz can significantly promote student engagement, as without the cues of body language, students may easily become distracted during small group discussion conducted online. Facilitators support students learning by asking open-ended and metacognitive questions, encouraging causal models with "what, why, and how" questions, and clarifying students' ideas, highlighting their significance, and gently guiding the discussion by repeating and rephrasing what they said. When discussion becomes unclear, asking students to summarize the group's

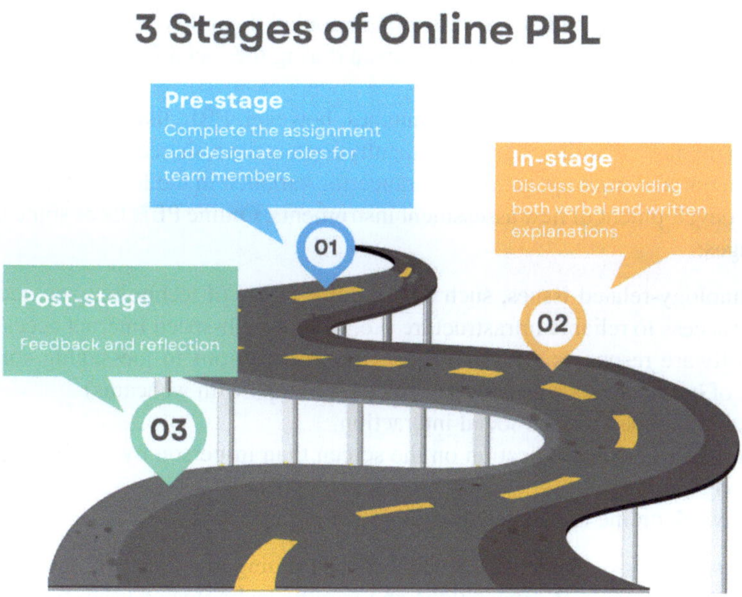

Fig. 8.1 The well-structured online PBL includes three stages: pre-stage (pre-class preparation), in-stage (in-class challenge), and post-stage (feedback and reflection)

current thinking can help them synthesize data, improve learning, and reveal facts that they consider significant (Hmelo-Silver & Barrows, 2006).

The post-stage includes both feedback and reflection. At the conclusion of each PBL session, students complete a brief formative evaluation (Blumberg, 2006). Participants evaluate the team's performance, monitor their progress toward problem resolution, comment on their collective and individual content mastery, and provide one another with feedback on their performance (Evensen & Hmelo, 2000). Students may voice concerns regarding individual contributions, encourage noncontributing members to participate more, and assist dominant students in allowing others to speak more. Using the design principle of continuous feedback enables the early avoidance of several problems with group performance (Felder et al., 2016). Plus, a constant feedback approach can lead to personal and professional growth.

8.1.2 Online PBL Pros and Cons

PBL has been embraced by many students as an active learning method. The PBL cases, though represent the genuine nature of clinical investigations in practice, are virtual in nature. Nevertheless, the cases are "authentic" enough in assisting students in developing a tolerance for uncertainty and/or ambiguity and developing the ability to approach difficult challenges. With the availability of technologies, migrating virtual cases online is not a challenging task, nor are synchronous live discussions about the cases. If implemented and supported appropriately, online PBL can be just as effective as in-person PBL. It offers unparalleled flexibility, saves travel time for everyone, and maximizes accessibility, even during the lockdowns of the pandemic (Fig. 8.2).

Online PBL has significant disadvantages, however. PBL, like other small-group teaching methods, requires significant faculty contact time, shared faculty and student commitment and training, greater tolerance for variance in the learning experience, and the development of new assessment instruments. Online PBL faces some unique challenges:

- Technology-related issues, such as difficulty in use of technology, no access or poor access to reliable infrastructure (i.e. lack of high-speed internet access, lack of software resources such as licenses or subscriptions to messaging software, lack of hardware such as laptops, tablets, desktops with webcams)
- Missing the face-to-face social interaction.
- Less effective communication on the screen than in-person by lacking the clues of body language.
- Teamwork online is more challenging than in-person.

To address the above challenges, students need training in online PBL techniques as well as an orientation of expectations and various technologies used. Faculty need specialized education and training in facilitation and in giving constructive online feedback.

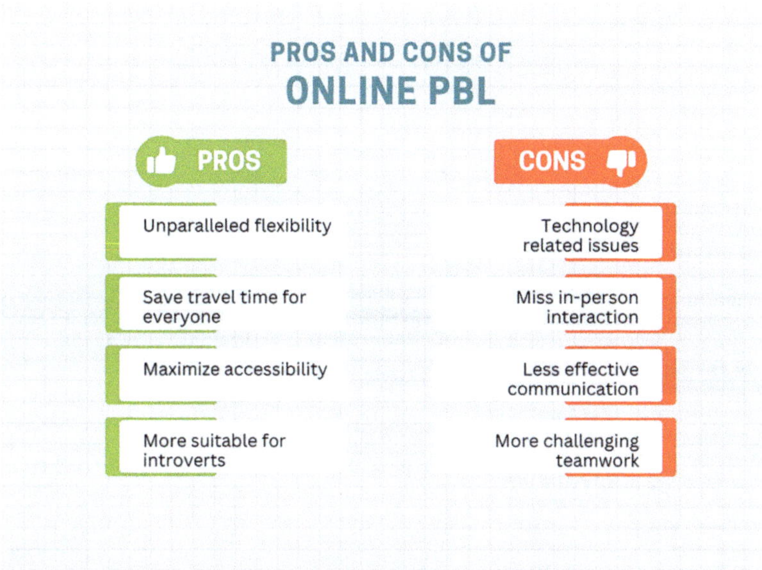

Fig. 8.2 Pros and cons of online PBL, which offers unparalleled flexibility but also faces certain challenges

8.2 Technologies in PBL

Digital technologies are ubiquitous in modern life including students learning. Personal computers, smartphones, tablet devices, wearable electronics, cloud computing, virtual reality, and augmented reality are components of the environment in which young adults grow and gain knowledge. However, the mere availability of technology and a strong push for "modernization" should not be the driving force behind the implementation of technology in education. This shift should be accompanied by strategies to enhance pedagogy and teaching practices, educator professional development, and the availability of superior web applications and peer-reviewed course content (OECD, 2016). In other words the educators need to use technology to their own advantage, using the strengths of this tool, to enhance and advance the act of leaning and not to use technology just for its own sake, as nod to "modernization" or being on the "cutting edge" (Fig. 8.3).

8.2.1 E-Learning

E-learning generally refers to the use of information and communications technology (ICT) in education to enhance and/or support learning (Giannakos et al., 2021). According to this definition, E-learning encompasses a vast array of modalities,

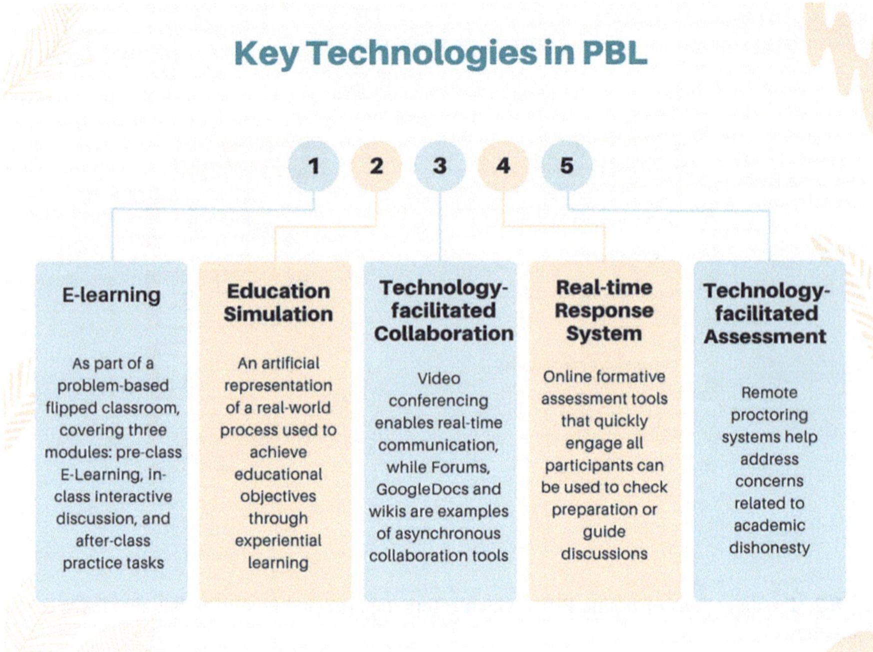

Fig. 8.3 Digital technologies used in PBL include E-learning, simulation, technology-facilitated collaboration, real-time response system and remote proctoring systems

ranging from on-campus courses with online access to coursework through a LMS (learning management system), content-based medical education platforms, online practice question banks, messaging and collaborative software (like Microsoft Teams and Pronto) and e-mail communication.

E-learning courses share two features: they are provided by a physical, campus-based institution, and they are connected to the Internet or another online network (OECD, 2016). From least intensive to most intensive, E-learning courses can be delivered in the following ways:

- Web-enhanced courses are now the standard for ICT presence in medical education in most nations. They refer to the use of the web for passive course elements and typically include some level of e-mail communication as well as an online communication platform or LMS for posting course information, materials, assignments, resources, and external links. Using e-learning in this way face-to-face time is not reduced.
- Web-dependent courses are those that incorporate an online component for key "active" course elements, such as online discussions, assessments, and project-based or collaborative work. As with web-enhanced courses, there is no reduction in face-to-face time; however, these online components are required for all students.

- Mixed mode courses gradually replace or supplement face-to-face time with online components, though classroom hours remain a significant component of all courses. Students are required to participate in online activities as an integral part of their coursework in these courses. The mixed mode course model may include asynchronous online course lectures followed by in-class discussions or learning seminars. Alternately, in-person lectures could be supplemented with online mini-seminars or tutorials. Mixed mode e-learning often exists at the program level and, in these instances, refers to a program of study that combines traditional and online courses. Another interpretation of mixed mode is that is a method of e-learning combining elements of team-based-learning, problem-based-learning and case-based learning, in variable proportions, from discipline to discipline and from school to school. This approach has the advantage of providing a customized e-learning experience according to the needs of that particular discipline or school.
- Fully online courses can be taken by students anywhere, provided that they have an interface (e.g., computer, tablet device, phone), the necessary software applications, and access to the Internet. With the exception of orientation, exams, and support services, this type of course is delivered entirely online with little to no face-to-face time.

As a promising education innovation E-learning is used mostly in "web-enhanced mode" in PBL promoting:

- Student learning. Published literature had shown that the amount of knowledge gained by students through E-learning and conventional methods is comparable. Web-based instruction has been shown in some studies to facilitate more effective learning (Chumley-Jones et al., 2002).
- Student satisfaction. Research has demonstrated that students are very satisfied with E-learning in terms of perceived ease of use and access, navigation, interactivity, and user-friendly interface design (Chumley-Jones et al., 2002). However, students view E-learning, as part of a blended-learning strategy, as a supplement rather than a replacement for traditional instruction, or as part of a problem-based flipped classroom, covering three modules: pre-class E-Learning, in-class interactive discussion, and after-class practice tasks.
- Customized learning experience for individuals, giving students more independence than they would have in a more traditional classroom setting. This capability of customize the learning experience can be extended, as needed, from the level of individual to the needs of a discipline or a school. In PBL, commercial learning platforms are widely used by students to assist the self-learning process.

8.2.2 Education Simulation

Authenticity of context is fundamental to problem-based learning, and such authenticity and real-world relevance of the scenario increases student engagement and promotes strategies for in-depth learning (De Leng et al., 2007). Students work at a more conceptual level to achieve learning outcomes. They critically review and synthesize new information with prior and current knowledge to apply understanding to novel situations (Bridges et al., 2015). Traditionally presented in the text format, the authenticity of PBL cases can be further enhanced by using educational simulation.

Simulation is a broad term referring to an artificial representation of a real-world process used to achieve educational objectives through experiential learning. Simulation-based education is any educational activity that employs simulation aids to mimic clinical scenarios (Flanagan et al., 2004). It offers a promising model for enhancing student learning by fostering improved content knowledge, motivation, critical thinking, and creativity (Cook, 2014). Incorporating simulations at an early stage, such as the preclinical PBL curriculum, facilitates the process of restructuring knowledge into higher-order concepts that can be directly applied to problem solving (Schmidt & Rikers, 2007).

Technology facilitated medical education simulations that can be adopted in PBL include manikin simulators, virtual reality, augmented reality, and mixed reality (Fig. 8.4).

Manikin simulators use full-size, anatomically correct, computer-controlled and/or human operator controlled patient models that display real-life vital signs like body temperature, heart rate, respiration rate and oxygen saturation (Ventre & Schwid,

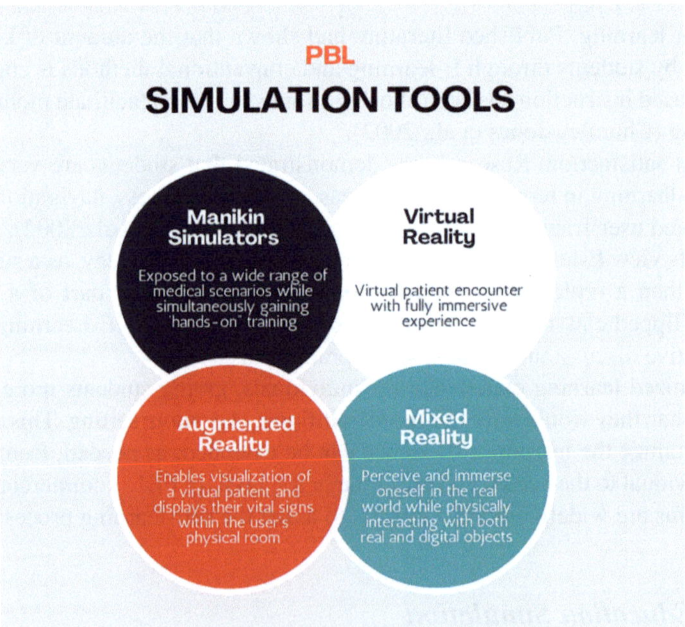

Fig. 8.4 Technology facilitated medical education simulations that can be adopted in PBL include manikin simulators, virtual reality, augmented reality, and mixed reality

2013). These models allow the practice of clinical procedures and diagnostic techniques without exposing a real patient to risk (Ypinazar & Margolis, 2006). These manikins can be programmed to display a variety of medical emergencies, such as a bleeding, convulsions, stroke, and cardiac arrest, and even react to medications administered. They can simulate medical, surgical, obstetrics and gynecological clinical scenarios. These human-like machines can even react to medications and inhaled anesthetic gases The patient model manikins can also be programmed or remote controlled by techs to enhance the interactivity even more, for example to react in real time to medications, administration of gases or medical procedures. The simulation can be recorded on video or can be watched in real time through closed circuit television or via one-way mirrors, depending on the simulation center infrastructure available. After simulation a debrief session will analyze what took place, with students participating in both acting in the simulation and then evaluating their peers and learning the pros and cons of every action taken, under the guidance of a medical educator. Used this way manikin simulation represents a powerful tool because it gives the students the opportunity to be WX in how to respond, adapt and learn from these experiences.

Virtual reality (VR) and virtual patient encounter (VPE) simulation is a fully immersive experience that deceives the user's senses into believing they are in an alternate environment distinct from the actual physical world (Pottle, 2019). Using a headpiece, the user can interact with digital objects using controllers. Interaction with the real world is limited while in a virtual reality environment (OECD, 2016). The system will record all user's actions, making it perfect for proving objective assessment and feedback (Deering & Auguste, 2013). They offer unmatched flexibility in terms of time and location, as they are conducted entirely in a computer-driven virtual environment (Ventre & Schwid, 2013). Some notable examples of VR simulators are the SimX platform (San Francisco, CA), which permits simultaneous participation by multiple users in the same simulation (SimX, n.d.). An example of how natural behavior can be leveraged on this platform: if a participant in a virtual reality environment moves the virtual stethoscope over the patient's precordium or lung, the user would hear what they would normally hear through a stethoscope on real patient (Vukanovic-Criley et al., 2008). Multiple studies demonstrated the efficacy of surgical VR simulators in training (e.g., Ahlberg et al., 2007; Grantcharov et al., 2004).

Augmented reality (AR) is a technology that superimposes digital information such as images, text, and characters onto the real world (Chang et al., 2019; Charnetski, 2019). It keeps the real world as the simulation's focal point but augments it with additional digital details that are unavailable without the computer additions, thereby enhancing reality (Dhar et al., 2021). So, while VR will remove you from your environment, AR will place digital objects in your environment via a handheld or head mounted device (Chang et al., 2019). Such system can be accessed via a head-mounted goggle system that enables visualization of a virtual patient and displays his or her vital signs within the user's physical room. Smartphones and tablets can also be used to access the system, with the onboard camera displaying the room and the virtual patient on the screen.

Mixed reality/haptic enabled VR combines physical and digital elements. Using head mounted stereo vision system and handheld haptic controllers, the user interacts with and manipulates physical and virtual objects (Rosen, 2013; Owens & Taekman, 2013). Mixed reality enables the user to perceive and be immersed in the real world while physically interacting with both real and digital objects. As a result, mixed reality eliminates distinctions between the real and the imagined. The VirtaMed ArthroS (VitraMed AG) (Zurich, Switzerland) is an example of a mixed reality system designed to provide orthopedic residents with interactive and autonomous simulations of actual surgical procedures (Mabrey et al., 2013). The system generates 3D images of the internal structures of the knee that interact with a virtual probe and arthroscope displayed on the monitor as the trainee performs an arthroscopic procedure on a manikin (VitraMed, n.d.) (Fig. 8.4).

Vertend (3D Immersive Collaboration Corp) (Maryland, United States) is a notable example of the use of simulation in PBL. It is a platform that enables the creation of virtual and immersive 3D collaborative spaces for content synthesis and sharing, allowing team members to utilize the group's knowledge and interact via voice, videos, text editors, the Internet, whiteboards, smartboards, and presentations (Vertend, 2022). The use of the platform has the potential to bring about several noteworthy improvements in team dynamics. It helps students feel more present in the classroom by allowing them to interact with each other's avatars. The use of a common online environment can help team work together more effectively. The time and energy of a team can be preserved through the archiving and subsequent retrieval of work, models, and recorded meetings. This innovative mode of operation could provide answers to pressing teamwork issues such as coordination, communication, knowledge creation, and dissemination (Fruchter, 2014; Araújo, 2019).

As a promising model for medical and health science education, simulations can facilitate:

- Proficiency by doing and redoing. Complex pre-clerkship and clinical concepts can be taught via educational simulations. Students can make mistakes and learn from them without fear of consequences (Galati & Williams, 2013). Simulations based on the real world make possible experiments that would otherwise be too expensive or risky to conduct on real patients (Ypinazar & Margolis, 2006).
- Engagement and motivation of students. Educational simulations can foster student engagement and motivation in various disciplines and education levels (Moll-Khosrawi et al., 2021).
- Students' critical thinking skills. Simulations have the potential to assist students in working hard, applying knowledge in creatively, and "thinking like a physician."

8.2.3 Technology-Facilitated Collaboration

Online collaboration tools can improve the interaction, engagement, learning, and critical thinking abilities of students (Mian & Khan, 2020). In addition, they can permit students from various institutions around the world to collaborate on various projects, thereby enhancing the flexibility, diversity of their educational experience, heightening their awareness of global challenges, and expanding their appreciation of other cultures (Soled et al., 2020). When combined with other learning strategies, technology-enabled collaboration can supplement problem-based learning or team-based learning (Resta & Laferrière, 2007). Models of collaboration made possible by technology may incorporate built-in assessment to measure team performance and individual collaborative actions. Technology-enabled collaboration models may include built-in assessment features taking into account team performance and/or collaborative activity (Ingram, 2009).

Current technologies allowing for real-time communication have made global collaboration much easier than in the past (OECD, 2016). Tools like video conferencing have paved the way to make online PBL possible.

As a promising model for medical education and other disciplines, technology-driven collaboration can lead to:

- Flexible collaboration: Online collaboration tools enable students to collaborate outside of traditional classroom hours and without geographical constraints (Alamro & Schofield, 2012; Lan et al., 2012).
- Cultural diversity: Online collaboration tools can promote intercultural interactions by extending the reach of collaborations to remote locations and even across continents (Soled et al., 2020; Annerstedt et al., 2010; Nerantzi, 2010).
- Enhanced learning. Although, not necessarily more effective than face-to-face interaction, learning, both individually and collectively, can benefit from the use of online collaboration tools (Kemp & Grieve, 2014). The positive effect of cooperative learning is contingent on team learning objectives and individual accountability (Kanthan & Mills, 2007).
- Increased interaction and engagement. Technology-enabled collaboration can enhance students' teamwork skills, and engagement (Mian & Khan, 2020). Cooperative learning has been linked to significantly more positive affective outcomes for students (Kanthan & Mills, 2007).
- Strengthened critical thinking: Online collaboration may improve higher order thinking even more than face-to-face collaboration by facilitating discussions that are more complex and cognitively demanding (Resta & Laferrière, 2007).

Forums, GoogleDocs and wikis are examples of asynchronous collaboration tools, whereas virtual conference platforms have been used widely in synchronous collaboration. Digital white board is slowly replacing traditional non-digital counterparts, thanks to its array of innovative features including multimedia integration and remote collaboration. All can be used for online PBL.

8.2.4 Real-Time Response System

Combining formative assessment in real time with PBL can improve the learning experience. Moreover, educators should consider using response systems to facilitate a more adaptive learning experience. Its instantaneous feedback enables professors to tailor their facilitations to the needs of students or student groups. These response systems can also guarantee that every student participates in classroom discussions, which is typically not the case in a large classroom due to time constraints or hesitation.

As a promising educational innovation, real-time response systems could enhance.

- Adaptive teaching. Real-time formative assessment enables teachers to monitor student learning in real time and better adapt facilitation to meet the unique needs of each student or group (Laird & Kuh, 2005).
- Student reflection. Real-time formative assessment can raise student achievement by empowering students to reflect on their learning needs and become actively involved in their own learning (Savary & Gifford, 2017; Gubbiyappa et al., 2016).
- Problem-solving skills. Real-time formative assessment allows for the evaluation of a variety of student activities and skills, such as problem-solving and creativity, thereby enhancing the acquisition of these abilities (Wu et al., 2011).

Many real-time response systems, like Poll Everywhere (Poll Everywhere (nd)), can be valuable online formative assessment tools that allow educators to add interactive questions to the class session and collect audience responses via QR code, URL link, or text message. Such tools can be exceptional beneficial in the context of online PBL, as they swiftly engage all participants. They can be used at the very beginning of the PBL session to check and encourage students' preparation, or it can be used to guide the group back on track when the discussion gets stuck.

8.2.5 Technology-Facilitated Assessment Tools

The fast evolvement of online education has introduced online exam as a prominent mode of assessment. There is a widespread fear, backed by some data, that the expansion of online tests poses a threat to academic integrity because they may present students with more opportunities to cheat than proctored, in-person exams. While academic dishonesty is an issue for any graduate's future career, it is especially concerning for physicians because of the potential for serious injury or death to patients (Azulay Chertok et al., 2014). An aspect of reducing cheating is authenticating the user and monitoring the user's activity during the examination using a remote proctoring system.

Before beginning an examination, students initiate the remote proctoring software on their computers. During the onboarding phase, the software uses a camera, webcam, or standalone device to confirm student identity by scanning their face and identification card, followed by an environment scan. Throughout the examination, the camera and microphone are used to monitor and record the student, the surroundings, and computer desktop activities. Session recordings are stored on a remote server following the examination. All videos are analyzed on the remote server for suspicious behavior using a specialized algorithm. The instructor and administrators can then evaluate each video to determine whether the anomaly represents an attempt to cheat. Exam irregularities include a student leaving his or her exam station, looking away from the exam, or utilizing additional resources like a second computer, tablet device, or reading materials.

Remote proctoring systems enable academics to address concerns pertaining to academic dishonesty. They do, however, raise a secondary concern regarding user security and privacy protection (EdSurge, 2022). Particularly, the use of video and monitoring of device activity allow for unintended sharing and/or unethical acquisition of data. In addition, large amounts of data are collected by these programs in order to execute their algorithms, which can encourage the unethical use of student-specific data.

Use of post hoc assessments, such as an oral exam or a viva voce, to validate results is an alternative strategy to address academic integrity in online examinations (Siddiqui et al., 2022). This, however, necessitates either an extensive time commitment to interview all students or creates equity issues regarding which students are interviewed and what should be done with the information gathered from a subset of the cohort. Alternately, rather than questioning students on their content knowledge using a post hoc oral examination, they could be questioned on their assessment strategy. This may be quite stressful for some students if they believe they are being "accused" of cheating, and it may impair their ability to recall their strategy and articulate their reasoning.

Assessment is essential for PBL, and it can be done online with appropriate tools. It can be formative, helping the facilitator to identify misconceptions or learning gaps across the cohort and individual students; it can be summative, verifying that students have acquired factual knowledge, clinical reasoning, communication skills, and higher order cognitive skills.

8.3 Key Messages for Technology in PBL Learning

In-depth research into promising ICT-integrated pedagogic models reveals the immense potential of digital technologies to enhance teaching in problem-based curricula. These cutting-edge technologically enhanced pedagogical models should be considered by educators as a means to better outcomes, including the development of higher order thinking skills and expanding the available learning opportunities for students.

- Technology-supported models, such as those based on simulations, online laboratory experiments, real-time response systems, and formative assessment tools, can enhance students' creativity, ambition, and problem-solving skills while enhancing their conceptual understanding and test performance.
- Technology-supported education can also expand learning opportunities for students. Online laboratories, for instance, enable a wider range of experimentation and experiential learning, which would be difficult without technology support.
- Additionally, technology expands the opportunities for intercultural collaboration, allowing students to experience the type of international collaboration that is prevalent in today's professional environments.
- Lastly, technology facilitates assessments that allow teachers to monitor student learning in real-time, adjust their instruction as necessary, and identify the skills students need to acquire in a more comprehensive manner than was previously possible.

The difficulty in adopting these models lies not in overcoming technological hurdles but rather in integrating new forms of instruction. Support from institutions is crucial to ensure their adoption by educators is long-lasting and successful. Teachers need access to materials and training to fully realize the potential of technology-supported models. It's true that teachers can monitor their students' progress in real time with the help of real-time formative assessment, but they're still responsible for incorporating that data into their lessons. Teachers can maximize the benefits of experiential learning by encouraging students to repeat their experiments and providing them with the support they need to understand them. To meet this pedagogical challenge, teachers need sufficient professional development. Lack of formal teacher training, as well as peer learning, is a frequent barrier to adopting new teaching methods and resources. Additionally, teachers need time to incorporate new technology-enhanced educational models into their pedagogy. While pedagogy is the driving force behind success, technology-supported models require certain equipment and basic devices, such as computers, tablets, and high-speed internet. The availability of peer-reviewed, teacher-friendly educational content and resources is an additional crucial factor for academic achievement. Teachers should assess the wealth of digital resources available for medical and health science education (Fig. 8.5).

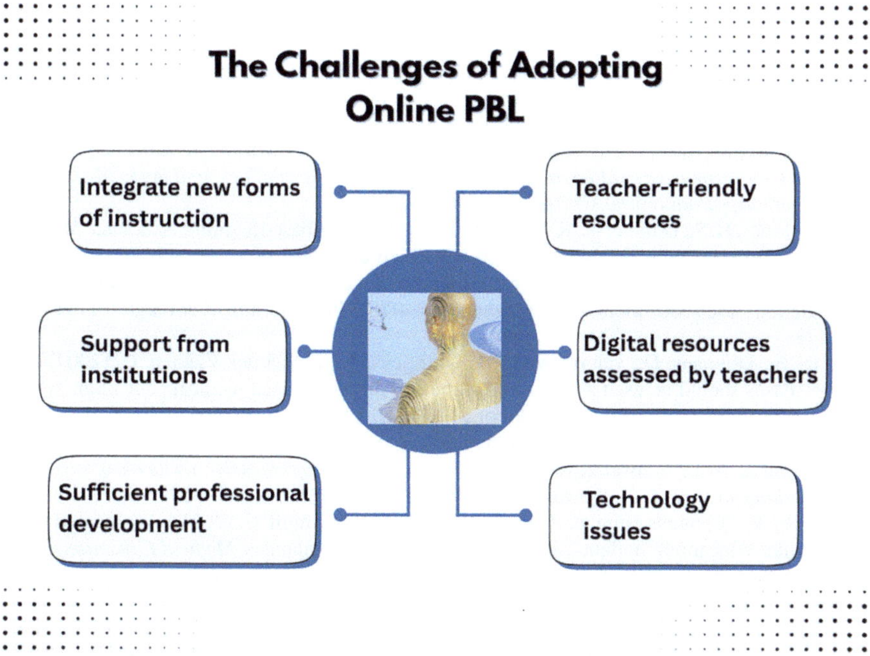

Fig. 8.5 Challenges in adopting online PBL include integrating new instructional methods, lack of institutional support, limited faculty development, resources accessibility and assessment by teachers, and technological issues

References

Ahlberg, G., Enochsson, L., Gallagher, A. G., Hedman, L., Hogman, C., McClusky, D. A., 3rd, Ramel, S., Smith, C. D., & Arvidsson, D. (2007). Proficiency-based virtual reality training significantly reduces the error rate for residents during their first 10 laparoscopic cholecystectomies. *American Journal of Surgery, 193*(6), 797–804. https://doi.org/10.1016/j.amjsurg.2006.06.050

Alamro, A. S., & Schofield, S. (2012). Supporting traditional PBL with online discussion forums: A study from Qassim Medical School. *Medical Teacher, 34*(Suppl 1), S20–S24. https://doi.org/10.3109/0142159x.2012.656751

Annerstedt, C., Huang-DeVoss, C., Lindh, J., Garza, D., & Rydmark, M. (2010). Research-able through problem-based learning. *Journal of the Scholarship of Teaching and Learning, 10*(2), 107–127.

Araújo, U. F. (2019). 3D immersive platforms and problem-based learning projects: A search for quality in education. In M. Moallem, W. Hung, & N. Dabbagh (Eds.), *The Wiley handbook of problem-based learning* (pp. 575–592). Wiley-Blackwell.

Azulay Chertok, I. R., Barnes, E. R., & Gilleland, D. (2014). Academic integrity in the online learning environment for health sciences students. *Nurse Education Today, 34*(10), 1324–1329. https://doi.org/10.1016/j.nedt.2013.06.002

Blumberg, P. (2006). Assessing students during the problem-based learning (PBL) process. *Medical Science Educator, 15*(2). Retrieved from http://www.iamse.org/mse-article/assessing-students-during-the-problem-based-learning-pbl-process/

Bridges, S., Chan, L. K., & Hmelo-Silver, C. E. (Eds.). (2015). *Educational technologies in medical and health sciences education* (Vol. 5). Springer.

Chang, T. P., Sherman, J. M., & Gerard, J. M. (2019). Overview of serious gaming and virtual reality. In D. Nestel, J. Hui, K. Kunkler, M. Scerbo, & A. Calhoun (Eds.), *Healthcare simulation research*. Springer. https://doi.org/10.1007/978-3-030-26837-4_5

Charnetski, M. D. (2019). Simulation methodologies. In S. Crawford, L. Baily, & S. Monks (Eds.), *Comprehensive healthcare simulation: Operations, technology, and innovative practice*. Springer. https://doi.org/10.1007/978-3-030-15378-6_3

Chumley-Jones, H. S., Dobbie, A., & Alford, C. L. (2002). Web-based learning. *Academic Medicine, 77*(Supplement), S86–S93. https://doi.org/10.1097/00001888-200210001-00028

Cook, D. A. (2014). How much evidence does it take? A cumulative meta-analysis of outcomes of simulation-based education. *Medical Education, 48*(8), 750–760. https://doi.org/10.1111/medu.12473

De Leng, B., Dolmans, D., van de Wiel, M., Muijtjens, A., & van der Vleuten, C. (2007). How video cases should be used as authentic stimuli in problem-based medical education. *Medical Education, 41*(2), 181–188. https://doi.org/10.1111/j.1365-2929.2006.02671.x

Deering, S., & Auguste, T. C. (2013). Simulation in obstetrics and gynecology. In A. I. Levine, S. DeMaria, A. D. Schwartz, & A. J. Sim (Eds.), *The comprehensive textbook of healthcare simulation* (pp. 437–452). Springer. https://doi.org/10.1007/978-1-4614-5993-4_30

Dhar, P., Rocks, T., Samarasinghe, R. M., Stephenson, G., & Smith, C. (2021). Augmented reality in medical education: Students' experiences and learning outcomes. *Medical Education Online, 26*(1). https://doi.org/10.1080/10872981.2021.1953953

EdSurge. (2022, August 25). *College's use of exam-proctoring software to 'scan' rooms violated privacy rights, judge finds—EdSurge News*. Retrieved November 26, 2022, from https://www.edsurge.com/news/2022-08-25-college-s-use-of-exam-proctoring-software-to-scan-rooms-violated-privacy-rights-judge-finds

Evensen, D. H., & Hmelo, C. E. (2000). *Problem-based learning: A research perspective on learning interactions* (1st ed., pp. 1–16). https://doi.org/10.4324/9781410604989

Felder, R. M., Brent, R., & Oakley, B. A. (2016). *Teaching and learning stem: A practical guide*. Jossey-Bass.

Flanagan, B., Nestel, D., & Joseph, M. (2004). Making patient safety the focus: Crisis resource management in the undergraduate curriculum. *Medical Education, 38*(1), 56–66. https://doi.org/10.1111/j.1365-2923.2004.01701.x

Fruchter, R. (2014). Transformative 3D immersive collaboration environment in support of AEC global teamwork. In I. Flood & R. Issa (Eds.), *Computing in civil and building engineering* (pp. 1425–1432). American Society of Civil Engineering.

Galati, M., & Williams, R. (2013). Business planning considerations for a healthcare simulation center. In A. I. Levine, S. DeMaria, A. D. Schwartz, & A. J. Sim (Eds.), *The comprehensive textbook of healthcare simulation*. Springer. https://doi.org/10.1007/978-1-4614-5993-4_46

Giannakos, M. N., Mikalef, P., & Pappas, I. O. (2021). Systematic literature review of E-learning capabilities to enhance organizational learning. *Information Systems Frontiers, 24*(2), 619–635. https://doi.org/10.1007/s10796-020-10097-2

Grantcharov, T. P., Kristiansen, V. B., Bendix, J., Bardram, L., Rosenberg, J., & Funch-Jensen, P. (2004). Randomized clinical trial of virtual reality simulation for laparoscopic skills training. *The British Journal of Surgery, 91*(2), 146–150. https://doi.org/10.1002/bjs.4407

Gubbiyappa, K., Barua, A., Das, B., Vasudeva Murthy, C., & Baloch, H. (2016). Effectiveness of flipped classroom with Poll Everywhere as a teaching-learning method for pharmacy students. *Indian Journal of Pharmacology, 48*(7), 41. https://doi.org/10.4103/0253-7613.193313

Hmelo-Silver, C. E., & Barrows, H. S. (2006). Goals and strategies of a problem-based learning facilitator. *Interdisciplinary Journal of Problem-Based Learning, 1*(1). https://doi.org/10.7771/1541-5015.1004

Hung, W., Moallem, M., & Dabbagh, N. (Eds.). (2019). *The Wiley handbook of problem-based learning*. Wiley-Blackwell.

Ingram, A. L. (2009). Measuring collaboration in online communication. In M. Khosrow-Pour (Ed.), *Encyclopedia of information science and technology* (Vol. 1, 2nd ed., pp. 2537–2541). Information Resources Management Association. https://doi.org/10.4018/978-1-60566-026-4

Kanthan, R., & Mills, S. (2007). Cooperative learning in the first year of undergraduate medical education. *World Journal of Surgical Oncology, 5*(1). https://doi.org/10.1186/1477-7819-5-136

Kemp, N., & Grieve, R. (2014). Face-to-face or face-to-screen? Undergraduates' opinions and test performance in classroom vs. online learning. *Frontiers in Psychology, 5*. https://doi.org/10.3389/fpsyg.2014.01278

Laird, T. F. N., & Kuh, G. D. (2005). Student experiences with information technology and their relationship to other aspects of student engagement. *Research in Higher Education, 46*(2), 211–233. https://doi.org/10.1007/s11162-004-1600-y

Lan, Y. F., Tsai, P. W., Yang, S. H., & Hung, C. L. (2012). Comparing the social knowledge construction behavioral patterns of problem-based online asynchronous discussion in e/m-learning environments. *Computers & Education, 59*(4), 1122–1135. https://doi.org/10.1016/j.compedu.2012.05.004

Mabrey, J. D., Atesok, K., Egol, K., Jazrawi, L., & Hall, G. (2013). Simulation in orthopedic surgery. In A. I. Levine, S. DeMaria, A. D. Schwartz, & A. J. Sim (Eds.), *The comprehensive textbook of healthcare simulation*. Springer. https://doi.org/10.1007/978-1-4614-5993-4_32

Mian, A., & Khan, S. (2020). Medical education during pandemics: A UK perspective. *BMC Medicine, 18*(1). https://doi.org/10.1186/s12916-020-01577-y

Moll-Khosrawi, P., Zöllner, C., Cronje, J. S., & Schulte-Uentrop, L. (2021). The effects of simulation-based education on medical students' motivation. *International Journal of Medical Education, 12*, 130–135. https://doi.org/10.5116/ijme.60c0.981e

Nerantzi, C. (2010). A case of problem-based learning for cross-institutional collaboration. *Electronic Journal of E-Learning, 10*, 306–314.

OECD. (2016). Innovating education and educating for innovation: The power of digital technologies and skills. Paris: OECD Publishing. https://doi.org/10.1787/9789264265097-en

Owens, R., & Taekman, J. M. (2013). Virtual reality, haptic simulators, and virtual environments. In A. I. Levine, S. DeMaria, A. D. Schwartz, & A. J. Sim (Eds.), *The comprehensive textbook of healthcare simulation*. Springer. https://doi.org/10.1007/978-1-4614-5993-4_16

Pearson, J. (2006). Investigating ICT using problem-based learning in face-to-face and online learning environments. *Computers & Education, 47*(1), 56–73. https://doi.org/10.1016/j.compedu.2004.09.001

Poll Everywhere. (n.d.). *Poll Everywhere*. Retrieved November 25, 2022, from https://www.polleverywhere.com

Pottle, J. (2019). Virtual reality and the transformation of medical education. *Future Healthcare Journal, 6*(3), 181–185. https://doi.org/10.7861/fhj.2019-0036

Resta, P., & Laferrière, T. (2007). Technology in support of collaborative learning. *Educational Psychology Review, 19*(1), 65–83. https://doi.org/10.1007/s10648-007-9042-7

Rosen, K. (2013). The history of simulation. In A. I. Levine, S. DeMaria, A. D. Schwartz, & A. J. Sim (Eds.), *The comprehensive textbook of healthcare simulation*. Springer. https://doi.org/10.1007/978-1-4614-5993-4_2

Savary, M. A., & Gifford, K. M. (2017). The benefits of a real-time web-based response system for enhancing engaged learning in classrooms and public science events. *Journal of Undergraduate Neuroscience Education, 15*(2), E13–E16.

Schmidt, H.G. and Rikers, R.M.J.P. (2007), How expertise develops in medicine: knowledge encapsulation and illness script formation. *Medical Education, 41*: 1133–1139. https://doi.org/10.1111/j.1365-2923.2007.02915.x

Siddiqui, N., Khan, R. N., Afifa, S., & Islam, Z. (2022). Perception and validity of online formative oral assessment in surgical trainees: A cross-sectional study. *Cureus*. https://doi.org/10.7759/cureus.24938

SimX. (n.d.). *SimX*. Retrieved November 24, 2022, from https://www.simxvr.com

Soled, D., Goel, S., Barry, D., Erfani, P., Joseph, N., Kochis, M., Uppal, N., Velasquez, D., Vora, K., & Scott, K. W. (2020). Medical student mobilization during a crisis: Lessons from a COVID-19 medical student response team. *Academic Medicine, 95*(9), 1384–1387. https://doi.org/10.1097/acm.0000000000003401

Ventre, K. M., & Schwid, H. A. (2013). Computer and web based simulators. In A. I. Levine, S. DeMaria, A. D. Schwartz, & A. J. Sim (Eds.), *The comprehensive textbook of healthcare simulation*. Springer. https://doi.org/10.1007/978-1-4614-5993-4_14

Vertend. (2022). *3D Immersive Collaboration Corp*. Retrieved December 12, 2022, from https://www.3dicc.com/product-details/

VitraMed. (n.d.). *VitraMed*. Retrieved December 31, 2022, from https://www.virtamed.com/en/

Vukanovic-Criley, J. M., Boker, J. R., Criley, S. R., Rajagopalan, S., & Criley, J. M. (2008). Using virtual patients to improve cardiac examination competency in medical students. *Clinical Cardiology, 31*(7), 334–339. https://doi.org/10.1002/clc.20213

Wu, P. H., Hwang, G. J., Milrad, M., Ke, H. R., & Huang, Y. M. (2011). An innovative concept map approach for improving students' learning performance with an instant feedback mechanism. *British Journal of Educational Technology, 43*(2), 217–232. https://doi.org/10.1111/j.1467-8535.2010.01167.x

Ypinazar, V., & Margolis, S. (2006). Clinical simulators: Applications and implications for rural medical education. *Rural and Remote Health*. https://doi.org/10.22605/rrh527

Chapter 9
Problem-Based Learning and Artificial Intelligence

Varna Taranikanti and Srineil Vuthaluru

9.1 Introduction

The integration of artificial intelligence (AI) into medical education represents a relatively recent phenomenon, yet its roots can be traced back to the early developments of AI in healthcare. Initially, the role of AI in medicine was primarily focused on enhancing diagnostic accuracy, optimizing treatment plans, and facilitating research. However, its potential for reshaping the dynamics in medical education began to gain recognition as the technology evolved. The recent era of digital technology has transmuted the healthcare landscape significantly, driven by changes in demographic needs, medical advancements, and shifts in federal policies. This transformation is paralleled in medical education, where new tools like AI are renovating teaching methodologies. The past decade has seen rapid advancements in AI and has heralded innovative applications in various domains and across a range of fields, with medicine and medical practice being two of the most notable beneficiaries (Fig. 9.1).

V. Taranikanti (✉)
Department of Foundational Medical Studies, Oakland University William Beaumont School of Medicine, Rochester, MI, USA
e-mail: taranikanti@oakland.edu

S. Vuthaluru
Department of Surgery, University of Nebraska Medical Center, Omaha, NE, USA
e-mail: svuthaluru@unmc.edu

S. Lorenzo and B. Zhang (eds.), *Mastering Problem-Based Learning in Health Profession Programs*, https://doi.org/10.1007/978-3-032-05405-0_9

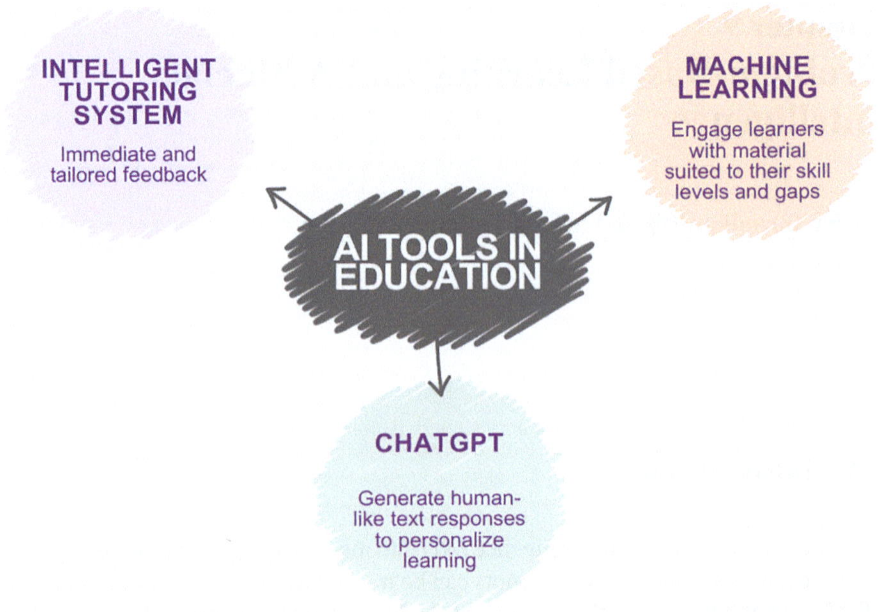

Fig. 9.1 Common AI tools used in education include intelligent tutoring system, machine learning and ChatGPT

9.1.1 Intelligent Tutoring Systems

Historically, the evolution of intelligent tutoring systems (ITS) from 1960 to 1990 marks a significant chapter in educational technology, particularly in relation to artificial intelligence (AI) and its application in problem-based learning, particularly for health professional education. The inception of ITS can be traced back to the 1970s, with the development of the first system, SCHOLAR, in 1970. This marked the beginning of harnessing AI to provide personalized, adaptive instruction (Carbonell, 1970). By the late 1970s and into the 1980s, other influential systems such as BIP, WUMPUS, and SOPHIE emerged, demonstrating the potential of ITSs in enhancing learning through tailored feedback and instruction (Auguste, 1985). The pedagogical effectiveness of these systems was noted to closely parallel that of human instructors (VanLehn, 2011). During the 1980s, advancements in AI, particularly in neural networks and knowledge tracing, spurred further development in ITSs (Rumelhart et al., 1986). One of the main advantages of ITS is its ability to provide immediate and tailored feedback to learners, which is essential in health professional education where understanding complex concepts can directly impact patient care and health outcomes. The interactive nature of ITS allows for a more engaging educational experience, making learning more effective compared to traditional methods. The authors reference the Technology Acceptance Model (TAM) to highlight how perceived usefulness and ease of use influence the acceptance of such technologies among educators and parents (Davis, 1989). There is growing importance of ITS in educational settings, particularly for health professional education. The authors, Manuel B. Garcia and Precious S. Garcia, argue that the integration of ITS into primary and health education can facilitate more personalized learning experiences, which are crucial for developing competencies in future health professionals (Garcia & Garcia, 2023). Thus, the history of ITS from 1960 to 1990 illustrates a foundational evolution that not only advanced educational methodologies but also laid the groundwork for AI applications in health professional training, emphasizing the importance of personalized, adaptive learning environments. This period also saw a growing intersection between cognitive science and educational research, emphasizing the importance of understanding learner needs and strategies for effective problem-solving (Andersson et al., 2022). By the 1990s, the integration of ITS in health professional education began to gain traction, leveraging AI to simulate real-world scenarios and enhance critical thinking skills for future practitioners. The relevance of ITS to problem-based learning lies in its ability to provide adaptive learning experiences that are crucial for the complexities of healthcare education. With evolution in technology such as Machine Learning, Al systems in the early 2000s started providing more personalized, adaptive learning experiences, responding to individual students' progress.

9.1.2 Machine Learning (ML)

In recent years Machine Learning (ML), a subset AI, is increasingly transforming health professional education by providing innovative solutions for personalized learning and assessment. ML algorithms analyse vast datasets without explicit programming to identify patterns and predict outcomes. The integration of machine learning and data analytics began to optimize curriculum development and personalized learning in the early twenty-first century, since then there has been rapid progress enabling educators to tailor curricula to meet individual learner needs (Chiu et al., 2024). Tools such as IBM Watson and Google Cloud AutoML are being utilized to develop adaptive learning platforms that assess student performance in real-time, adjusting the difficulty and type of content presented based on individual progress (Sayed et al., 2023; Bodonhelyi et al., 2025). This personalized approach supports PBL by ensuring that learners engage with material relevant to their current skill levels and knowledge gaps, thereby enhancing their critical thinking and problem-solving abilities.

Moreover, ML can aid in the evaluation of clinical skills and competencies. Automated assessment tools, such as those utilizing natural language processing (NLP) through platforms like Microsoft Azure Text Analytics, can analyze student interactions during simulated patient encounters, providing immediate feedback and identifying areas for improvement (Katz et al., 2021). By integrating ML into medical education, institutions can not only improve learning outcomes but also foster a more efficient and effective educational environment. As the integration of AI and

ML continues to evolve, it is essential for medical educators to understand and embrace these technologies to better prepare future healthcare professionals for the complexities of modern practice.

9.1.3 ChatGPT

The growing phenomenon of artificial intelligence has escalated in 2022 when ChatGPT was released by Open Al and has become the first widely available large language model (LLM) (Mesko, 2023). ChatGPT is a specific example of an AI chatbot that utilizes advanced machine learning models (like Large Language Models (LLMs)) to generate human-like text responses. With further emergence of this resource and other Al-powered research tools allowed educators, students and researchers to engage with technology and simulations in more efficient ways, while predictive analytics began to further personalize the learning process (Zhang & Aslan, 2021; Javaid et al., 2022). Since then, there was a shift in the world's perception of AI and these technologies are well-accepted by the general public and academicians because of their accessibility and user-friendly interface (Fig. 9.2) Since then, they have been integrated into various sectors and has propelled advancements in efficiency, accuracy, and personalization.

In healthcare, AI tools are revolutionizing not only patient care but also the education of future healthcare professionals. As AI technologies evolve, their intersection with PBL presents a unique opportunity to enhance educational practices. AI can

AI tools, their origin, and guidelines for creating resources for AI-generated case scenarios or simulations for PBL

AI Tool	Origin	Guidelines for Use
ChatGPT (GPT-3.5 / GPT-4)	Open AI	Generates text-based case scenarios, clinical vignettes, and problem-solving questions
DALL·E 2	OpenAI	Generates images from text prompts
CLIP	Open AI	Generates relevant visuals to accompany case scenarios and integrates into text
MedPaLM	Google	Medical content generation and Q&A. Text-based scenarios and support multimodal approaches by integrating clinical data.
DeepMind's AlphaFold	Google	Specially for simulating molecular biology cases or generating complex biological data and images.
Synthesia	Synthesia AI	Video-based learning materials, including simulations of patient interactions, medical procedures
RAG (Retrieval augmented generation)	OpenAI, Google	Generates real-time, context-rich, relevant output and integrates retrieval capabilities into the generative model.
Runway ML	Runway AI	Text-to-image, image-to-text, and multimodal integrations to enhance the realism of case scenarios
Stable Diffusion	Stability AI	Integrates detailed prompts to create high-quality medical images for PBL

Fig. 9.2 An overview of some of the key AI tools, their origins, and guidelines for use in preclinical education within the framework of PBL in medical education

facilitate personalized learning experiences, provide immediate feedback, and simulate complex clinical scenarios. This chapter aims to provide an in-depth analysis of resources as how AI can transform PBL to create more effective and personalized learning experiences. It also explores the transformative potential of AI in PBL, examining its role, benefits, challenges, and future directions in health professional education.

9.2 Integration of AI into Problem-Based Learning

Problem-based learning (PBL) has emerged as a prominent pedagogical approach in health professional education (HPE). PBL is a student-centered method that encourages learners to engage with real case scenarios, develops critical thinking and collaborative skills. This shift towards self-directed learning, working with peers in analysing problems are essential for practical application when presented with real world problems and for effective healthcare delivery. Health professional education has traditionally relied on an apprenticeship model, where students and trainees learn through observation and hands-on experience under the guidance of experienced practitioners. While this model has served the field well for decades, it faces significant challenges in the contemporary landscape of healthcare, including the increasing complexity of clinical practices, heightened expectations for proficiency, and regulations that limit trainee autonomy. Moreover, the traditional model may not adequately address the urgent need for objective assessment and feedback in competency evaluation across various healthcare professions. The integration of AI into health professional education presents a unique opportunity to enhance this framework through a PBL approach. By leveraging AI, educators can create more individualized learning experiences, facilitate the development of critical thinking skills, and provide timely feedback, ultimately improving the readiness of health professionals to meet the demands of modern healthcare (Fig. 9.3).

The components of PBL include (1) Generating open ended problems that are relevant and applicable to real-life situations. (2) Student-centered learning where students work collaboratively to explore the problem and share ideas, discuss concepts and learn from each other. (3) Self-directed learning (SDL) where students are responsible for their own learning by identifying what they need to know, seeking out resources to fill those gaps, and reflecting on their learning process (Atta & Alghamdi, 2018; Leary et al., 2019; Loyens et al., 2008).

9.2.1 Generation of Case Scenarios

Case scenarios serve as the cornerstone of PBL, providing students with the context necessary to apply their theoretical knowledge to practical situations. Effective case scenarios are characterized by their authenticity, complexity, and relevance to

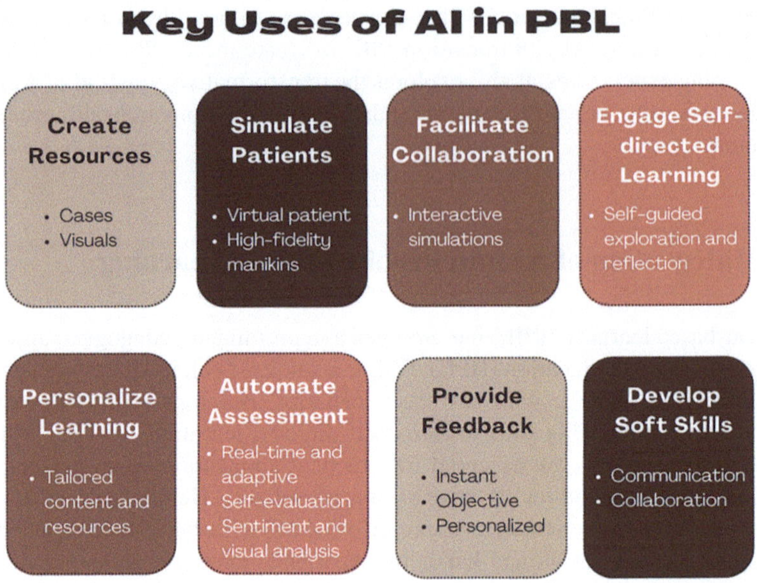

Fig. 9.3 A diverse range of AI applications in PBL includes creating resources, simulating patients, facilitating collaboration, engaging self-directed learning, personalizing learning, automating assessment, providing feedback and developing soft skills

the curricula. They should mimic real-life clinical situations, allowing students to explore various dimensions of patient care, including diagnosis, treatment, and ethical considerations. In medical and healthcare education, the effectiveness of PBL can be significantly enhanced through the integration of Natural Language Processing (NLP) and Machine Learning (ML) techniques. These technologies offer innovative methods for generating case scenarios that are relevant, diverse, and grounded in current medical knowledge and practices. The challenge lies in creating a sufficient variety of these scenarios that encompass a wide range of medical conditions, patient demographics, and socio-economic and cultural contexts. NLP can analyze vast datasets, including clinical guidelines, medical literature, and electronic health records (EHRs), to extract relevant information and generate coherent narratives. By using NLP, educators can automate the creation of case scenarios that reflect current medical knowledge and practice.

The first step involves training AI. This can be done using the vast number of case reports and available medical literature. AI-assisted computer-generated patient scenarios speed up case development with specific learning objectives. A number of crucial procedures must be followed while creating a clinical case scenario for PBL in order to guarantee that the scenario is pertinent, interesting, and instructive. Start by outlining the learning goals in detail, such as improving diagnostic abilities, comprehending available treatments, or taking ethical considerations into account. This clarity aids in directing the course of the scenario. The scenario should then be contextualized by including particular patient demographics, medical histories, and presenting symptoms. Using multimedia features such as AI-generated images, radiographs and videograph could enhance diversity and would provide a more realistic representation (Bakkum et al., 2024). The prompt should help framing the scenario in a way that promotes inquiry. Although using optimized prompts is simple and repeatable, the procedure itself requires computer abilities that not all teachers have (Kıyak & Emekli, 2024).

9.2.2 *Evolving Resources for Generating Clinical Cases Scenarios for PBL*

The generation of AI driven clinical case scenarios for PBL relies on a diverse array of resources and methodologies each contributing unique strengths to the educational process.

AI tools such as large language models (e.g., ChatGPT), require careful prompt crafting to create realistic scenarios based on health science knowledge (Nahass et al., 2024). Multimodal networks (e.g., DALL.E2), are useful for creating visual simulations of clinical scenarios, anatomical diagrams, or clinical imaging for case-based learning (Sun et al., 2024). CLIP is used for integrating multimodal content into the text, and for generating relevant visuals to accompany case scenarios (Farinacci, 2024). Specialized systems (e.g., MedPaLM, AlphaFold) can assist educators in developing diverse educational resources by generating text-based case scenarios, anatomical or procedural images, and also simulate patient interactions (Synthesia AI), thereby fostering experiential learning and allowing students to engage in self-paced, problem-solving activities (Wong et al., 2024). Additionally, AI tools integrate with Retrieval-Augmented Generation (RAG) systems by pulling real-time, contextually relevant data from large medical databases that could be used for the curricular needs of the institution (Lopez et al., 2025). Runaway ML and Stable Diffusion are other platforms that enhance realism by creating tools such as text-to-text images or image-to-text images that integrate detailed prompts to create high-quality medical images for PBL. These tools leverage sophisticated algorithms to facilitate a deeper understanding of medical concepts and improve the overall learning experience.

9.2.3 *AI-Evolving Simulation Technology*

AI-driven virtual patient simulation technology is an important resource that provides interactive and immersive environments for PBL. These chatbots can simulate patient interactions, allowing learners to practice their clinical skills in a safe environment.

Moreover, AI-driven simulations allow students to engage with a dynamic and realistic range of clinical scenarios, complex in nature enabling them to apply theoretical knowledge in practice. These simulations allow students to develop critical thinking and decision-making skills in a controlled environment. Research by Zhang et al. (2021) highlights the effectiveness of AI simulations in improving diagnostic accuracy and enhancing students' clinical reasoning abilities. The scenarios can range from simple routine check-ups to complex medical emergencies, allowing students to practice and improve their diagnostic, treatment, practical, and communication skills while boosting their abilities to provide compassionate care. It includes virtual patients and high-fidelity manikins that provide an authentic, interactive and wide range of behaviour and emotions. The AI generated-patient may boost their abilities to provide empathetic treatment (Tagliaferri et al., 2025).

9.2.4 Simulation Integration

Since then, there has been rapid progress in virtual and augmented reality systems (that revolutionized training by offering immersive, hands-on learning environments (Won et al., 2023; Tang et al., 2020). AI-powered video-based simulations, such as virtual reality (VR) simulators like SimNow, provide immersive environments where trainees can practice essential skills without the pressures of real-life patient interactions. These simulations allow learners to engage in realistic scenarios, enhancing their clinical reasoning and decision-making capabilities in a controlled setting. These days, many hospitals and simulation centers use a range of human patient simulators, from low-fidelity to high-fidelity mannequins. The most advanced of these can react to learner stimuli like voice, compressions, drug administration, physical examinations, and even procedural interventions (Davila & Price, 2025). Other recent advances in AI are transforming peer-to-peer mental health support by enhancing empathic communication through human–AI collaboration. The development of HAILEY, an AI-in-the-loop agent, illustrates how AI can provide just-in-time feedback to peer supporters, enabling them to respond more empathetically to those in need. A randomized controlled trial on TalkLife demonstrated a 19.6% increase in conversational empathy, particularly among peer supporters who struggled with providing support. This feedback-driven approach empowers participants, fostering self-efficacy without creating dependency on AI. Integrating such AI tools into a PBL framework can enhance collaborative learning experiences (Sharma et al., 2023). By simulating real-world scenarios where empathy is crucial, PBL can leverage AI feedback to improve empathetic skills in health professional education, preparing trainees for complex interpersonal interactions in their future practice.

By incorporating AI, these platforms can adapt to the learner's skill level, offering personalized feedback that is crucial for developing competence in various health professions Research indicates that simulation-based training can significantly improve procedural skills and confidence among healthcare trainees (McGaghie et al., 2024). Mastery learning in health professions education, emphasizing the principle of "excellence for all." It outlines the historical roots of mastery learning and its foundation in behavioral, constructivist, and social cognitive paradigms. The model is defined through five key components that balance the time spent learning with the time needed for mastery. Integrating mastery learning with PBL can enhance the acquisition of procedural skills, as PBL's emphasis on real-world problem-solving aligns well with mastery principles. Furthermore, incorporating AI into this framework can offer personalized feedback and adaptive learning pathways, ensuring that learners achieve proficiency in procedural skills while receiving the necessary support to overcome challenges. This synergy between mastery learning, PBL, and AI can lead to more effective training outcomes in health professions education.

The use of VR technology in health education not only facilitates the acquisition of technical skills but also fosters teamwork and communication in multidisciplinary settings. A published study evaluates the effectiveness of virtual reality (VR) in nursing education, focusing on knowledge, skills, satisfaction, confidence, and performance time. A meta-analysis of 12 studies involving 821 participants revealed that VR significantly improved knowledge (SMD = 0.58), but showed no notable advantages over control methods in enhancing skills, satisfaction, confidence, or performance time (Chang, 2017). Integrating VR into a PBL framework can enhance its effectiveness by providing immersive, real-world scenarios that foster critical thinking and application of knowledge. Additionally, leveraging AI can personalize learning experiences within VR environments, offering tailored feedback and adaptive learning pathways. This combination has the potential to better support skill development and overall learner satisfaction in nursing education, warranting further research to explore these synergies.

As health professionals face increasingly complex patient needs, integrating AI-driven simulation into curricula can better prepare them to deliver high-quality care in real-world scenarios.

AI can generate a diverse range of hypothetical clinical cases, allowing trainees to engage in case-based discussions. For instance, a large language model (LLM) can simulate complex clinical scenarios, prompting trainees to diagnose, plan, and propose interventions in a collaborative environment. By embedding these simulations into PBL modules, trainees can face challenging scenarios and receive immediate AI-driven feedback. Students can also use AI tools to analyse large datasets from clinical trials or patient records. This helps them learn how to interpret data, identify trends, and make evidence-based decisions. Natural language processing (NLP) algorithms enable AI systems to understand and interpret human language, making it possible to interact with students in real-time during simulated patient encounters. For instance, AI-powered virtual patients can communicate with students using natural language, simulating realistic patient-doctor interactions (Zidoun & Mardi, 2024). These systems analyse the student's questions, diagnoses, and treatment plans, providing immediate feedback on their communication skills, clinical reasoning, and decision-making (Ferguson et al., 2016). This real-time assessment helps identify specific areas for improvement while enhancing the learning experience. This approach aligns with the PBL philosophy by Virtual Patients like "Body

Interact" and "i-Human Patients" simulate patient interactions, presenting students with evolving clinical scenarios that require real-time decision-making (Lok & Foster, 2019; Gilbert et al., 2024). High-Fidelity advanced Manikins such as "SimMan" by Laerdal and "HAL" by Gaumard (Meguerdichian, 2021) can mimic physiological responses, allowing students to perform physical examinations, diagnose conditions, and administer treatments. During a high-fidelity simulation of a cardiac arrest scenario, an AI system could provide real-time feedback on the student's CPR technique, including compression depth and rate, improving their proficiency in life-saving procedures IBM Watson for Health uses NLP to provide real-time responses and feedback to health professional students during virtual patient interactions (Sparling & Cooper, 2024). The system can analyze the context of the conversation, understand medical terminology, and offer feedback on the student's diagnostic questions and proposed treatments (Ferguson et al., 2016). Machine learning algorithms analyze large datasets of clinical interactions to identify patterns and best practices. During a simulated patient encounter, these algorithms can compare a student's performance against established benchmarks, providing real-time feedback on their clinical skills. For example, an AI system might analyze a student's physical examination technique, diagnostic accuracy, or treatment decisions, offering specific suggestions for improvement based on data from expert clinicians (Amato et al., 2019) (Fig. 9.4).

Resource	Type	Description
Body Interact	Virtual Patient	Simulates patient interactions with evolving clinical scenarios
i-Human Patients	Virtual Patient	Presents students with dynamic and realistic clinical scenarios for real-time decision-making
SimMan (Laerdal)	High-Fidelity Manikin	Mimics physiological responses, allows physical examinations, diagnosis, and treatments
HAL (Gaumard)	High-Fidelity Manikin	Mimics physiological responses, enables students to practice clinical skills in a realistic environment
IBM Watson for Health	AI/NLP Technology	Provides real-time feedback during virtual patient interactions; analyzes conversation context; understands medical terminology.
Simulated Patient Encounters (SPEs)	Performance Assessment Platform	Uses machine learning to assess student performance and provide real-time feedback on areas where the student's approach deviates from best practices
Intelligent Tutoring Systems (ITS)	Adaptive Learning System	Tracks student progress; identifies struggling areas; offers targeted feedback and adjusts simulation complexity

Fig. 9.4 Simulation technologies as a resource for Problem-Based Learning (PBL)

9.3 Student Engagement and Self-Directed Learning

Group collaboration is essential in PBL, as it fosters a dynamic learning environment where students can share knowledge, challenge assumptions, and engage in meaningful discussions. Research has shown that the integration of AI technology, such as ChatGPT can significantly enhance participants' confidence and self-efficacy, thereby promoting active involvement throughout the PBL process (Li et al., 2025; Wang et al., 2024). By encouraging students to ask more questions during discussions, these AI tools can create an atmosphere conducive to inquiry and exploration, vital components of effective collaborative learning. This interactive engagement aligns well with the theoretical foundations of PBL, which are rooted in constructivist theories emphasizing experiential learning and active participation (Sinha et al., 2015; Hmelo-Silver & Eberbach, 2012).

AI can uniquely integrate the active, social, and experiential aspects of learning by offering interactive simulations that engage students in problem-solving activities. These simulations not only allow for the exploration of complex clinical scenarios but also promote collaborative interactions among students as they work together to analyze problems and formulate solutions. For instance, a bot can present a clinical case that requires input from each group member, prompting them to draw from their individual knowledge and experiences. Such collaborative efforts enhance critical thinking and encourage diverse perspectives, ultimately leading to richer learning outcomes (Kumar et al., 2023).

Furthermore, the incorporation of AI in PBL creates opportunities for students to engage in reflective practices, as they can revisit discussions and review feedback provided by chatbots. This iterative process supports deeper understanding and retention of knowledge while reinforcing the importance of teamwork and communication skills essential in healthcare settings. By facilitating group collaboration through AI technology, educators can create an enriched learning experience that prepares students for real-world challenges in their future professional environments. The synergy between group collaboration and AI technology in PBL not only enhances student engagement and confidence but also aligns with constructivist principles that promote active learning. By fostering an environment where inquiry and exploration thrive, AI tools like chatbots can significantly contribute to the development of critical skills necessary for students in the health professions.

The theoretical underpinnings of PBL are rooted in constructivist theories, emphasizing the importance of experiential learning and active participation in the learning process (Hmelo-Silver & Eberbach, 2012). AI can integrate the active, social, and experiential aspects of learning by offering interactive, dynamic simulations that engage students in problem-solving while encouraging collaboration. The integration of artificial intelligence in education not only enhances the learning experience but also fosters essential skills such as self-directed learning and critical thinking. Tools such as ChatGPT, powered by OpenAI's GPT-3 technology, exemplify the capabilities of AI to support self-directed and self-paced learning in a safe environment. This pedagogy encourages active engagement, which is a crucial and invaluable asset within the PBL framework (Hui et al., 2025). These advanced language models allow users, whether health professional students or seasoned healthcare practitioners, to access precise, real-time information, and receive continuous guidance by working through complex case scenarios. Such process helps to refine both their knowledge base and clinical reasoning skills, mirroring the experiential and social learning elements found in PBL. AI can also support constructivist learning by adapting to individual students' needs, and fostering deeper understanding through self-guided exploration and reflection. By facilitating active participation in knowledge exploration, these systems empower students to engage more deeply with complex medical concepts and to seek out solutions independently. For example, a study by Mohammad-Rahimi et al. (2024) revealed that students using AI-assisted tools performed significantly better in clinical assessments compared to their peers relying solely on traditional methods. PBL requires students to take ownership of their learning by investigating complex issues, collaborating with peers, and applying knowledge to solve problems. This shift promotes deeper understanding and retention of information, ultimately preparing learners for the challenges they will face in clinical practice. Thus AI has proven effective in helping health professional students develop the competencies needed for real-world clinical practice. PBL in health professional programs can be significantly enhanced through the integration of AI into educational strategies, and has gained momentum in recent years (Chen et al., 2024; Divito et al., 2024; Hui et al., 2025) AI, defined as systems capable of performing tasks traditionally requiring human intelligence, has the potential to significantly enhance learning outcomes in PBL.

9.4 Role of AI Chatbots in PBL

Research indicates that PBL enhances not only knowledge acquisition but also the development of essential skills such as communication, teamwork, and adaptability (Kavadella et al., 2024). These competencies are particularly critical in healthcare, where professionals must navigate complex clinical scenarios and collaborate effectively with interdisciplinary teams. The integration of AI into PBL is exemplified through various applications that enhance interactive learning experiences. Case studies have demonstrated the successful implementation of AI chatbots in medical education. Chatbots have emerged as innovative tools in the realm of education, particularly in Problem-Based Learning (PBL) environments. By leveraging artificial intelligence, chatbots can facilitate more interactive and engaging learning experiences, enhancing students' critical thinking and problem-solving skills. In PBL, students are often presented with complex, real-world problems that require them to collaborate and explore multiple solutions. Chatbots can assist in this process by providing instant access to relevant information, resources, and guidance tailored to each student's needs (Chua & Annamalai, 2025).

AI chatbots can adapt to individual learning styles, offering tailored content and resources that cater to diverse learner needs. They serve as virtual tutors, providing personalized feedback and guidance as students engage with clinical cases (Taranikanti & Davidson, 2023). In addition to providing information, chatbots can also simulate patient interactions, enabling students to practice clinical reasoning in a safe environment. For instance, a medical student might interact with a chatbot designed to mimic a patient presenting a set of symptoms. This interaction encourages the student to think critically about differential diagnoses and treatment options, fostering a deeper understanding of clinical practice. The ability to role-play these scenarios allows students to gain valuable experience in a low-stakes setting, preparing them for real-world clinical encounters.

Machine learning algorithms are utilized to tailor educational experiences to individual learners. These algorithms analyse student data, preferences, and learning styles to generate customized learning paths and content recommendations. By giving healthcare personnel improved skills and knowledge, the application of AI in education has the potential to improve patient outcomes. Studies have shown potential benefits of personalized learning, such as increased engagement, improved retention, and enhanced academic outcomes (Nagi et al., 2023).

One of the primary advantages of using chatbots in PBL is their ability to deliver immediate feedback. When students pose questions or seek clarification on specific topics, chatbots can respond in real time with accurate information, helping to clarify concepts and reinforce learning. This rapid feedback loop enables learners to stay engaged and motivated, as they can quickly address their uncertainties without waiting for traditional instructor-led responses. Moreover, chatbots can facilitate self-directed learning by prompting students to explore additional resources, ask deeper questions, and reflect on their understanding. Another significant benefit of chatbots is their capacity to gather and analyse data on student interactions. By tracking how students engage with the chatbot, educators can gain insights into common misconceptions, areas of difficulty, and overall engagement levels. This data can inform curriculum adjustments and help instructors tailor their teaching strategies to better meet students' needs. Additionally, chatbots can provide personalized learning paths, adapting to the unique strengths and weaknesses of each student, thereby enhancing the overall learning experience.

9.4.1 Personalized Learning Experiences Through AI Chatbots

One of the most significant advantages of integrating AI into PBL is the potential for personalized learning experiences (Fig. 9.5). A pedagogical approach known as "adaptive learning" uses AI to modify course material, pace, and evaluations according to each student's development, level of skill, and preferred method of learning. In contrast to conventional static curriculum, adaptive learning environments change as the student does, guaranteeing that the learning process smoothly fits their aptitudes and comprehension. Beyond personalization, AI actively engages students with content at their ideal level of difficulty to avoid boredom or dissatisfaction. This flexibility reflects the individualized character of one-on-one training, resulting in a dynamic and responsive learning environment that is not only efficient but also sensitive to the learner's ever-evolving needs. AI systems can analyze data from students' interactions, identifying strengths and weaknesses to tailor educational content accordingly. This customization is particularly beneficial in healthcare education, where learners come from diverse backgrounds and encounter varied clinical scenarios (Agrawal et al., 2025). Furthermore, personalized learning experiences facilitated by AI can bridge the gap between theoretical knowledge and practical application. By providing learners with tailored resources and support, AI tools can enhance the overall effectiveness of PBL, ensuring that students are well-prepared for the challenges they will face in clinical practice (Kavadella et al., 2024).

The integration of AI chatbots in medical education offers a transformative approach to personalized learning, particularly through PBL. According to Taranikanti and Davidson (2023), AI technologies can tailor educational content to individual student needs, enabling them to focus on specific areas requiring additional practice. This customization is vital for mastering complex medical concepts

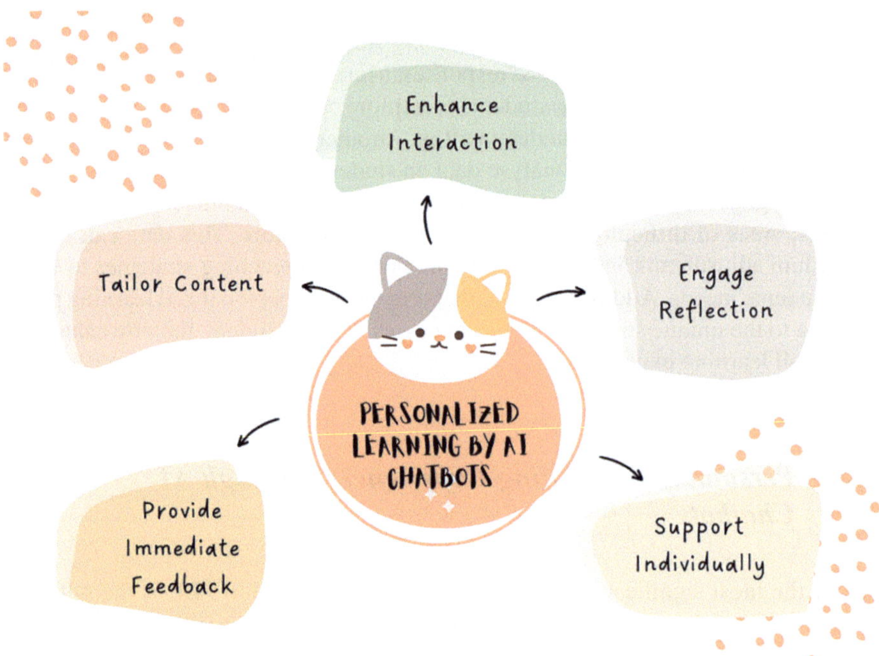

Fig. 9.5 AI chatbots personalize learning through tailoring content, enhancing interaction, encouraging reflection, providing individual support, and delivering immediate feedback

at a self-directed pace, which is essential for the learning environment of today's students, especially those from Generation Z.

AI chatbots promote active engagement by allowing students to explore concepts in real-time and collaboratively solve clinical problems. This interactive format not only enhances critical thinking but also fosters metacognitive skills, which are crucial for effective learning. By reflecting on their understanding and assessing their learning strategies, students can identify their strengths and weaknesses, ultimately leading to more effective study habits and improved retention of knowledge. One of the key advantages of incorporating AI chatbots into PBL is the provision of immediate feedback. When students engage with clinical scenarios, they receive tailored prompts that guide them towards correct diagnoses and treatment plans. This iterative questioning process helps correct misconceptions and reinforces learning, thereby improving clinical reasoning skills essential for future practitioners. Furthermore, the flexible nature of AI chatbots aligns well with the preferences of Gen Z learners, who value personalized and gamified educational experiences. By offering self-paced learning opportunities, AI can accommodate diverse learning styles and needs, making education more accessible and effective.

Hence, integration of AI chatbots within PBL frameworks in medical education provides a significant opportunity for personalized learning. By facilitating immediate feedback, fostering metacognitive awareness, and tailoring educational experiences, AI technologies can enhance students' mastery of complex concepts (Nissen et al., 2025; Hui et al., 2025).

However, the implementation of chatbots in PBL is not without challenges. Concerns about the accuracy and reliability of information provided by chatbots persist, particularly in medical education where up-to-date knowledge is critical. There is a need for robust mechanisms to evaluate and validate the information that chatbots deliver, ensuring that it aligns with current medical guidelines and evidence-based practices (Beck et al., 2024). Furthermore, educators must be cautious about over-reliance on AI tools; while chatbots can be powerful resources, they should complement, not replace, human instructors and the interpersonal aspects of learning.

9.5 AI in Generating Assessments and Automated Evaluation

As educational methodologies continue to evolve, the integration of AI in assessment practices is becoming increasingly significant. AI offers innovative ways to create assessments, provide real-time evaluations, and enhance the overall learning experience for students. One of the most notable advantages of AI in this context is its ability to facilitate self-evaluation, enabling students to gain insights into their own strengths and weaknesses. This self-awareness is critical for fostering a growth mindset and promoting lifelong learning.

For example, AI can provide adaptive assessments that adjust the difficulty level based on a student's performance. Research indicates that personalized learning environments foster greater engagement and motivation, leading to improved educational outcomes (Lee et al., 2024). Additionally, AI tools can offer immediate feedback, allowing learners to correct misunderstandings and reinforce their knowledge in real time. In the health professional education context, AI tools like ChatGPT have revolutionized the preparation process for high-stakes exams like the USMLE (United States Medical Licensing Examination) by offering personalized, on-demand learning assistance. They enable health professional students to access vast amounts of information quickly, clarify complex concepts, and receive tailored feedback based on their strengths and weaknesses. Studies have revealed that ChatGPT's performance on licensure board exams such as USMLE Steps 1, 2, and 3 sample items shows promise, with scores above 60% on Steps 1 and 2, indicating its potential as a learning tool for medical students (Yaneva et al., 2024; Liu et al., 2024; Gilson et al., 2023). This synergy between AI and PBL aligns with the demands of high-stakes exams and realistic professional needs, fostering a deeper, more integrated understanding of medical practice.

AI can automatically generate evaluation reports by analysing various aspects of student performance, including engagement levels, the quality of contributions, and problem-solving skills. By comparing the solutions provided by all participants in a PBL setting, AI can offer a comprehensive analysis that highlights individual and group dynamics. Such evaluations provide teachers with unbiased assessment standards, allowing for more equitable grading practices. Furthermore, students receive immediate feedback on their assignments, which is essential for timely improvement and deeper learning (Divito et al., 2024).

Platforms like Simulated Patient Encounters (SPEs) use machine learning to assess student performance. By comparing student actions to a database of expert clinician actions, the system provides real-time feedback on areas where the student's approach deviates from best practices (Wang et al., 2022). Intelligent Tutoring Systems use AI to provide personalized instruction and feedback. During a simulated patient encounter, ITS can track a student's progress, identify areas where they struggle, and offer targeted feedback and hints. These systems can adapt the simulation's difficulty and complexity based on the student's performance, ensuring that they are appropriately challenged and supported throughout the learning process (VanLehn, 2011). The Cognitive Tutor system by Carnegie Learning is an example of an ITS that offers real-time feedback to students. While traditionally used in other domains, adaptations for health professional education can guide students through complex clinical scenarios, providing hints and explanations tailored to their performance (Koedinger & Aleven, 2007). During a simulated patient encounter, ITS can track a student's progress, identify areas where they struggle, and offer targeted feedback and hints. These systems can adapt the simulation's difficulty and complexity based on the student's performance, ensuring that they are appropriately challenged and supported throughout the learning process (VanLehn, 2011).

9.5.1 *AI-Powered OSCE's in Healthcare Education*

The integration of AI in OSCEs has the potential to transform healthcare education, enabling learners to develop the observation, communication, and evaluation skills necessary for delivering exceptional patient care. By harnessing the power of AI, educators can create a more immersive, interactive, and effective learning experience, ultimately enhancing the quality of care and improving patient outcomes. Platforms like "OSCE AI" use machine learning algorithms to create personalized clinical scenarios, adapting the difficulty and content based on student performance. Natural Language Processing (NLP) can analyze and synthesize vast amounts of clinical data to generate detailed and contextually accurate case scenarios. Tools like IBM's Watson for Health use NLP to provide evidence-based case studies (Bhatt & Peddoju, 2017). Collaborative networks and open access resources enable educators to share and access a wide range of clinical case scenarios, fostering a community of practice and continuous improvement. Open Educational Resources (OER) like MERLOT provide free access to educational materials, including clinical case scenarios developed by educators worldwide (Orr et al., 2015). Professional Network organizations such as the Society for Simulation in Healthcare (SSH) and the International Association for Health Professional Education (AMEE) offer resources and forums for sharing best practices in developing clinical case scenarios (Lyons et al., 2021; Armijo-Rivera et al., 2021). AI driven collaborative networks and open access resources foster a community of practice, ensuring continuous innovation and improvement in the development of clinical case scenarios. By leveraging these resources, educators can create rich and engaging PBL experiences that prepare students for the complexities of clinical practice.

The capability of AI to perform sentiment and visual analysis on students' responses and reactions adds another layer of insight into their learning experiences. By analyzing facial expressions, body language, and even verbal cues, AI can gauge levels of attentiveness and engagement during assessments. This data can be instrumental in predicting future academic outcomes, allowing educators to identify students who may require additional support or targeted interventions (Kurni et al., 2023). Such predictive analytics can lead to timely and effective strategies to help struggling students, ensuring that no one is left behind in the learning process.

9.6 Feedback Mechanisms in PBL

AI's ability to analyze large datasets enables a more individualized approach to medical education, improving the efficiency and equity of assessments. This integration can be particularly beneficial within PBL frameworks, where students engage in real-world scenarios requiring critical thinking and collaboration. By leveraging AI, educators can offer tailored feedback and adaptive learning pathways that align with each student's needs, thus enhancing the PBL experience. The feedback provided by

AI tools grounded in machine learning and computer vision permits a move away from subjective evaluations traditionally employed by mentors.

9.6.1 Objective and Personalized Feedback

Natural language processing tools can analyze trainees' communication patterns, assisting instructors in providing structured, objective assessments of their soft skills—an area traditionally fraught with subjective biases.

AI systems can provide immediate automated feedback on student performance in real-time (Samsonovich et al., 2024). For example, after a simulated patient encounter, AI can analyse the student's approach and suggest areas for improvement. Trainees can receive tailored feedback on their technical skills, allowing them to track progress and focus on specific competencies. This reinforces the PBL methodology of self-directed learning and assessment. Assessments in health professional education face numerous challenges, such as data complexity, resource constraints, and inherent biases, often leading to stressful and inequitable learning environments. In a recent study in academic medicine introduces precision education, a data-driven approach that personalizes the educational experience for each learner. It highlights how AI, including ML and deep learning (DL), can enhance this model by providing consistent, objective assessments and facilitating personalized coaching for at-risk trainees. AI is unbelievably powerful for identifying deep-rooted patterns and limiting beliefs that even good coaches and therapists can miss (CET AI Journal Lisa Turner).

AI-driven feedback systems provide immediate, specific, and actionable feedback, helping students understand their strengths and weaknesses. This immediate feedback is crucial for effective learning, as it allows students to correct mistakes and refine their skills in real-time. For example, if a student misdiagnoses a condition during a simulation, the AI system can provide instant feedback if they miss a critical step in the diagnostic process, explaining the importance of that step and offering guidance on how to correct the error (Kononowicz et al., 2016) or why the diagnosis was incorrect and guide the student toward the correct diagnosis (Braun et al., 2019), notify a student immediately. Simulated patient encounters with AI-driven feedback help students develop and hone their clinical skills in a safe and controlled environment. The immediate feedback provided by AI systems helps students learn from their mistakes and build confidence in their clinical abilities (Cook et al., 2013).

Personalized Learning Pathways: AI-driven systems can create personalized learning pathways for each student based on their performance and learning needs. By analyzing a student's interactions during simulated patient encounters, AI systems can identify specific areas where the student needs improvement and provide tailored resources and practice opportunities. This personalized approach ensures that each student receives the support they need to succeed, enhancing their overall learning experience (Strielkowski et al., 2024). An AI system might track a student's performance over multiple simulations, identifying trends in their clinical reasoning errors and suggesting targeted exercises to address these gaps (Holmes & Tuomi, 2022).

This incorporation encourages a more comprehensive approach to skill assessment within the PBL framework.

9.7 Developing Soft Skills and Communication Through Generative AI

9.7.1 Leveraging AI into Massive Open Online Courses (MOOCs)

The COVID-19 pandemic has catalyzed a significant transformation in medical education, highlighting the urgent need for scalable learning solutions. AI-driven PBL offers a compelling framework to accommodate large numbers of students without a proportional increase in faculty workload. Platforms like Coursera can leverage AI to deliver scalable PBL courses, ensuring consistent quality and personalized feedback for thousands of students simultaneously. During the pandemic, many medical schools faced unprecedented challenges, particularly in low- and middle-income countries where resources are limited. The introduction of Massive Open Online Courses (MOOCs) emerged as a vital educational resource, enabling medical students to access critical knowledge and skills remotely. A study evaluating a COVID-19 MOOC demonstrated that 83% of registered medical students completed the course, reflecting high levels of engagement and satisfaction (Yilmaz et al., 2021). This suggests that MOOCs can effectively reach and educate large student cohorts, particularly when traditional classroom settings are compromised.

The RE-AIM framework (reach, effectiveness, adoption, implementation, maintenance) provides a robust methodology for assessing the impact of educational interventions like MOOCs. In the aforementioned study, the course reached 16,237 unique visitors, underscoring the potential of online platforms to disseminate knowledge on a broad scale. The high completion rates, coupled with positive feedback, indicate that students found the MOOC well-organized and beneficial for their learning.

Furthermore, AI-driven PBL can facilitate collaboration among students from diverse backgrounds and geographical locations. By engaging in project-based activities, students develop critical thinking and problem-solving skills while working in teams. AI can assist in forming balanced groups, ensuring that diverse perspectives are represented and enhancing the overall learning experience. The impact of AI-driven PBL extends beyond immediate educational outcomes; it also plays a crucial role in standardizing educational quality across institutions. In a field where discrepancies in training can have serious implications for patient care, AI-driven solutions can ensure that all students receive the same foundational knowledge, regardless of their institution's resources.

An essential aspect of health professional training includes the mastery of effective communication and interpersonal skills, which are often overlooked. AI-driven real-time feedback in simulated patient encounters offers significant benefits for both students and teachers in medical education. For students, these systems provide immediate, personalized feedback that enhances their learning experience, improves their clinical skills, and supports self-directed learning. Generative AI, particularly LLMs, can play a pivotal role in addressing this gap encouraging teamwork and critical analysis. Generative AI can help create role playing scenarios that simulate patient interactions or team collaborations, allowing trainees to practice their communication skills in a low-risk environment. As trainees navigate these situations, AI can evaluate their responses and provide constructive feedback on their interpersonal skills, enhancing the PBL experience.

9.8 Benefits of Integrating Generative AI into PBL for Facilitators

For teachers, AI-driven feedback systems offer efficient assessment and feedback processes, data-driven insights, and enhanced teaching effectiveness.

9.8.1 Efficient Assessment and Feedback

AI-driven feedback systems can significantly reduce the workload for teachers by automating the assessment and feedback process. Instead of manually reviewing each student's performance during a simulation, teachers can rely on AI systems to provide detailed and accurate feedback highlighting areas of strength and opportunities for improvement, which the teacher can then review and discuss with the student (Guan et al., 2020). AI can enhance the effectiveness of PBL by enabling personalized learning experiences. For example, AI algorithms can analyze students' interactions and performance metrics to identify areas where they struggle, providing tailored resources and feedback. This level of customization not only improves individual learning outcomes but also fosters a sense of engagement and ownership among students. As highlighted in the MOOCs study (Yilmaz et al., 2021), students reported gaining valuable insights into pandemic management, diagnostic algorithms, and health care worker safety, which are all crucial for their future careers.

This efficiency allows teachers to focus on more complex instructional tasks, such as facilitating discussions, providing mentorship, and addressing individual student needs (Tan et al., 2025).

Data-Driven Insights: The vast amounts of data from simulated patient encounters, provides teachers with valuable insights into student performance and learning outcomes.

AI has been used by educationists for automatic recognition of student emotions from facial expressions. In a study (Tonguc et al.) the authors used a software with Microsoft Emotion Recognition API and analyzed different emotions such as sadness, happiness, contempt, anger etc. in a lecture which provided valuable feedback to educators that enabled them to adjust their teaching strategies to enhance student engagement and learning outcomes. These insights can help teachers identify common areas of difficulty, track student progress over time, helping teachers quickly identify trends and make informed decisions about curriculum design, instructional renovation and intervention strategies (Siemens, 2013).

Enhanced Teaching Effectiveness: By providing real-time feedback and personalized learning pathways, AI systems enhance teaching effectiveness by allowing teachers to focus their efforts on areas where they can have the greatest impact. For instance, teachers can use AI-generated insights or iterative AI chatbots to build metacognitive skills and identify students who are struggling and provide targeted interventions, such as additional practice opportunities or one-on-one coaching (Holstein & Aleven, 2022; Taranikanti & Davidson, 2023).

Scalability: The integration of AI in PBL presents a transformative opportunity for medical education. AI-driven PBL can be scaled to accommodate large numbers of students without a proportional increase in faculty workload. This scalability makes it possible to offer high-quality ethics education to more students (Holstein & Aleven, 2022). An online platform like "Coursera" could use AI to deliver scalable PBL courses on medical ethics, providing consistent quality and individualized feedback to thousands of students simultaneously. By leveraging platforms like Coursera, educational institutions can deliver scalable, high-quality learning experiences that not only meet the immediate needs of students during crises but also prepare them for future challenges in healthcare. As we continue to navigate the complexities of modern education, embracing AI-driven solutions will be essential in ensuring that medical students are well-equipped to serve their communities effectively.

9.9 Ethical Considerations and Other Limitations of AI in PBL

Incorporating health AI ethics into PBL is essential as artificial intelligence increasingly influences healthcare practices. This integration allows students to engage with key ethical issues such as informed consent, bias, safety, transparency, patient privacy, and resource allocation in a real-world context. By utilizing case studies that highlight these ethical challenges, PBL can effectively prepare future healthcare professionals to navigate the complexities of health AI, fostering a deep understanding of the ethical implications and responsibilities associated with AI technologies in clinical practice.

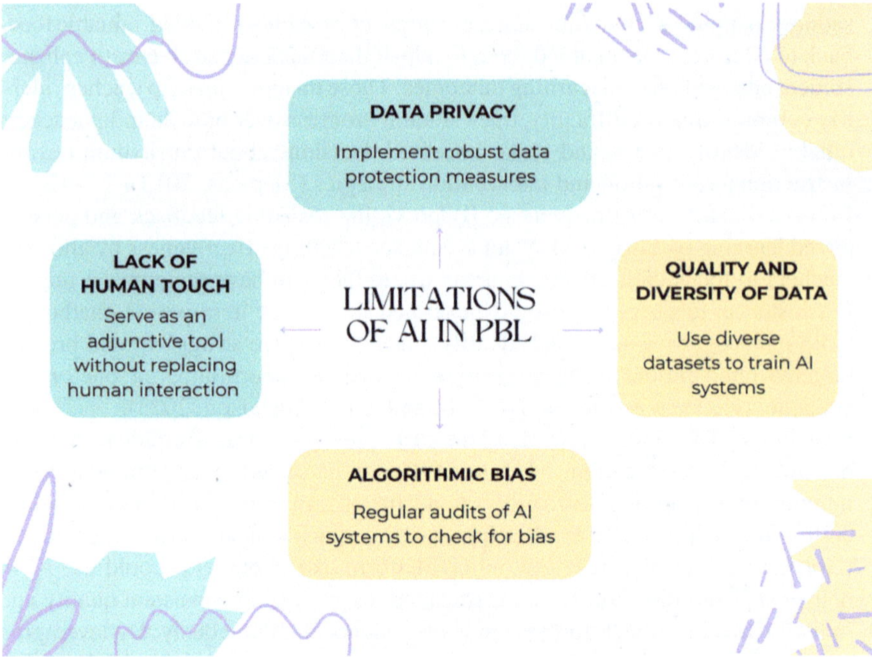

Fig. 9.6 Challenges of adopting AI in PBL include data privacy concerns, the quality and diversity of data, algorithmic bias and the absence of human touch

Despite the potential benefits, there are challenges associated with using AI to provide real-time feedback in simulated patient encounters. These challenges include data privacy concerns, the need for high-quality and diverse datasets, and the potential for algorithmic bias (Fig. 9.6). Addressing these challenges requires ongoing research and collaboration between educators, technologists, and policymakers.

9.9.1 Data Privacy

Educators should address important ethical considerations, including algorithmic transparency and data privacy, which must be carefully managed to avoid bias and ensure fairness. Embracing AI in medical education assessment not only promises to create a more personalized and effective learning environment but also necessitates collaborative and ethical oversight to uphold educational goals and social justice. The integration of AI with PBL represents a strategic opportunity to revolutionize health professions education while addressing the complexities of contemporary learning environments. As educators continue to explore the integration of AI technologies in the classroom, it is essential to address concerns regarding accuracy and reliability, ensuring that these tools serve as effective companions in the learning journey. Ultimately, the successful incorporation of chatbots into PBL can prepare students to navigate the complexities of clinical practice with confidence and competence.

Ensuring the privacy and security of student data is paramount. AI systems often require access to large amounts of data to function effectively, raising concerns about data privacy and security. Educational institutions must implement robust data protection measures and comply with relevant regulations, such as the General Data Protection Regulation and the Family Educational Rights and Privacy Act (FERPA) (Jeelani et al., 2024). Institutions can employ encryption and anonymization techniques to protect student data while allowing AI systems to analyze performance and provide feedback.

9.9.2 Quality and Diversity of Data

AI systems rely on high-quality, diverse datasets to function effectively. Ensuring that these datasets are representative of all student populations is crucial to avoid biases and ensure equitable learning outcomes. It could lead to skewed feedback and reinforcement of unethical practices if the training data is not representative of diverse ethical perspectives. Continuous monitoring and evaluation of AI algorithms are necessary to identify and mitigate biases, ensuring fair and equitable learning experiences for all students. Developers can use diverse datasets that include a wide range of patient cases and student interactions to train AI systems, reducing the risk of bias and ensuring the system is effective across different demographic groups (Holstein et al., 2019).

9.9.3 Algorithmic Bias

AI systems can inadvertently perpetuate existing biases in educational systems. Continuous monitoring and evaluation of AI algorithms are necessary to identify and mitigate biases, ensuring fair and equitable learning experiences for all students. Techniques such as fairness-aware machine learning and bias detection algorithms can help mitigate these issues. Implementing regular audits of AI systems to check for bias and adjusting algorithms as needed can help ensure equitable treatment of all students (Chin et al., 2023).

9.9.4 Limitations in Healthcare Education

Despite its promising accuracy in certain domains, AI's performance in the context of healthcare education is not without limitations, particularly when it comes to the complexity and variability inherent in real-world clinical decision-making. This is especially evident in high-stakes examinations that incorporate simulation components, where nuanced understanding and adaptability are crucial. The variability in AI's accuracy across different question types raises questions about how effectively these resources can be utilized in educational settings, particularly within medical school curricula focused on practice-based learning. This highlights the necessity for expert validation and a nuanced approach to integrating AI into health professional education, ensuring that the technology complements rather than replaces critical thinking and clinical judgment.

Curriculum designers face significant challenges when attempting to balance the integration of generative AI within academia, particularly in health professional education. The contentious nature of AI usage raises ethical concerns regarding potential misuse, cheating, and privacy issues, compelling educators to carefully consider the implications of AI in their teaching practices. The use of AI in this context is contentious, with ethical concerns about misuse, potential abuse, cheating, and privacy issues prompting educators to consider the best ways to incorporate this technology into their teaching practice (Bohler et al., 2024). As this chapter explores the current applications of AI in preclinical medical education and surgical training, it also investigates the future directions of AI-enhanced PBL. By addressing these challenges, the chapter aims to provide an in-depth analysis of how AI can transform PBL, creating more effective and personalized learning experiences while maintaining ethical standards and fostering critical thinking among students.

9.9.5 Technical Limitations

An AI system trained on a limited set of ethical scenarios might not adequately cover the full range of issues students need to understand, leading to gaps in their education. AI systems are only as good as the data they are trained on and the algorithms that power them. Inaccurate or biased data can lead to flawed simulations and feedback, potentially reinforcing incorrect ethical principles (Andersson et al., 2022). For example, an AI system trained on a limited set of ethical scenarios might not adequately cover the full range of issues students need to understand, leading to gaps in their education. Developing and maintaining AI-driven PBL systems requires significant resources, including technological infrastructure, skilled personnel, and ongoing maintenance. These requirements can be a barrier for some educational institutions.

9.9.6 Lack of Human Touch

While AI can simulate many aspects of ethical decision-making, it lacks the nuanced understanding and empathy that human educators provide. The absence of a human touch in ethical discussions can limit the depth and richness of the learning experience (Ghosh & Jermsittiparsert, 2024). AI might struggle to fully appreciate and respond to the emotional complexities involved in scenarios like end-of-life care decisions, which require deep empathy and understanding. As AI becomes more integral to medical and surgical education, it is critical to address the ethical implications and limitations of these technologies. The introduction of AI should never replace the essential mentorship and human interaction that is foundational to training. Instead, AI should serve as an adjunctive tool to augment existing curricula, ultimately leading to the development of safe, competent, and compassionate surgeons.

9.9.7 Conclusion

The incorporation of AI into education represents an exciting frontier that can enrich the traditional apprenticeship model. Through the lens of PBL, AI technologies can enhance the educational experience by providing objective assessments, personalized feedback, and opportunities to practice essential soft skills. By combining the strengths of PBL with AI's ability to provide personalized, on-demand learning, educators can help students refine their clinical reasoning and problem-solving skills more effectively, preparing them for the complexities of modern medical practice. Therefore, while AI can be a valuable supplementary tool in PBL, educators must combine it with expert validation and active learning strategies to ensure students develop the critical thinking and clinical reasoning.

As we continue to explore these advancements, its integration into medical education will likely become increasingly sophisticated, further improving the quality and effectiveness of clinical training. A thoughtful approach to ethics and mentorship will ensure that we foster the next generation of leaders who are equipped not only with knowledge, clinical and technical skills but also with the communication and empathy needed in patient care (Fig. 9.7).

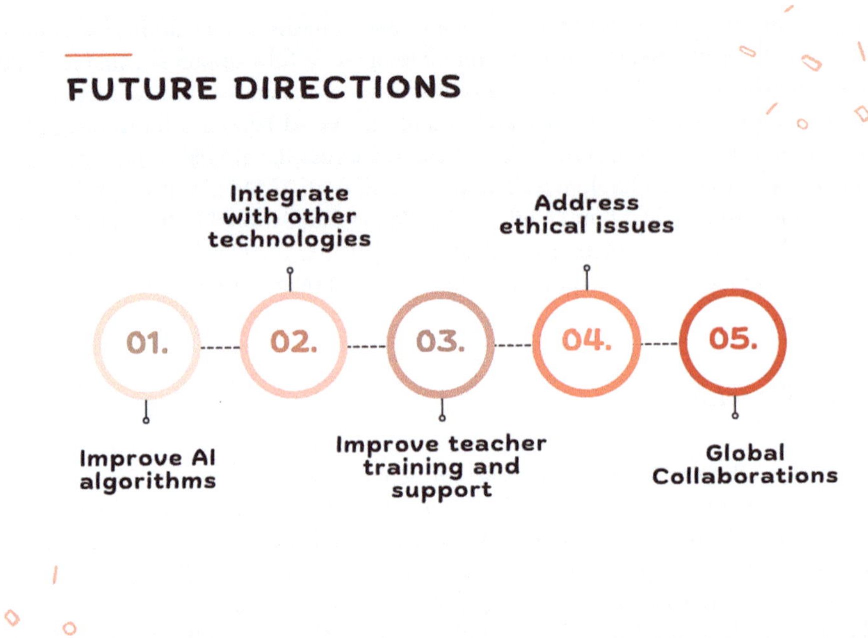

Fig. 9.7 Future directions for AI use in PBL will focus on enhancing AI algorithms, integrating with other emerging technologies, improving teacher training and support, addressing ethical issues, and promoting global collaboration

References

Agrawal, A., Gupta, G., Agrawal, A., & Gupta, H. (2025). Evaluating diversity and stereotypes amongst AI generated representations of healthcare providers. *Frontiers in Digital Health, 7*, 1537907. https://doi.org/10.3389/fdgth.2025.1537907

Amato, F., Marrone, S., Moscato, V., Piantadosi, G., Picariello, A., & Sansone, C. (2019). HOLMeS: eHealth in the big data and deep learning era. *Information, 10*(2), 34. https://doi.org/10.3390/info10020034

Andersson, H., Svensson, A., Frank, C., Rantala, A., Holmberg, M., & Bremer, A. (2022). Ethics education to support ethical competence learning in healthcare: An integrative systematic review. *BMC Medical Ethics, 23*(1), 29. https://doi.org/10.1186/s12910-022-00766-z

Armijo-Rivera, S., Machuca-Contreras, F., Raul, N., De Oliveira, S. N., Mendoza, I. B., Miyasato, H. S., & Díaz-Guio, D. A. (2021). Characterization of simulation centers and programs in Latin America according to the ASPIRE and SSH quality criteria. *Advances in Simulation, 6*(1), 41. https://doi.org/10.1186/s41077-021-00188-8

Atta, I. S., & Alghamdi, A. H. (2018). The efficacy of self-directed learning versus problem-based learning for teaching and learning ophthalmology: A comparative study. *Advances in Medical Education and Practice, 9*, 623–630. https://doi.org/10.2147/AMEP.S171328

Auguste, D. (1985). Intelligent tutoring systems. *Artificial Intelligence, 26*(2), 233–238. https://doi.org/10.1016/0004-3702(85)90033-5

Bakkum, M. J., Hartjes, M. G., Piët, J. D., Donker, E. M., Likic, R., Sanz, E., de Ponti, F., Verdonk, P., Richir, M. C., van Agtmael, M. A., & Tichelaar, J. (2024). Using artificial intelligence to create diverse and inclusive medical case vignettes for education. *British Journal of Clinical Pharmacology, 90*(3), 640–648. https://doi.org/10.1111/bcp.15977

Beck, S., Kuhner, M., Haar, M., Daubmann, A., Semmann, M., & Kluge, S. (2024). Evaluating the accuracy and reliability of AI chatbots in disseminating the content of current resuscitation guidelines: A comparative analysis between the ERC 2021 guidelines and both ChatGPTs 3.5 and 4. *Scandinavian Journal of Trauma, Resuscitation and Emergency Medicine, 32*(1), 95. https://doi.org/10.1186/s13049-024-01266-2

Bhatt, C. M., & Peddoju, S. K. (Eds.). (2017). *Cloud computing systems and applications in healthcare*. IGI Global. https://doi.org/10.4018/978-1-5225-1002-4

Bodonhelyi, A., Thaqi, E., Özdel, S., Bozkir, E., & Kasneci, E. (2025). From passive watching to active learning: Empowering proactive participation in digital classrooms with AI video assistant. In *Proceedings of the 2025 CHI Conference on Human Factors in Computing Systems* (pp. 1–21). https://doi.org/10.1145/3706598.3713513

Bohler, F., Aggarwal, N., Peters, G., & Taranikanti, V. (2024). Future implications of artificial intelligence in medical education. *Cureus, 16*(1), e51859. https://doi.org/10.7759/cureus.51859

Braun, L. T., Borrmann, K. F., Lottspeich, C., Heinrich, D. A., Kiesewetter, J., Fischer, M. R., & Schmidmaier, R. (2019). Guessing right—Whether and how medical students give incorrect reasons for their correct diagnoses. *GMS Journal for Medical Education, 36*(6), Doc85. https://doi.org/10.3205/zma001293

Carbonell, J. (1970). AI in CAI: An artificial-intelligence approach to computer-assisted instruction. *IEEE Transactions on Man Machine Systems, 11*(4), 190–202. https://doi.org/10.1109/TMMS.1970.299942

Chang, E. Y. (2017). DeepQ: Advancing healthcare through artificial intelligence and virtual reality. In *Proceedings of the 25th ACM International Conference on Multimedia* (p. 1068). https://doi.org/10.1145/3123266.3130875

Chen, Y., Qi, H., Qiu, Y., Li, J., Zhu, L., Gao, X., Wang, H., & Jiang, G. (2024). Artificial intelligence in medical problem-based learning: Opportunities and challenges. *Global Medical Education*. https://doi.org/10.1515/gme-2024-0015

Chin, M. H., Afsar-Manesh, N., Bierman, A. S., Chang, C., Colón-Rodríguez, C. J., Dullabh, P., Duran, D. G., Fair, M., Hernandez-Boussard, T., Hightower, M., Jain, A., Jordan, W. B., Konya, S., Moore, R. H., Moore, T. T., Rodriguez, R., Shaheen, G., Snyder, L. P., Srinivasan, M., et al. (2023). Guiding principles to address the impact of algorithm bias on racial and ethnic disparities in health and health care. *JAMA Network Open, 6*(12), e2345050. https://doi.org/10.1001/jamanetworkopen.2023.45050

Chiu, M.-C., Chiang, Y.-H., & Chiu, J.-E. (2024). Developing an explainable hybrid deep learning model in digital transformation: An empirical study. *Journal of Intelligent Manufacturing, 35*(4), 1793–1810. https://doi.org/10.1007/s10845-023-02127-y

Chua, H. W., & Annamalai, N. (2025). A bibliometric analysis and systematic review in AI chatbots in language teaching and learning. *International Journal of Technology in Education, 8*(2), 274–331. https://doi.org/10.46328/ijte.1035

Cook, D. A., Brydges, R., Zendejas, B., Hamstra, S. J., & Hatala, R. (2013). Technology-enhanced simulation to assess health professionals: A systematic review of validity evidence, research methods, and reporting quality. *Academic Medicine, 88*(6), 872–883. https://doi.org/10.1097/ACM.0b013e31828ffdcf

Davila, U., & Price, A. (2025). Past present and future of simulation in pediatrics. In *StatPearls*. StatPearls Publishing. Retrieved from http://www.ncbi.nlm.nih.gov/books/NBK559082/

Davis, F. D. (1989). Perceived usefulness, perceived ease of use, and user acceptance of information technology. *MIS Quarterly, 13*(3), 319. https://doi.org/10.2307/249008

Divito, C. B., Katchikian, B. M., Gruenwald, J. E., & Burgoon, J. M. (2024). The tools of the future are the challenges of today: The use of ChatGPT in problem-based learning medical education. *Medical Teacher, 46*(3), 320–322. https://doi.org/10.1080/0142159X.2023.2290997

Farinacci, E. (2024). Film and audiovisual education in the artificial intelligence era: Approaches and challenges. *Cinergie—Il Cinema e Le Altre Arti, 13*(26), 121–133. https://doi.org/10.6092/ISSN.2280-9481/19386

Ferguson, J. S., Van Wert, R., Choi, Y., Rosenbluth, M. J., Smith, K. P., Huang, J., & Spira, A. (2016). Impact of a bronchial genomic classifier on clinical decision making in patients undergoing diagnostic evaluation for lung cancer. *BMC Pulmonary Medicine, 16*(1), 66. https://doi.org/10.1186/s12890-016-0217-1

Garcia, M. B., & Garcia, P. S. (2023). Intelligent tutoring system as an instructional technology in learning basic nutrition concepts: An exploratory sequential mixed methods study. In M. B. Garcia, M. V. Lopez Cabrera, & R. P. P. De Almeida (Eds.), *Advances in medical education, research, and ethics* (pp. 265–284). IGI Global. https://doi.org/10.4018/978-1-6684-7164-7.ch012

Ghosh, U. K., & Jermsittiparsert, K. (2024). Personalised learning systems and the human touch in society 5.0. In K. Jermsittiparsert, I. S. Wekke, & P. Suanpang (Eds.), *Practice, progress, and proficiency in sustainability* (pp. 211–232). IGI Global. https://doi.org/10.4018/979-8-3693-7989-9.ch012

Gilbert, A., Carnell, S., Lok, B., & Miles, A. (2024). Using virtual patients to support empathy training in health care education: An exploratory study. *Simulation in Healthcare: The Journal of the Society for Simulation in Healthcare, 19*(3), 151–157. https://doi.org/10.1097/SIH.0000000000000742

Gilson, A., Safranek, C. W., Huang, T., Socrates, V., Chi, L., Taylor, R. A., & Chartash, D. (2023). How does ChatGPT perform on the United States Medical Licensing Examination (USMLE)? The implications of large language models for medical education and knowledge assessment. *JMIR Medical Education, 9*, e45312. https://doi.org/10.2196/45312

Guan, C., Mou, J., & Jiang, Z. (2020). Artificial intelligence innovation in education: A twenty-year data-driven historical analysis. *International Journal of Innovation Studies, 4*(4), 134–147. https://doi.org/10.1016/j.ijis.2020.09.001

Hmelo-Silver, C. E., & Eberbach, C. (2012). Learning theories and problem-based learning. In S. Bridges, C. McGrath, & T. L. Whitehill (Eds.), *Problem-based learning in clinical education* (pp. 3–17). Springer. https://doi.org/10.1007/978-94-007-2515-7_1

Holmes, W., & Tuomi, I. (2022). State of the art and practice in AI in education. *European Journal of Education, 57*(4), 542–570. https://doi.org/10.1111/ejed.12533

Holstein, K., & Aleven, V. (2022). Designing for human–AI complementarity in K-12 education. *AI Magazine, 43*(2), 239–248. https://doi.org/10.1002/aaai.12058

Holstein, K., Wortman Vaughan, J., Daumé, H., Dudik, M., & Wallach, H. (2019). Improving fairness in machine learning systems: What do industry practitioners need? In *Proceedings of the 2019 CHI Conference on Human Factors in Computing Systems* (pp. 1–16). https://doi.org/10.1145/3290605.3300830

Hui, Z., Zewu, Z., Jiao, H., & Yu, C. (2025). Application of ChatGPT-assisted problem-based learning teaching method in clinical medical education. *BMC Medical Education, 25*(1), 50. https://doi.org/10.1186/s12909-024-06321-1

Javaid, M., Haleem, A., Pratap Singh, R., Suman, R., & Rab, S. (2022). Significance of machine learning in healthcare: Features, pillars and applications. *International Journal of Intelligent Networks, 3*, 58–73. https://doi.org/10.1016/j.ijin.2022.05.002

Jeelani, O. F., Njie, M., & Korzhuk, V. (2024). Methods and algorithms of ensuring data privacy in AI-based healthcare systems and technologies. *Studies in Health Technology and Informatics, 316*, 1260–1261. https://doi.org/10.3233/SHTI240640

Katz, A., Norris, M., Alsharif, A., Klopfer, M., Knight, D., & Grohs, J. (2021). Using natural language processing to facilitate student feedback analysis. In *2021 ASEE Virtual Annual Conference Content Access Proceedings* (p. 37994). https://doi.org/10.18260/1-2-37994

Kavadella, A., Dias Da Silva, M. A., Kaklamanos, E. G., Stamatopoulos, V., & Giannakopoulos, K. (2024). Evaluation of ChatGPT's real-life implementation in undergraduate dental education: Mixed methods study. *JMIR Medical Education, 10*, e51344. https://doi.org/10.2196/51344

Kıyak, Y. S., & Emekli, E. (2024). ChatGPT prompts for generating multiple-choice questions in medical education and evidence on their validity: A literature review. *Postgraduate Medical Journal, 100*(1189), 858–865. https://doi.org/10.1093/postmj/qgae065

Koedinger, K. R., & Aleven, V. (2007). Exploring the assistance dilemma in experiments with cognitive tutors. *Educational Psychology Review, 19*(3), 239–264. https://doi.org/10.1007/s10648-007-9049-0

Kononowicz, A. A., Woodham, L., Georg, C., Edelbring, S., Stathakarou, N., Davies, D., Masiello, I., Saxena, N., Tudor Car, L., Car, J., & Zary, N. (2016). Virtual patient simulations for health professional education. *Cochrane Database of Systematic Reviews*. https://doi.org/10.1002/14651858.CD012194

Kumar, T., Soozandehfar, S. M. A., Hashemifardnia, A., & Mombeini, R. (2023). Self vs. peer assessment activities in EFL-speaking classes: Impacts on students' self-regulated learning, critical thinking, and problem-solving skills. *Language Testing in Asia, 13*(1), 36. https://doi.org/10.1186/s40468-023-00251-3

Kurni, M., Mohammed, M. S., & K G, S. (2023). *A beginner's guide to introduce artificial intelligence in teaching and learning*. Springer International Publishing. https://doi.org/10.1007/978-3-031-32653-0

Leary, H., Walker, A., Lefler, M., & Kuo, Y. (2019). Self-directed learning in problem-based learning: A literature review. In M. Moallem, W. Hung, & N. Dabbagh (Eds.), *The Wiley handbook of problem-based learning* (1st ed., pp. 181–198). Wiley. https://doi.org/10.1002/9781119173243.ch8

Lee, H.-Y., Chen, P.-H., Wang, W.-S., Huang, Y.-M., & Wu, T.-T. (2024). Empowering ChatGPT with guidance mechanism in blended learning: Effect of self-regulated learning, higher-order thinking skills, and knowledge construction. *International Journal of Educational Technology in Higher Education, 21*(1), 16. https://doi.org/10.1186/s41239-024-00447-4

Li, P.-H., Lee, H.-Y., Lin, C.-J., Wang, W.-S., & Huang, Y.-M. (2025). InquiryGPT: Augmenting ChatGPT for enhancing inquiry-based learning in STEM education. *Journal of Educational Computing Research, 62*(8), 1937–1966. https://doi.org/10.1177/07356331241289824

Liu, M., Okuhara, T., Chang, X., Shirabe, R., Nishiie, Y., Okada, H., & Kiuchi, T. (2024). Performance of ChatGPT across different versions in medical licensing examinations worldwide: Systematic review and meta-analysis. *Journal of Medical Internet Research, 26*, e60807. https://doi.org/10.2196/60807

Lok, B., & Foster, A. E. (2019). Can virtual humans teach empathy? In A. E. Foster & Z. S. Yaseen (Eds.), *Teaching empathy in healthcare* (pp. 143–163). Springer International Publishing. https://doi.org/10.1007/978-3-030-29876-0_9

Lopez, I., Swaminathan, A., Vedula, K., Narayanan, S., Nateghi Haredasht, F., Ma, S. P., Liang, A. S., Tate, S., Maddali, M., Gallo, R. J., Shah, N. H., & Chen, J. H. (2025). Clinical entity augmented retrieval for clinical information extraction. *Npj Digital Medicine, 8*(1), 45. https://doi.org/10.1038/s41746-024-01377-1

Loyens, S. M. M., Magda, J., & Rikers, R. M. J. P. (2008). Self-directed learning in problem-based learning and its relationships with self-regulated learning. *Educational Psychology Review, 20*(4), 411–427. https://doi.org/10.1007/s10648-008-9082-7

Lyons, K. M., Cain, J. J., Haines, S. T., Gasevic, D., & Brock, T. P. (2021). The clinical educator's guide to fostering learner motivation: AMEE Guide No. 137. *Medical Teacher, 43*(5), 492–500. https://doi.org/10.1080/0142159X.2020.1837764

McGaghie, W. C., Barsuk, J. H., Wayne, D. B., & Issenberg, S. B. (2024). Powerful medical education improves health care quality and return on investment. *Medical Teacher, 46*(1), 46–58. https://doi.org/10.1080/0142159X.2023.2276038

Meguerdichian, D. A. (2021). Mannequin simulators. In C. Strother, Y. Okuda, N. Wong, & S. McLaughlin (Eds.), *Comprehensive healthcare simulation: Emergency medicine* (pp. 123–144). Springer International Publishing. https://doi.org/10.1007/978-3-030-57367-6_12

Mesko, B. (2023). The ChatGPT (Generative Artificial Intelligence) revolution has made artificial intelligence approachable for medical professionals. *Journal of Medical Internet Research, 25*, e48392. https://doi.org/10.2196/48392

Mohammad-Rahimi, H., Sohrabniya, F., Ourang, S. A., Dianat, O., Aminoshariae, A., Nagendrababu, V., Dummer, P. M. H., Duncan, H. F., Nosrat, A. (2024). Artificial intelligence in endodontics: Data preparation, clinical applications, ethical considerations, limitations, and future directions. *International Endodontic Journal, 57*(11), 1566–1595. https://doi.org/10.1111/iej.14128. Epub 2024 Jul 29. PMID: 39075670.

Nagi, F., Salih, R., Alzubaidi, M., Shah, H., Alam, T., Shah, Z., & Househ, M. (2023). Applications of artificial intelligence (AI) in medical education: A scoping review. *Studies in Health Technology and Informatics, 305*, 648–651. https://doi.org/10.3233/SHTI230581

Nahass, G. R., Chin, S. W., Scharf, I. M., Kazmouz, S., Kaplan, N., Chiu, R., Yang, K., Bou Zeid, N., Corcoran, J., & Alkureishi, L. W. T. (2024). Prompt engineering to increase GPT3.5's performance on the Plastic Surgery In-Service Exams. *Journal of Plastic, Reconstructive & Aesthetic Surgery, 98*, 158–160. https://doi.org/10.1016/j.bjps.2024.09.001

Nissen, L., Rother, J. F., Heinemann, M., Reimer, L. M., Jonas, S., & Raupach, T. (2025). A randomised cross-over trial assessing the impact of AI-generated individual feedback on written online assignments for medical students. *Medical Teacher*, 1–7. https://doi.org/10.1080/0142159X.2025.2451870

Orr, D., Rimini, M., Van Damme, D., & Organisation for Economic Co-operation and Development. (2015). *Open educational resources: A catalyst for innovation.* OECD Publishing.

Rumelhart, D. E., Hinton, G. E., & Williams, R. J. (1986). Learning representations by back-propagating errors. *Nature, 323*(6088), 533–536. https://doi.org/10.1038/323533a0

Samsonovich, A. V., Kitsantas, A., Wahidi, S., & Dolgikh, A. A. (2024). Self-regulated learning (SRL) with AI in problem-based learning. In A. V. Samsonovich & T. Liu (Eds.), *Biologically inspired cognitive architectures 2024* (Vol. 477, pp. 345–357). Springer Nature. https://doi.org/10.1007/978-3-031-76516-2_34

Sayed, W. S., Noeman, A. M., Abdellatif, A., Abdelrazek, M., Badawy, M. G., Hamed, A., & El-Tantawy, S. (2023). AI-based adaptive personalized content presentation and exercises navigation for an effective and engaging E-learning platform. *Multimedia Tools and Applications, 82*(3), 3303–3333. https://doi.org/10.1007/s11042-022-13076-8

Sharma, A., Lin, I. W., Miner, A. S., Atkins, D. C., & Althoff, T. (2023). Human–AI collaboration enables more empathic conversations in text-based peer-to-peer mental health support. *Nature Machine Intelligence, 5*(1), 46–57. https://doi.org/10.1038/s42256-022-00593-2

Siemens, G. (2013). Learning analytics: The emergence of a discipline. *American Behavioral Scientist, 57*(10), 1380–1400. https://doi.org/10.1177/0002764213498851

Sinha, S., Rogat, T. K., Adams-Wiggins, K. R., & Hmelo-Silver, C. E. (2015). Collaborative group engagement in a computer-supported inquiry learning environment. *International Journal of Computer-Supported Collaborative Learning, 10*(3), 273–307. https://doi.org/10.1007/s11412-015-9218-y

Sparling, J. L., & Cooper, J. B. (2024). Teamwork and communication simulation to improve safety in the OR. In J. J. Hoballah, H. M. Kaafarani, & G. Tsoulfas (Eds.), *Principles of perioperative safety and efficiency* (pp. 229–250). Springer International Publishing. https://doi.org/10.1007/978-3-031-41089-5_14

Strielkowski, W., Grebennikova, V., Lisovskiy, A., Rakhimova, G., & Vasileva, T. (2024). AI-driven adaptive learning for sustainable educational transformation. *Sustainable Development*, sd.3221. https://doi.org/10.1002/sd.3221

Sun, H., Song, Y., Liu, J., Hu, J., Chen, Y.-W., & Lin, L. (2024). *One framework to rule them all: Unifying multimodal tasks with LLM neural-tuning (Version 2).* arXiv: https://doi.org/10.48550/ARXIV.2408.03001.

Tagliaferri, L., Fionda, B., Casà, C., Cornacchione, P., Scalise, S., Chiesa, S., Marconi, E., Dinapoli, L., Di Capua, B., Chieffo, D. P. R., Marazzi, F., Frascino, V., Colloca, G. F., Valentini, V., Miccichè, F., & Gambacorta, M. A. (2025). Allies not enemies—Creating a more empathetic and uplifting patient experience through technology and art. *Strahlentherapie Und Onkologie, 201*(3), 316–332. https://doi.org/10.1007/s00066-024-02279-7

Tan, X., Cheng, G., & Ling, M. H. (2025). Artificial intelligence in teaching and teacher professional development: A systematic review. *Computers and Education: Artificial Intelligence, 8*, 100355. https://doi.org/10.1016/j.caeai.2024.100355

Tang, F. M. K., Lee, R. M. F., Szeto, R. H. L., Cheung, J. C. T., & Ngan, O. M. Y. (2020). Experiential learning with virtual reality: Animal handling training. *Innovation and Education, 2*(1), 2. https://doi.org/10.1186/s42862-020-00007-3

Taranikanti, V., & Davidson, C. J. (2023). Metacognition through an iterative anatomy AI Chatbot: An innovative playing field for educating the future generation of medical students. *Anatomia, 2*(3), 271–281. https://doi.org/10.3390/anatomia2030025

VanLehn, K. (2011). The relative effectiveness of human tutoring, intelligent tutoring systems, and other tutoring systems. *Educational Psychologist, 46*(4), 197–221. https://doi.org/10.1080/00461520.2011.611369

Wang, M., Sun, Z., Jia, M., Wang, Y., Wang, H., Zhu, X., Chen, L., & Ji, H. (2022). Intelligent virtual case learning system based on real medical records and natural language processing. *BMC Medical Informatics and Decision Making, 22*(1), 60. https://doi.org/10.1186/s12911-022-01797-7

Wang, X.-M., Huang, X.-T., Han, Y.-H., & Hu, Q.-N. (2024). Promoting students' creative self-efficacy, critical thinking and learning performance: An online interactive peer assessment approach guided by constructivist theory in maker activities. *Thinking Skills and Creativity, 52*, 101548. https://doi.org/10.1016/j.tsc.2024.101548

Won, M., Ungu, D. A. K., Matovu, H., Treagust, D. F., Tsai, C.-C., Park, J., Mocerino, M., & Tasker, R. (2023). Diverse approaches to learning with immersive virtual reality identified from a systematic review. *Computers & Education, 195*, 104701. https://doi.org/10.1016/j.compedu.2022.104701

Wong, L.-W., Tan, G. W.-H., Ooi, K.-B., Hew, J.-J., & Dwivedi, Y. K. (2024). Editorial: Generative artificial intelligence in the creator economy. *Online Information Review, 48*(7), 1515–1521. https://doi.org/10.1108/OIR-11-2024-694

Yaneva, V., Baldwin, P., Jurich, D. P., Swygert, K., & Clauser, B. E. (2024). Examining ChatGPT performance on USMLE sample items and implications for assessment. *Academic Medicine, 99*(2), 192–197. https://doi.org/10.1097/ACM.0000000000005549

Yilmaz, Y., Sarikaya, O., Senol, Y., Baykan, Z., Karaca, O., Demiral Yilmaz, N., Altintas, L., Onan, A., & Sayek, İ. (2021). RE-AIMing COVID-19 online learning for medical students: A massive open online course evaluation. *BMC Medical Education, 21*(1), 303. https://doi.org/10.1186/s12909-021-02751-3

Zhang, K., & Aslan, A. B. (2021). AI technologies for education: Recent research & future directions. *Computers and Education: Artificial Intelligence, 2*, 100025. https://doi.org/10.1016/j.caeai.2021.100025

Zhang, S. M., Wang, Y. J., & Zhang, S. T. (2021). Accuracy of artificial intelligence-assisted detection of esophageal cancer and neoplasms on endoscopic images: A systematic review and meta-analysis. *Journal of Digestive Diseases, 22*(6), 318–328. https://doi.org/10.1111/1751-2980.12992

Zidoun, Y., & Mardi, A. E. (2024). Artificial intelligence (AI)-based simulators versus simulated patients in undergraduate programs: A protocol for a randomized controlled trial. *BMC Medical Education, 24*(1), 1260. https://doi.org/10.1186/s12909-024-06236-x

Chapter 10
Implementation of Problem-Based Learning: Challenges and Successes

Mark Coty

10.1 Introduction to Problem-Based Learning Implementation

Embarking on the journey of implementing Problem-Based Learning (PBL) is akin to navigating uncharted waters, replete with both exhilarating opportunities and formidable obstacles. PBL, as an educational approach, distinguishes itself by prioritizing the cultivation of skills through focused engagement (Ungaretti et al., 2014). The core tenet of PBL lies in empowering students to collaboratively explore and construct projects that showcase their understanding, thereby fostering autonomy, constructive inquiry, goal-setting, communication, and reflection within authentic, real-world contexts (Bell, 2010; Kokotsaki et al., 2016). Within the realm of professional education, medical schools stand out as pioneers in embracing PBL, demonstrating its extensive and enduring application (Ungaretti et al., 2014). Nonetheless, this learning approach can be adapted to any educational program, including those in health professions such as dental, pharmacy, nursing, physical therapy and physician assistant.

Amidst the growing enthusiasm for PBL, researchers have meticulously examined its implementation in diverse settings, from primary to higher education. However, despite the recognized potential of PBL, its widespread adoption and successful implementation have been hampered by various challenges, necessitating a thorough examination of both the impediments and the pathways to realizing its full promise. In contrast to traditional curricula where teachers act as the main source of information, PBL necessitates that instructors encourage critical thinking, foster self-directed learning, monitor group progress, and create a learning environment that stimulates teamwork and generates deep understanding (Azer, 2005). The success of PBL hinges on careful planning, committed faculty, suitable resources, and a

M. Coty (✉)
Orlando College of Osteopathic Medicine, Winter Garden, FL, USA
e-mail: mcoty@ocom.org

S. Lorenzo and B. Zhang (eds.), *Mastering Problem-Based Learning in Health Profession Programs*, https://doi.org/10.1007/978-3-032-05405-0_10

supportive institutional culture, necessitating institutions to confront practical and conceptual challenges (Azer, 2011). Overcoming these challenges is essential to harness the power of PBL in fostering critical thinking, problem-solving, and lifelong learning skills among students.

This chapter examines the nuanced landscape of PBL implementation, exploring both the challenges and triumphs that have emerged from various scholarly investigations, to help institutions seeking to realize the transformative potential of this learner-centered approach and adopt a meaningful PBL program.

10.2 The Integral Role of Leadership Commitment in PBL Implementation

The successful implementation of PBL is heavily reliant on strong leadership commitment, which serves as the bedrock for fostering a culture of innovation and collaboration (Azer, 2011). This commitment must permeate all levels of the institution, from administrators to faculty members, to ensure that PBL is not viewed as a mere add-on but rather as an integral component of the educational ecosystem. Sustained support from leadership provides the necessary resources, infrastructure, and incentives for faculty to embrace PBL, invest in professional development, and collaborate effectively (Rehman et al., 2024).

Good leaders direct, and great leaders empower and support. The commitment of leadership entails providing sufficient time and resources for faculty training, curriculum development, and assessment design, which are essential for the effective implementation of PBL (Kokotsaki et al., 2016). In addition, leaders must champion PBL by recognizing and rewarding faculty contributions to PBL initiatives, showcasing successful PBL projects, and fostering a culture of continuous improvement. Leadership support is also essential for navigating institutional barriers and garnering buy-in from stakeholders, including students, parents, faculty, staff, and the wider community. To ensure that PBL implementation aligns with institutional objectives and to track its effectiveness, leaders must also establish well-defined goals, metrics, and accountability frameworks (Pinthong & Chaisongmuang, 2019). Moreover, leadership should proactively cultivate and incentivize interdisciplinary collaboration among faculty members, acknowledging that real-world problems often transcend disciplinary boundaries and necessitate a synthesis of diverse perspectives and specialized knowledge (Fig. 10.1).

Without strong leadership support, a PBL initiative is likely to face a domino effect that undermines faculty motivation, impedes resource allocation, and ultimately compromises the sustainability of the program. The lack of leadership commitment can trigger erosion of faculty motivation, restriction of resources, and ultimately jeopardize the long-term viability of the PBL initiatives. This could lead to pressures from both faculty and students, causing the new PBL curriculum to revert to conventional teaching practices and negating any progress that has been made. The

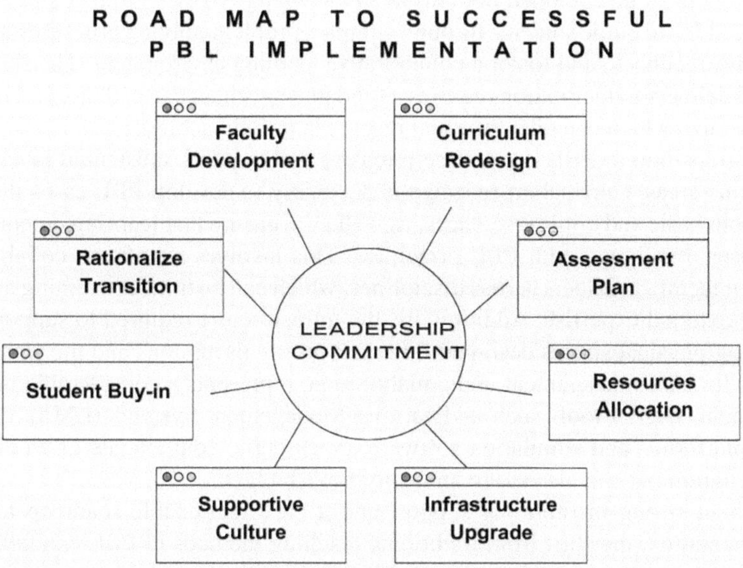

Fig. 10.1 Leadership commitment is crucial to the success of PBL, encompassing various aspects such as curriculum design and assessment, resources allocation, infrastructure upgrades, and engaging of both faculty and students

reversion to the competing norms in curricula would occur due to the loss of leadership support, which would diminish faculty motivation, restrict resource allocation, and ultimately jeopardize the sustainability of the PBL initiatives. Faculty look to leadership for guidance and faculty buy-in is imperative for true curricular change. Thus loss of leadership buy-in would result in the failure of PBL, leading to the program's stagnation and eventual abandonment, thereby undermining the potential benefits of this learner-centered approach (Abraham & Ramnarayan, 2016).

Some institutions have encountered significant challenges in implementing PBL effectively, particularly due to resistance from faculty who are accustomed to traditional, lecture-based teaching methods. This resistance can stem from a variety of factors, including faculty members' reluctance to relinquish their role as the primary source of knowledge. In traditional settings, faculty act as the "sage on the stage," delivering content in a top-down manner. In contrast, PBL requires faculty to shift to a more facilitative role, guiding students through inquiry, problem-solving, and collaborative learning. For many instructors, this shift can feel uncomfortable and unfamiliar, leading to hesitancy or outright resistance to adopting the new model.

Faculty members may struggle with the transition to a student-centered approach, particularly if they have not been adequately trained in PBL methods. The need for faculty development is one of the most significant challenges in PBL adoption, as instructors must be equipped not only with knowledge of their subject area but also with the skills to guide students through complex problem-solving processes, provide formative feedback, and foster a collaborative learning environment. The shift from content delivery to facilitation requires a fundamental change in pedagogical mindset and practice, which can take time and resources to fully achieve.

The transition to PBL is resource-intensive and requires substantial investments in various areas. Curriculum redesign is necessary to develop PBL cases that integrate both basic and clinical sciences, as well as to ensure that learning outcomes are appropriately aligned with PBL principles. This involves significant collaboration between faculty members across disciplines, which can be time-consuming and may require external expertise. Additionally, the infrastructure required to support PBL, including physical spaces designed for small-group discussions and the technology needed for case management and collaboration, represents a considerable financial investment. Digital tools such as Learning Management Systems (LMS), collaborative platforms, and simulation software are essential components of an effective PBL program but can also strain an institution's budget.

Without strong institutional support and a clear, actionable roadmap for PBL implementation, the shift from traditional teaching methods to PBL can falter. The lack of consistent support from leadership can lead to inconsistencies in how PBL is delivered across different departments or courses, reducing its effectiveness and hindering its full potential. Institutions may struggle to maintain the commitment of faculty if the necessary resources and training are not provided in a timely and ongoing manner. This can result in faculty feeling unsupported or underprepared, further exacerbating resistance and limiting the success of PBL initiatives.

In essence, leadership commitment is the linchpin of successful PBL implementation. Strong leadership provides the vision, direction, and support necessary to overcome these challenges. Leaders must champion the adoption of PBL, ensuring that adequate resources are allocated for faculty development, curriculum redesign, and infrastructure upgrades. Furthermore, they must communicate a clear and compelling case for the value of PBL, engaging stakeholders at all levels of the institution, from faculty to students to administrators. A committed leadership team fosters a culture of collaboration, innovation, and continuous improvement, which is essential for the sustainable implementation and success of PBL. By prioritizing these efforts, institutions can create an environment where PBL thrives, enabling students to benefit from an active, student-centered learning experience that prepares them for the complex, ever-evolving demands of their future professions.

Informed leadership relies on assessment, both programmatic and Institutional. The assessment of student learning in a PBL environment can pose unique challenges. While traditional summative assessments may capture acquired knowledge of learners, they may not effectively capture the development of critical thinking, problem-solving, self-direction, and collaborative skills that are the hallmarks of PBL (Bahri & Idris, 2018). Developing robust and reliable assessment strategies that align with PBL's learning objectives is crucial but can be complex and time-consuming. Implementing assessment strategies that differ from traditional methods could result in resentment in the program by faculty members who are unwilling

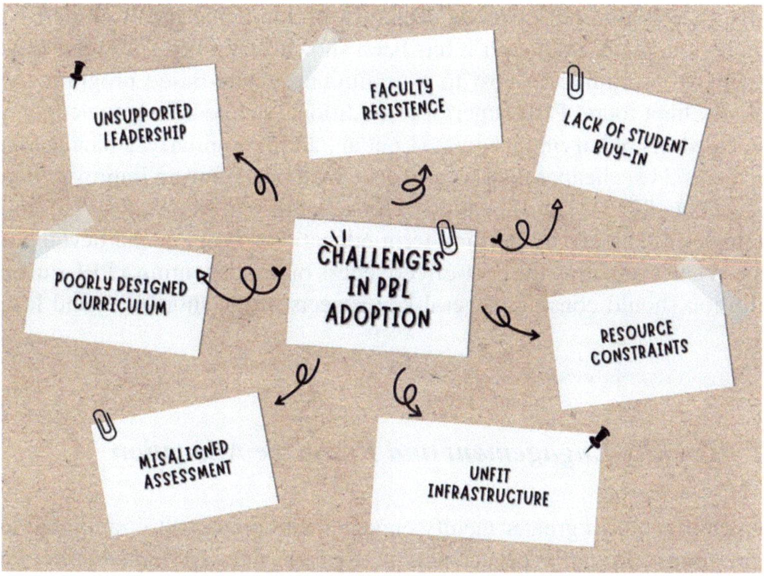

Fig. 10.2 The multifaceted challenges of implementing PBL include faculty resistance, student disengagement, limited leadership support, restricted resources, and a poorly designed curriculum with misaligned assessment

or hesitant to alter former assessment methods. Faculty organizations could pose a threat to implementation with a demand for leadership to return to traditional methods, which would cause the program's failure. For this reason, leadership must be committed to the curricular change and support the faculty along the journey.

Ultimately, the successful implementation of PBL requires a comprehensive and sustained effort that addresses the multifaceted challenges (Fig. 10.2) inherent in this transformative approach to education. Institutions must be prepared to invest in faculty development, curricular redesign, and assessment strategies that support the effective integration of PBL while also addressing the concerns and barriers faced by faculty and students. Without a concerted and well-planned effort, the potential benefits of PBL may remain elusive, and the institution may struggle to achieve its desired learning outcomes.

10.3 Financial Resources Required to Implement a PBL Curriculum

PBL implementation necessitates a substantial financial investment in diverse areas, including faculty training, curriculum development, infrastructure upgrades, and ongoing student support services. It is important to determine whether it is more expensive than traditional methods. The cost of additional faculty for PBL facilitation may be a factor, although it has been shown that a PBL program is actually less expensive or similar in cost to a traditional lecture-based program. A meta-analysis in China found PBL superior to traditional methods in knowledge mastery and clinical skills, justifying its costs (Li et al., 2022). Similarly, a blended learning approach was 24% cheaper than face-to-face methods, offering improved outcomes (Maloney et al., 2015). The allocation of financial resources towards PBL initiatives is a strategic investment in the long-term educational success and development of students. When evaluating the cost-effectiveness of implementing a PBL curriculum, an institution should consider several key aspects of the short-term and long-term costs.

10.3.1 Faculty Engagement and Resource Allocation

PBL typically requires greater faculty engagement compared to traditional lecture-based programs, primarily due to its small-group, tutor-facilitated structure. In a traditional lecture-based approach, faculty often deliver content in a one-directional format, with little to no immediate feedback from students. However, in PBL, faculty members take on more dynamic roles as facilitators, guiding students through the process of inquiry, problem-solving, and collaborative learning. This increased involvement is one of the key distinguishing factors of PBL, requiring a shift in how faculty allocate their time and resources.

In some programs, it may be beneficial that two facilitators, one clinical expert and one basic science expert, should co-facilitate each PBL session. This approach stems from the idea that students benefit from learning from both perspectives simultaneously. For example, clinical experts bring real-world, patient-centered insights, while basic science experts provide the foundational knowledge necessary to understand the physiological, biochemical, or anatomical principles involved. The belief is that these complementary expertise areas help students better connect theoretical knowledge with practical applications. However, this dual-facilitator approach has its challenges. For one, it may seem resource-intensive, as it necessitates more faculty time and commitment. While some institutions believe in the added value of having both experts, there are also institutions where a single facilitator, well-versed in both clinical and basic science topics, manages the entire PBL process. This more streamlined approach can be more cost-effective, as it reduces the number of faculty involved per group. Nevertheless, the importance of a well-trained, capable facilitator cannot be overstated. The facilitator's role in fostering group discussions, encouraging critical thinking, and maintaining student engagement is pivotal in the success of PBL.

A study comparing PBL with traditional curricula found that while faculty costs remained similar, PBL involved broader educational roles for instructors, such as tutoring, curriculum development, and regular assessments of both student progress and the effectiveness of PBL cases (Hamdy & Agamy, 2011). This suggests that while PBL might not require a significant increase in the number of faculty, the nature of faculty engagement is more resource-intensive. Facilitators in PBL are not simply delivering content, they are actively involved in mentoring students, guiding group dynamics, and supporting student-driven learning. They need to be adept at asking thought-provoking questions, promoting self-directed learning, and providing continuous feedback on both group and individual performance.

In addition to the increased faculty engagement, the integration of PBL into existing educational infrastructures requires investments in both technology and physical space (Fig. 10.3). PBL sessions rely heavily on interactive, collaborative learning environments, which can pose challenges for institutions with limited resources. For example, classrooms need to be flexible and designed for group-based work, with moveable chairs and tables that allow for collaborative discussions. This might require significant renovation or reconfiguration of existing lecture halls or classrooms.

Moreover, the use of technology plays a key role in supporting PBL. Learning management systems (LMS) are essential for managing the delivery of PBL cases, tracking student progress, and providing resources for research and collaboration. Additionally, digital platforms may be needed to facilitate asynchronous collaboration among students or to enable virtual PBL sessions for remote learning environments. The cost of acquiring, implementing, and maintaining these technologies can

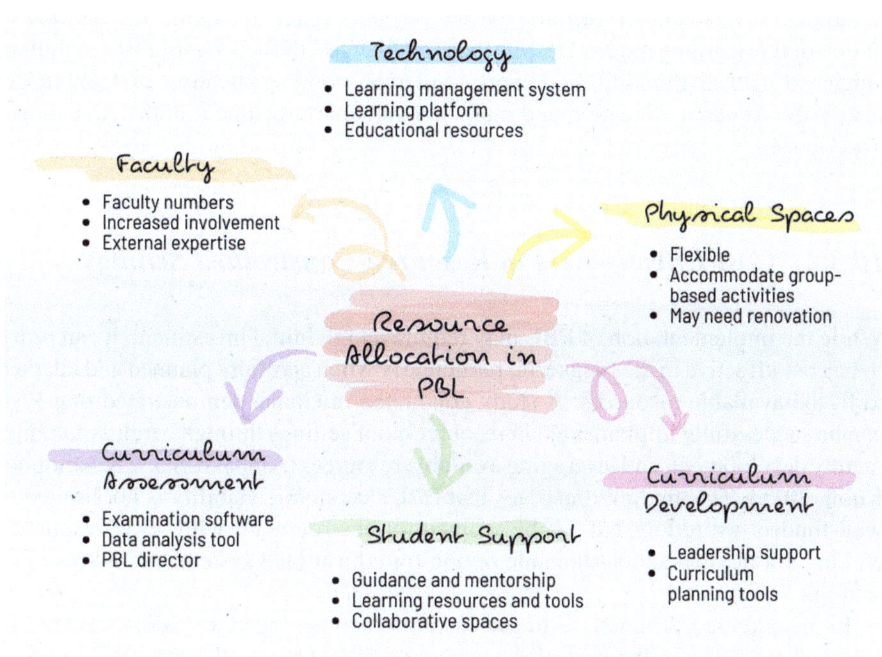

Fig. 10.3 Resources allocation in PBL include increased faculty engagement, curriculum redesign, adoption of technology, renovation of physical space and enhanced student support

add up, particularly when institutions are transitioning from traditional methods to PBL-based models.

For example, one institution may decide to invest in a collaborative online platform where students can work together in virtual study groups, access resources, and submit reflective reports. Additionally, digital tools such as video conferencing software may be required to facilitate discussions when students cannot meet in person. The cost of training faculty to effectively use these platforms adds another layer of financial investment.

Additionally, PBL demands faculty time for curriculum development, as PBL cases must be carefully designed to align with educational goals and ensure that the content challenges students to think critically while integrating knowledge from multiple disciplines. This often involves collaboration between faculty members across various departments, such as clinical faculty working with basic science instructors to create realistic and interdisciplinary cases. These cases require ongoing refinement and adjustment to stay relevant and engaging for students, which can be time-consuming for faculty members.

While PBL may not necessarily require a higher number of faculty members compared to traditional lecture-based methods, it demands a more intensive and multifaceted form of faculty engagement. Faculty members take on roles as facilitators, mentors, and curriculum developers, all of which require time, training, and expertise. The integration of PBL into an institution's infrastructure also requires significant investments in technology and physical space to support the interactive nature of this learning model. Despite these challenges, the benefits of PBL, including enhanced critical thinking, teamwork, and real-world application of knowledge, justify the resource allocation and make it a valuable investment in the educational experience.

10.3.2 Cost-Effectiveness in Resource-Constrained Settings

While the implementation of PBL may require a high initial investment, it can prove to be cost-effective in the long term, particularly when carefully planned and adapted to fit the available resources. A study conducted in Ghana demonstrated that PBL can be successfully implemented in resource-poor settings through careful planning, faculty development, and leveraging available resources (Amoako-Sakyi & Amonoo-Kuofi, 2015). This finding illustrates that PBL's economic viability is not limited to well-funded institutions but can be adapted for environments with fewer resources, making it a flexible and sustainable option for educational systems in low-resource settings.

In resource-constrained settings, institutions may need to adopt alternative approaches to ensure the cost-effectiveness of PBL. One such approach is a tutorless model of PBL, which has been shown to be a cost-effective alternative in certain settings (Walsh, 2013). Instead of having dedicated faculty members for each small group, this model allows students to engage with the material independently or with minimal guidance from facilitators. In this setup, faculty members act as a support system rather than direct instructors, providing occasional guidance and feedback when necessary. This approach reduces the need for multiple facilitators, which can be costly, while still maintaining the core principles of PBL: student-driven learning, critical thinking, and collaborative problem-solving.

Additionally, institutions in low-resource settings can maximize the use of existing faculty by encouraging them to take on multiple roles, such as facilitator, curriculum developer, and assessor. Faculty can be trained to integrate PBL methodologies into their existing teaching practices without requiring significant additional investment in new hires. This helps institutions minimize costs while ensuring that faculty development remains a priority. For example, a medical school might train their existing faculty to co-facilitate PBL sessions, focusing on their strengths in either clinical or basic science knowledge. This allows the institution to make the best use of its available faculty without incurring the cost of hiring specialized PBL tutors.

Moreover, optimizing the use of existing infrastructure is crucial in resource-constrained environments. Instead of building entirely new facilities for PBL, institutions can adapt existing lecture halls and classrooms to accommodate group-based activities. Simple changes, such as rearranging desks into smaller clusters, can create an environment conducive to collaborative learning without requiring expensive renovations. Technology can also be utilized creatively to enhance PBL in low-resource settings. For instance, online learning platforms or open-access educational resources can be used to supplement face-to-face PBL sessions, reducing the need for expensive textbooks or printed materials.

A good example of this is the use of low-cost digital tools and platforms to facilitate collaborative learning. Institutions can use free or low-cost software for group discussions, sharing resources, and submitting assignments. This can significantly reduce costs compared to more expensive proprietary systems, while still allowing students to engage in meaningful, technology-enhanced learning.

While initial costs for implementing PBL in low-resource settings may still be a consideration, these adaptive strategies allow institutions to make the most of their existing resources and implement PBL in a sustainable way. By focusing on faculty development, leveraging technology, and optimizing available infrastructure, institutions can deliver high-quality, student-centered education that is both economically viable and educationally effective.

Although PBL implementation typically requires a higher initial financial commitment, it can be cost-effective in resource-constrained environments with careful planning and strategic resource allocation. The success of PBL in low-resource settings, as demonstrated in studies like those conducted in Ghana (Amoako-Sakyi & Amonoo-Kuofi, 2015), highlights its potential for educational systems worldwide. By adopting tutor-less models, maximizing the use of existing faculty, and optimizing infrastructure, institutions can ensure that PBL is not only feasible but also sustainable in the long term.

10.3.3 Indirect Cost Savings Through Improved Outcomes

In addition to the direct costs associated with implementing PBL, there are significant indirect cost savings that can arise from improved learning outcomes and the development of professional competencies. One of the most compelling arguments for adopting PBL lies in its potential to enhance essential skills such as critical thinking, problem-solving, and self-directed learning. Research has consistently shown that students in PBL environments develop these skills to a greater extent compared to their peers in traditional lecture-based programs (Bashith & Amin, 2017). These enhanced competencies are not only valuable in an academic setting but also have profound implications for students' future professional performance, particularly in clinical practice.

The improvement in critical thinking and problem-solving skills directly impacts clinical decision-making. PBL students are trained to approach problems with a systematic, analytical mindset, which is crucial when diagnosing and treating patients. This enhanced ability to think critically and adaptively may reduce the likelihood of medical errors, which is an area where substantial costs are incurred in healthcare. Medical errors can lead to patient harm, prolonged hospital stays, legal liabilities, and financial burdens on the healthcare system. Studies have shown that PBL can significantly improve diagnostic accuracy by enhancing critical thinking and clinical reasoning skills. For instance, a meta-analysis by Wang et al. (2016) found that PBL in physical diagnostics education in China led to significant improvements in students' knowledge and skills compared to traditional teaching methods. This suggests that the competencies developed through PBL may contribute to improved diagnostic accuracy. Similarly, an umbrella review by Ge et al. (2025) indicated that PBL effectively enhances students' clinical skills and critical thinking abilities, which are essential for accurate diagnosis and may indirectly reduce diagnostic errors. These findings indicate that the development of critical thinking through PBL can play a pivotal role in minimizing diagnostic errors, leading to better patient care.

Moreover, the self-directed learning component of PBL is particularly important in fostering lifelong learning habits, which are essential for healthcare providers. In the rapidly evolving field of medicine, new treatments, technologies, and best practices emerge regularly. PBL encourages students to take responsibility for their learning, continually seek new information, and adjust their understanding as necessary. This capacity for self-directed learning enables healthcare providers to stay current with advancements in their fields, reducing the risk of outdated practices and enhancing overall patient care.

Another indirect cost savings comes from the potential for improved teamwork and collaboration among healthcare professionals. PBL is inherently collaborative, as students work in small groups to solve clinical cases. This collaborative approach helps students build interpersonal and communication skills that are vital in healthcare settings, where teamwork is often key to successful patient outcomes. Effective communication among healthcare teams has been linked to fewer patient complications, better patient satisfaction, and more efficient delivery of care. For example, a hospital that implements PBL-based training might see improved collaboration between physicians, nurses, and allied health professionals, leading to faster decision-making and better coordinated patient care. The cost savings here stem from reduced redundancy, more efficient care, and fewer miscommunications that could lead to adverse outcomes.

Finally, the overall improvement in clinical performance and professional competencies can lead to better patient outcomes, which directly impacts the financial sustainability of healthcare systems. Hospitals and clinics that train their staff using PBL methods may see reductions in patient readmissions, unnecessary tests, and extended hospital stays, all of which contribute to lower healthcare costs. In the long term, as PBL-trained healthcare providers advance in their careers, the cumulative impact of improved skills and patient outcomes can lead to significant cost savings for healthcare institutions and systems.

While the direct costs of implementing PBL can be considerable, the indirect cost savings generated by improved learning outcomes and professional competencies are equally significant. Enhanced critical thinking, problem-solving, self-directed learning, and collaboration all contribute to better performance in clinical practice, which in turn can reduce the costs associated with medical errors, patient complications, and inefficient healthcare delivery. By fostering these skills early in medical education, PBL has the potential to create long-term savings for healthcare systems, making it a financially viable investment for institutions focused on improving both the quality and efficiency of care.

10.3.4 Factors Influencing Cost-Effectiveness

10.3.4.1 Curriculum Design and Integration

Integrating PBL with traditional lecture-based methods can enhance cost-effectiveness by combining the strengths of both approaches. A study conducted in China found that combining PBL with lecture-based teaching not only improved student performance but also increased student satisfaction without significantly raising costs (Zhan et al., 2023). This hybrid approach offers a balanced solution, allowing institutions to preserve the structure and efficiency of traditional teaching while reaping the benefits of PBL's active learning model. However, some studies have shown that learning outcomes from such hybrid programs are often similar to those of traditional lecture-based programs (Lim, 2012). As a result, it is essential for institutions to carefully design and integrate curricula to maximize the advantages of PBL while ensuring it remains cost-effective. This may involve strategically blending lecture sessions with PBL activities, ensuring that the overall instructional time and resources are efficiently utilized without compromising the educational outcomes.

10.3.4.2 Technology and Blended Learning

Blended learning, which combines PBL with digital tools and online platforms, has proven to be a cost-effective way to deliver PBL while reducing infrastructure and operational costs. A recent study on ChatGPT-assisted PBL highlighted how the use of AI-driven tools can lead to improved learning outcomes while lowering costs, primarily due to the reduction in infrastructure needs (Zeng et al., 2025). By incorporating virtual components into PBL, institutions can minimize the need for physical classroom space and logistics associated with in-person sessions. Virtual PBL platforms allow for asynchronous learning, which further reduces the costs of scheduling, faculty time, and physical resources. This flexibility makes virtual or blended PBL a highly cost-efficient option, especially in resource-constrained environments, as it allows for broader access to educational opportunities without the significant investments typically associated with traditional face-to-face learning environments.

A well-designed curriculum that integrates PBL with traditional teaching methods, alongside the adoption of digital tools for blended learning, can significantly improve the cost-effectiveness of PBL programs. By leveraging technology and optimizing curriculum structures, educational institutions can offer high-quality, interactive learning experiences that are financially sustainable in the long term.

10.3.5 Cost-Effectiveness Analysis

10.3.5.1 Comparative Studies

A meta-analysis in China found PBL superior to traditional methods in knowledge mastery and clinical skills, justifying its costs (Li et al., 2022). Similarly, a blended learning approach was 24% cheaper than face-to-face methods, offering improved outcomes (Maloney et al., 2015). These findings suggest that the enhanced educational outcomes of PBL can offset its costs. While initial investments in PBL could be high, long-term benefits include improved student competencies and reduced costs over time. A blended learning model achieved cost-effectiveness after three iterations, highlighting the importance of sustained implementation (Maloney et al., 2015). These long-term gains make PBL a worthwhile investment.

10.3.6 Challenges and Considerations

10.3.6.1 Resource Constraints

Implementing PBL in resource-poor settings presents unique challenges that require careful planning, creative solutions, and flexibility. The experience of the University of Cape Coast in Ghana provides valuable insights into how PBL can be successfully implemented in such contexts. In their study, Amoako-Sakyi and Amonoo-Kuofi (2015) explored the challenges and strategies involved in integrating PBL into the medical curriculum in a resource-limited environment. They highlighted the importance of aligning PBL with available resources and investing in faculty development to address the challenges inherent in such settings.

The study emphasized that for PBL to be effective in resource-constrained environments, institutions must tailor the approach to the specific needs and limitations of their context. At the University of Cape Coast, the faculty worked to adapt the PBL model by drawing on existing resources, such as classroom space, teaching staff, and technological tools, to ensure that the PBL approach could be integrated successfully. Rather than attempting to replicate PBL models used in wealthier institutions with more resources, the university designed a model that worked within their existing framework, ensuring that the learning objectives could still be met. A key finding from the study was the importance of investing in faculty development. The successful implementation of PBL requires that instructors are not only familiar with the theoretical aspects of PBL but also skilled in the practical facilitation of student-centered learning. Amoako-Sakyi and Amonoo-Kuofi (2015) noted that faculty training was essential to equip teachers with the skills to guide students through the iterative process of inquiry, self-directed learning, and group problem-solving, which are central to PBL. The study found that by focusing on faculty development and providing ongoing support for instructors, the University of Cape Coast was able to overcome some of the typical barriers to PBL, such as resistance to change and a lack of experience with student-centered methods.

The integration of PBL at the University of Cape Coast was not without challenges. For instance, the initial lack of resources posed logistical challenges, including limited access to medical simulation equipment, digital resources, and spaces conducive to small-group work. However, the study highlighted how strategic planning allowed the institution to overcome these barriers. Faculty worked to incorporate low-cost technological solutions, such as online discussion platforms and digital learning materials, to supplement traditional teaching methods and support collaborative learning in a more cost-effective manner. This creative approach to resource use allowed the university to adopt PBL without requiring significant financial investment, demonstrating that PBL can be viable even in low-resource settings with thoughtful planning.

Furthermore, the study emphasized that the benefits of PBL, such as enhanced student engagement, critical thinking, and problem-solving abilities, were evident even in a resource-limited context. Students reported a high level of satisfaction with the learning approach, noting that PBL helped them develop a deeper understanding of clinical concepts and better prepared them for real-world medical practice. The experience of the University of Cape Coast underscores the importance of adopting bespoke strategies for PBL integration, carefully aligning the curriculum with available resources, and investing in faculty development. The study also demonstrates that PBL is not an educational approach reserved for well-funded institutions; with creativity and careful resource management, it can be successfully implemented in

Table 10.1 Different PBL models and their cost-effectiveness factors

Model type	Cost-effectiveness factors	Citation
Traditional PBL	High initial costs, resource-intensive, requires faculty training	Finucane et al. (2009)
Blended PBL	Reduces infrastructure costs, leverages technology	Zeng et al. (2025), Maloney et al. (2015)
Virtual PBL	Minimizes physical infrastructure, flexible and cost-efficient	Shrivastava and Shrivastava (2023)
Hybrid PBL	Combines PBL with lectures, balances cost and effectiveness	Zhan et al. (2023)

resource-poor settings, providing students with an enriched learning experience that prepares them for their future roles in healthcare.

While implementing PBL in resource-constrained environments requires significant planning and adaptability, the University of Cape Coast's experience proves that it is a feasible and highly beneficial educational model. By focusing on faculty development, leveraging existing resources, and integrating low-cost technological solutions, institutions can successfully adopt PBL and reap its long-term benefits.

10.3.6.2 Comparative Table of PBL Models

Table 10.1 highlights how different PBL models address cost-effectiveness, emphasizing the role of technology and integration in optimizing resources.

The analysis of these models underscores the importance of selecting the appropriate PBL approach based on institutional needs and available resources, ultimately aiming to enhance educational outcomes while managing costs effectively. Selecting the right model not only influences the financial implications but also impacts student engagement, learning experiences, and overall success in achieving educational objectives. Understanding the unique strengths and challenges of each PBL model can empower educators to make informed decisions that align with their specific goals and contexts.

10.4 Examining the Educational Journey: The Merits and Drawbacks of PBL

The implementation of Problem-Based Learning represents a transformative shift in the educational landscape, offering a multitude of potential benefits while also presenting unique challenges that must be carefully considered. PBL excels at fostering active learning, where students are not passive recipients of information but actively engaged in constructing their own understanding through problem-solving and critical inquiry (Dolmans et al., 2005). Students cultivate essential skills in research, collaboration, and communication as they work together to analyze complex scenarios and develop viable solutions (Savery, 2015). This active engagement leads to deeper understanding and better retention of knowledge, empowering students to apply what they learn in real-world contexts (Chang, 2016).

While PBL offers many advantages, it also presents significant challenges that require careful planning and mitigation strategies (Azer, 2011; Savery, 2015). One common concern is the potential for increased resource demands, as PBL often requires more faculty time for facilitating group discussions, developing authentic problems, and providing individualized feedback to students (Albanese & Mitchell, 1993). This increased demand is often viewed as a deterrent to initiating a PBL program (Hamdy & Agamy, 2011). Institutions may also need to invest in additional resources, such as technology infrastructure, learning spaces, and library materials, to support PBL activities effectively. A significant impediment to the successful adoption of PBL lies in the realm of faculty development, which requires a comprehensive and sustained investment in training and support (Azer, 2011). Many instructors may feel inadequately prepared to facilitate student-led discussions, assess problem-solving skills, and provide guidance without resorting to traditional lecture-based approaches. Overcoming these obstacles necessitates a concerted effort to equip faculty with the pedagogical knowledge and skills necessary to thrive in a PBL environment (Hamdy & Agamy, 2011).

Another challenge associated with PBL is the potential for student resistance, especially among those accustomed to traditional lecture-based instruction, which often leads to student dissatisfaction. Some students may feel uncomfortable with the ambiguity and open-ended nature of PBL problems, while others may struggle to manage their time effectively or work collaboratively in groups (Bahri & Idris, 2018). Addressing these concerns requires clear communication about the goals and expectations of PBL, as well as providing students with sufficient scaffolding and support to develop the necessary skills for success (Albanese & Mitchell, 1993). Students should be encouraged to recognize that the skills they acquire through PBL will benefit them well beyond graduation (Pinthong & Chaisongmuang, 2019). Furthermore, addressing the diverse learning needs of students in a PBL environment requires instructors to possess a nuanced understanding of differentiated instruction and individualized support strategies. This includes the ability to provide targeted feedback, adapt instructional approaches, and create flexible learning opportunities that cater to the unique strengths, weaknesses, and learning preferences of each student. By employing differentiated instruction, instructors can ensure that all students, regardless of their background or aptitude, are actively engaged and supported in the PBL process. This level of individualized attention is crucial for fostering student success and promoting equitable learning outcomes in a PBL setting.

10.5 Developing the Rationale Behind Curricular Change: The Why?

Before embarking on the implementation of PBL, institutions must develop a compelling rationale for curricular change, clearly articulating the benefits of PBL in addressing specific learning objectives and institutional goals. This rationale should be grounded in evidence-based research demonstrating the effectiveness of PBL in promoting critical thinking, problem-solving, collaboration, and self-directed learning (Dolmans et al., 2005). Faculty members can cultivate a shared understanding of PBL's value and garner support from diverse stakeholders by actively involving faculty, students, administrators, and external partners in the development of the rationale. The process of developing a rationale can reveal the motivations and values of stakeholders, which will lead to greater acceptance of the program. In addition to articulating the pedagogical benefits of PBL, the rationale should also address the practical considerations of implementation, such as resource allocation, faculty development, and assessment strategies.

The administration of a health profession program must provide leadership for the change to a PBL curriculum using current metrics such as curricular outcome, national board licensing examination data, and residency placement. The administrators should ask questions such as, are we reaching our curricular goals to support the mission and vision of the institution? Are we graduating students prepared for the demands of the profession that may include collaboration, knowledge, critical thinking, and professionalism? Would converting to a PBL program improve some or all of these attributes? Once the data is collected, the stakeholders should decide how the data compares to the mission and vision. Once this is completed, the group should decide if curricular change is in order, using the data from the assessment metrics. The communication of the rationale must be transparent, persuasive, and tailored to the specific concerns and interests of different stakeholders.

The administration should initiate a comprehensive needs assessment, employing surveys, focus groups, and individual interviews to gather detailed perspectives from students, faculty, and staff regarding their expectations, concerns, and perceived resource requirements for a successful PBL transition.

Outcome data alone is not enough, in a PBL curriculum, students learn much more than just traditional knowledge facts, they also learn critical thinking skills, collaboration, mastery of material vs memorization, self-directed learning, and working in teams, all of which are characteristics in high demand in today's healthcare professions. The Institution should weigh the importance of these factors as they rationalize a curricular change to a PBL program. This will also build faculty and student support of the change. Moreover, the rationale should align with the institution's mission, values, and strategic priorities, ensuring that PBL implementation contributes to the overall success and reputation of the institution. A concise and well-articulated rationale is crucial for fostering faculty and student buy-in to the curricular change, facilitating a smoother transition and greater adoption of PBL principles throughout the institution.

Pros and cons of a PBL student from the first day of matriculation through the clerkships and beyond should be clearly outlined to provide all parties involved with a comprehensive understanding of the implications and value proposition associated with this pedagogical approach. By conducting thorough research and presenting a well-reasoned argument, institutions can address potential objections and demonstrate the compelling advantages of PBL in enhancing student learning and preparing them for future success. This rationale serves as a compass, guiding the implementation process and ensuring that all stakeholders are working towards a common goal, which will improve success and lessen the risk of program failure (Albanese & Mitchell, 1993).

10.6 Essential Faculty Development Training

A pivotal aspect of effective PBL implementation lies in comprehensive faculty development and training programs (Fig. 10.4) that equip instructors with the skills and knowledge necessary to facilitate student-centered learning experiences. Faculty development programs should focus on the core principles of PBL, including case design, the "art" of facilitation, assessment strategies, and the creation of a supportive learning environment. These programs should emphasize the importance of shifting from a traditional lecture-based approach to a facilitative role, where instructors guide students through the problem-solving process rather than providing direct answers (Pinthong & Chaisongmuang, 2019). To accomplish this, faculty teams should be assembled to identify successful PBL programs at other schools and ask to visit the schools to learn successful strategies for delivering a PBL program. Ideally, these programs would collaborate and offer instructors structured opportunities to rehearse PBL methodologies in simulated classroom environments, enabling them to refine their learner-centered techniques, assimilate constructive criticism from both seasoned peers and subject matter experts, and participate in introspective analyses of their instructional efficacy through video recordings and feedback sessions (Pinthong & Chaisongmuang, 2019).

Effective faculty development also involves ongoing mentorship and peer support, where experienced PBL practitioners guide and support their colleagues in implementing PBL in their own courses (Azer, 2005). Moreover, faculty training should extend to the strategic integration of technology to augment PBL experiences, encompassing platforms for online discussions that foster collaborative knowledge construction, sophisticated collaborative writing tools that facilitate group report generation and feedback exchange, and immersive virtual simulations that replicate real-world. Once trained in PBL, the faculty team should report their observations back to other faculty members and administrators. In addition, faculty development initiatives must stress the significance of reflective practice, prompting instructors to critically assess their PBL facilitation approaches, glean insights from student feedback, and iteratively refine their techniques to optimize student learning outcomes. Prior to starting a PBL program, faculty should hold mock PBL sessions with

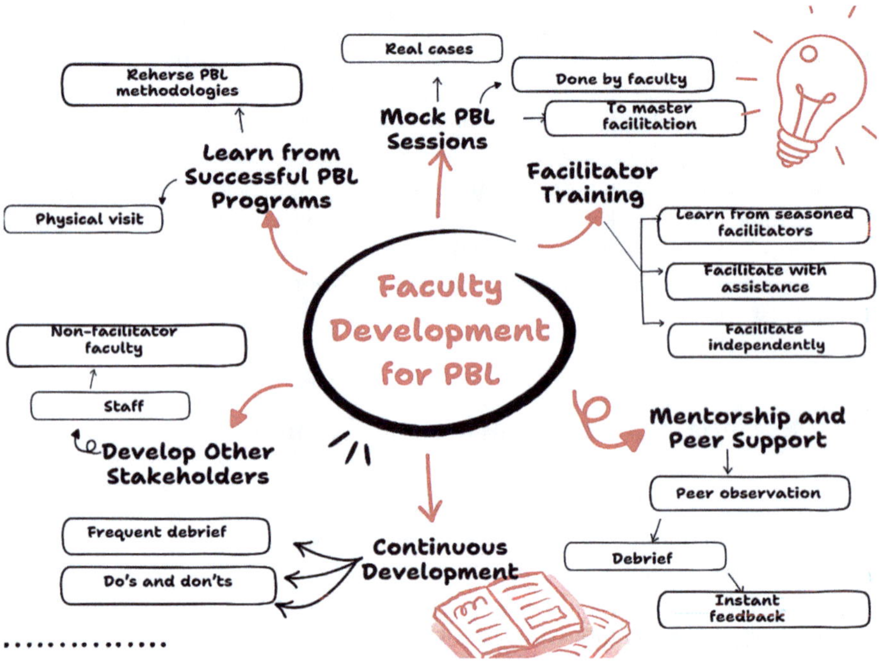

Fig. 10.4 The comprehensive faculty development program for PBL begins with learning from successful PBL implementations and participating in mock PBL sessions, followed by facilitator training, mentoring, and peer support. It also includes ongoing professional development and the development of other stakeholders beyond faculty members who serve as facilitators

real cases using interactive classroom activities, small group discussions, and self-directed learning modules to enhance their mastery of PBL facilitation. These mock PBL sessions should leverage interactive classroom activities, small group discussions, and self-directed learning modules to enhance the faculty's mastery of PBL facilitation techniques. There should be frequent debriefing sessions with faculty to discuss the pros and cons of the group process. Ultimately, sustained investment in faculty development fosters a community of practice where instructors can learn from each other, share best practices, and collectively enhance the quality of PBL implementation across the institution (Kober, 2015).

Continuous faculty development is also required to maintain the curriculum. Without it, dysfunctional tutorial groups can arise (Dolmans et al., 2005). Continuous faculty development not only improves PBL implementation but also helps in building a community of faculty dedicated to improving teaching and learning (Kober, 2015). One effective approach to continual faculty development is frequent faculty debrief sessions. During these sessions, faculty facilitators discuss what went well and what could have been improved. They also discuss do's and don'ts of the PBL curricular model. Facilitators utilize this forum to discuss solutions among other facilitators, thus providing some commonality in the tutorial process within the institution.

A successful program involves all institutional stakeholders, not just faculty facilitators. The institution should develop institution-wide training and development sessions for non-facilitator faculty and staff. It is imperative that every member of the institution be committed to the program and that every member has some knowledge of the tenets of PBL and how this program differs from traditional learning modalities. It is important to remember that a new PBL program may be met with resistance from within the institution due to various reasons, including concerns about increased workload, lack of familiarity with PBL methods, or skepticism about its effectiveness (Hamdy & Agamy, 2011). In particular, learning specialists and student advisors should have a clear understanding of the program to help students navigate this territory. Often, faculty advisors, learning specialists, mental health specialists, and other staff members were trained in a traditional pathway, thus they will offer advice that may not help a student struggling to find their way in a PBL program. The institution should provide support for these individuals and clearly explain the curriculum and pedagogy that is being employed.

Along with mock sessions for facilitators, prior to starting a new PBL curriculum, staff members, learning specialists, and mental health support personnel should be involved with philosophical training sessions and mock PBL sessions. They should also hold mock advising appointments to prepare them for the new modality. Often, the students who have the most difficulty in a PBL program have a difficult time with self-directed learning. A health professions program applicant has developed a strong proficiency in an environment where objectives are provided, the student masters these objectives, takes an examination on them, and then repeats the process. This is not self-directed learning. Students in a PBL environment may find themselves feeling deprived of direction and confused about how to learn in a PBL environment. They may feel as though the institution is not providing what they need. For this reason, all student support service providers must be involved with training to provide useful advice (Kober, 2015). Before the course begins, instructors must explain the concepts, objectives, methods, and practice of PBL to the students and facilitators (Pinthong & Chaisongmuang, 2019).

10.7 Assessment of PBL Programs at Other Schools

Perhaps as a very first step in the PBL implementation process, a faculty team should be assembled to visit other schools that offer PBL programs and learn from their experiences, successes, and failures. This will provide invaluable insights into effective PBL implementation. By observing PBL in action at different institutions, faculty and administrators will gain a deeper understanding of the nuances of PBL's learner-centered approach, including problem design, facilitation techniques, assessment strategies, student enquiry of information, and creating a supportive learning environment. Additionally, visiting other schools will help to identify potential challenges and pitfalls in PBL implementation and will lead to the development of strategies for mitigating these risks. Such visits offer opportunities to engage in discussions with faculty, students, and administrators involved in PBL, allowing for the exchange of ideas, best practices, and lessons learned. By learning from other institutions' experiences, schools can avoid common mistakes and improve the likelihood of successful PBL implementation (Azer, 2011).

Furthermore, observing how other institutions have adapted PBL to their specific contexts and disciplines can provide inspiration for tailoring PBL to the unique needs and characteristics of one's own institution. Specifically, visits should concentrate on observing the PBL process itself and not just reviewing documents. By engaging with the PBL community at other schools, institutions can build networks of support and collaboration that can be invaluable in sustaining and improving PBL implementation over time. These observations should be strategically channeled toward the overarching goal of enhancing student learning outcomes, focusing on learner-centered techniques and assessment methods that demonstrably foster deeper understanding, critical thinking, and problem-solving capabilities.

10.8 Institutional Culture Supportive of the PBL Program

PBL thrives in institutional cultures that encourage collaboration, innovation, and continuous improvement. For PBL to be successfully implemented and widely adopted, it is essential to create a supportive institutional culture that shapes the attitudes, beliefs, and behaviors of both faculty and students (Kober, 2015). This culture should emphasize the value of teamwork, creative teaching approaches, and ongoing professional development, fostering an environment where faculty members feel empowered to experiment with new methods, share best practices, and engage in reflective teaching practices.

Building such a culture requires several key strategies. First, providing opportunities for faculty to collaborate on PBL projects is crucial. These collaborative efforts help faculty members learn from one another, pool resources, and share insights that enhance the overall effectiveness of the PBL approach. Creating communities of practice such as spaces where faculty can discuss challenges, successes, and innovations, further supports the exchange of ideas and encourages the continuous refinement of teaching practices. Recognizing and rewarding faculty contributions to PBL is also essential to acknowledge their efforts and sustain enthusiasm for teaching innovation.

The faculty community is integral to improving both teaching and learning, as their collective efforts contribute to the ongoing success of the PBL program (Kober, 2015). In addition to these practical strategies, fostering a culture of trust and mutual respect is vital. Faculty members must feel safe to take risks, try new approaches, and learn from their mistakes without fear of judgment. When faculty feel supported and respected, they are more likely to engage deeply in PBL and contribute meaningfully to its evolution within the institution. Furthermore, intense faculty involvement at every level of the PBL implementation process is critical to ensuring a positive outcome. Faculty must be actively engaged not only in the design and delivery of PBL but also in the continuous evaluation and adaptation of the program. This involvement ensures that the PBL program remains relevant, effective, and responsive to the needs of students and the broader educational community.

The success of a PBL program depends on a supportive institutional culture that promotes collaboration, innovation, and professional growth. By creating an environment where faculty feel empowered to experiment, share ideas, and learn from one another, institutions can lay the groundwork for a successful PBL implementation that benefits both faculty and students alike.

10.9 Navigating the Labyrinth: Challenges in PBL Implementation

The successful integration of PBL into educational frameworks is often hindered by a complex interplay of challenges, ranging from faculty preparedness to curriculum design and institutional support (Glew, 2003). One of the most significant obstacles to PBL implementation is the inadequate support from basic science departments. Faculty members in these departments may prioritize traditional, passive learning techniques over more learner-centered, innovative approaches. This preference can impede the adoption of PBL, as faculty may feel unfamiliar or uncomfortable with the active, student-driven learning model (Glew, 2003). Furthermore, some faculty members may have reservations about the PBL concept itself, viewing it as an unproven or time-consuming method that complicates their already demanding roles. Additionally, faculty who place a greater emphasis on research rather than student engagement may inadvertently undermine the effective implementation of PBL, focusing more on their scholarly work than on the necessary adjustments to teaching practices.

Another critical barrier to successful PBL implementation is poor oversight and insufficient assessment of the PBL curriculum. Administrators and faculty who do not fully understand or appreciate the nuances of PBL may fail to provide the necessary guidance and support to ensure its success. This lack of oversight can result in inconsistencies in how PBL is executed across different departments or courses, leading to a failure in capturing the true essence of PBL, which is its ability to foster deep learning and critical thinking in students (Glew, 2003).

A study examining the early implementation of PBL in Asian medical schools highlighted how students initially faced difficulties in adapting to this new learning model. However, through a period of adjustment and with the support of open-minded tutors, these challenges were eventually overcome (Khoo, 2003). This finding underscores the importance of having tutors and instructors who are not only trained in PBL methods but who also embrace a flexible and supportive attitude toward students' transition into this active learning model. Tutors who are willing to provide guidance, address student concerns, and adapt to the evolving needs of their learners play a pivotal role in overcoming the challenges associated with the early stages of PBL implementation.

To mitigate these challenges, it is crucial to focus on improving assessment strategies within PBL settings. Specifically, enhancing continuous formative assessment is essential to monitor students' progress and provide timely feedback. Traditional summative assessments, such as final exams, are less suited to the PBL approach, which emphasizes ongoing learning and the development of critical thinking skills. Nendaz and Tekian (1999) emphasize the importance of integrating formative assessments that are aligned with the iterative and collaborative nature of PBL. These assessments should be designed to evaluate not only the knowledge students acquire but also their problem-solving abilities, teamwork, and communication skills (Nendaz & Tekian, 1999).

Moreover, a comprehensive approach should be adopted to prepare both students and instructors for the unique demands of PBL. It is essential to clarify the core concepts, objectives, methods, and practical applications inherent in PBL, ensuring that all participants understand how PBL differs from traditional learning models and how they can contribute to its success (Pinthong & Chaisongmuang, 2019). Faculty must receive adequate training and ongoing professional development to facilitate PBL effectively, while students need clear guidance on how to navigate the self-directed, collaborative learning environment that PBL fosters. Preparing both groups for the shifts in teaching and learning that PBL requires can help overcome resistance and confusion, ultimately leading to a more successful integration of this transformative educational approach.

While the implementation of PBL presents several challenges such as those related to faculty support, curriculum design, and assessment, these barriers can be overcome with careful planning, faculty development, and a commitment to fostering a supportive learning environment. By addressing these complexities and providing adequate resources and training for both faculty and students, institutions can effectively navigate the labyrinth of PBL implementation and unlock its full potential as a powerful educational tool.

10.10 Student Buy-In: The Cornerstone of PBL Success

Enthusiastic student participation is crucial to the success of PBL, but many students initially resist the shift from traditional lecture-based learning to the more self-directed and collaborative nature of PBL (Dolmans et al., 2005). Some students find the open-ended nature of PBL problems disconcerting, while others may lack the self-directed learning skills necessary to thrive in a PBL environment. Addressing student resistance requires a multifaceted approach that includes clearly communicating the benefits of PBL, providing students with adequate support and resources, and creating a positive and supportive learning environment (Fig. 10.5). One potential solution involves the introduction of a "foundation course" designed to cultivate essential learning abilities, including problem-solving skills, teamwork dynamics,

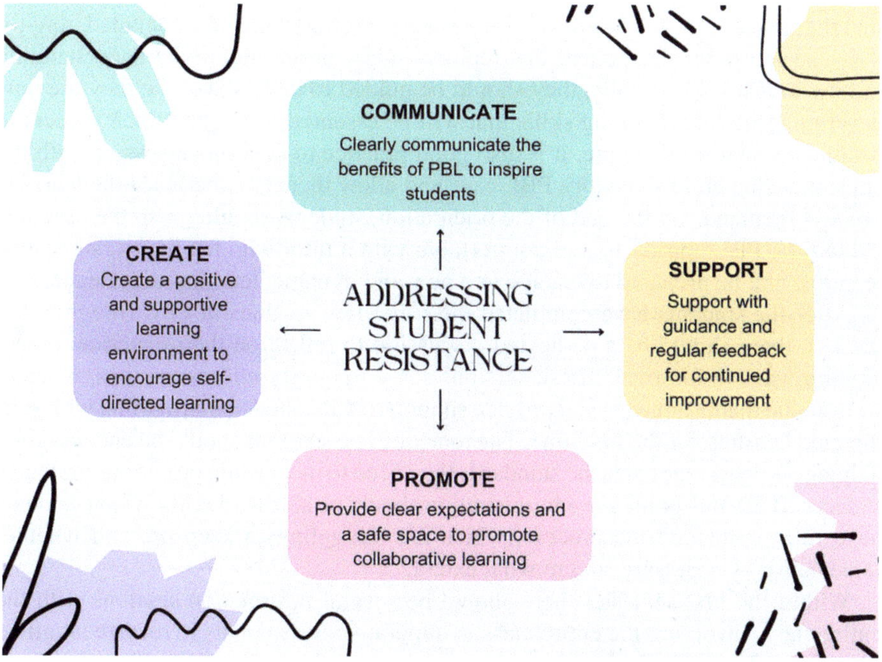

Fig. 10.5 Addressing student resistance to PBL involves multiple approaches, such as communicating the benefits of PBL, providing students with adequate support and resources, and cultivating a positive and supportive learning environment

information-seeking expertise, and self-assessment techniques (Azer, 2005). This introductory course should be meticulously crafted to equip students with the foundational skills necessary to succeed in a PBL environment. By explicitly teaching students how to learn effectively in a PBL context, institutions can empower them to become more active, engaged, and self-directed learners.

Student training for a PBL program begins with interviews. With social media and discussion groups, students find information and misinformation relative to a program in which they have no familiarity. It is important that students hear all aspects of the program at the interview. During this introduction, students should be made aware of the differences between a PBL curriculum and what they are accustomed to from their prior academic career. They must also be made aware of any misconceptions that they might have obtained from social media. During the interview information session, students should also be introduced to the benefits of learning in a PBL environment that will facilitate a deeper understanding, critical thinking, and problem-solving capabilities. During this session, students should be advised about the challenges of transitioning to a self-directed curriculum, which may require changing their learning habits.

During orientation, students should be given an in-depth introduction to the PBL process, including the "nuts" and "bolts" of how to find issues to learn, where to find them, and how to learn them. The instruction should include a detailed, day-to-day instruction for the student that replaces their current traditional understanding of how to learn. Essentially, they should be guided to understand that they are now developing lifelong learning skills that will be essential throughout their careers in healthcare. During this time, it is also good practice to do a mock session with the students using an introductory PBL case and allow them to experience the learning process firsthand. By the end of the orientation, students should grasp the rationale behind the PBL approach, feel comfortable with a tutor who facilitates rather than lectures, and be prepared to engage in a new and dynamic learning experience.

After the students have completed their first few sessions in PBL (roughly 2–3 weeks), there should be a dedicated discussion to reflect on their experiences and explore ways to improve. These sessions serve to clarify misconceptions, whether from social media or peers, and provide support to those students struggling with self-directed learning for the first time. The tone of these sessions should be encouraging, helping students recognize the standards they need to meet while providing strategies to succeed. By this point, the administration should be able to identify which students have fully embraced the process, which are struggling to keep up, and whether remediation is necessary, and to what extent.

Within the first semester there should be several information sessions with the entire class. Involving the entire class is imperative for students to receive a unified message and one that can be openly discussed in a group environment. These sessions may be best administered following an exam to point out what was learned, why the method of learning was important to the topic in that case, and to point out the utility of the information for years to come. For each semester thereafter, PBL information sessions should continue. It is important to maintain student buy-in throughout their academic career (Fig. 10.6).

10.11 Summary and Conclusion

PBL is a method of self-directed learning that is built upon the foundation of an enthusiastic faculty, an excited and understanding student body, and a commitment from the administration to maintain the integrity of the experience throughout the curriculum. Implementing a PBL curriculum presents both significant challenges and unique opportunities for fostering deeper learning, critical thinking, and problem-solving skills (Chang, 2016). Addressing challenges such as faculty development, resource allocation, and student buy-in requires a multifaceted approach that includes careful planning, ongoing support, and a commitment to continuous improvement (Azer, 2011). Institutions that successfully navigate these challenges can create a more engaging, relevant, and effective learning environment for their students, preparing them to become lifelong learners and innovative problem-solvers in an ever-changing world. By embracing the principles of PBL and addressing the inherent challenges, institutions can transform their educational programs and empower students to reach their full potential (Azer, 2005, 2011; Dolmans et al., 2005; Hamdy & Agamy,

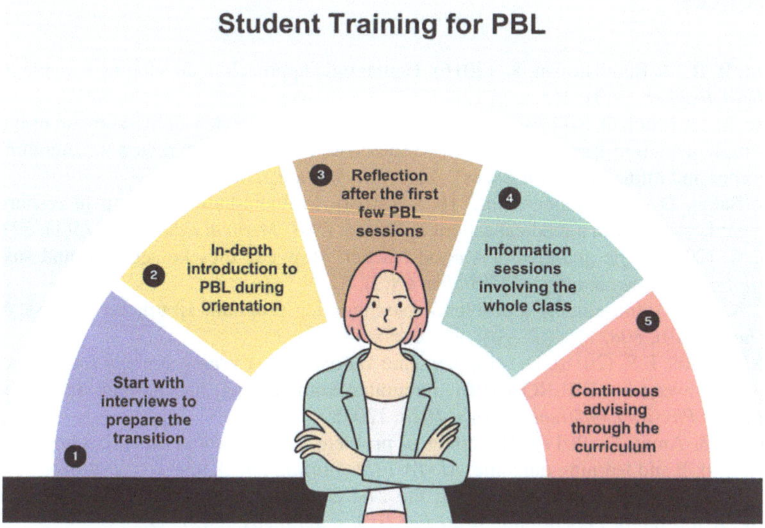

Fig. 10.6 Training students using multiple approaches to familiarize and engage them in PBL. It is a progressive process starting from an interview, followed by orientation, reflection after the initial PBL session, information sessions and ongoing advising by facilitators throughout the curriculum

2011). Ultimately, the success of PBL implementation hinges on a collaborative effort between faculty, students, and administrators, all working together to create a vibrant and supportive learning community. Worldwide, many universities are adapting their curricula by implementing integrated problem-based learning programs; however, the introduction of a PBL program is a demanding process and necessitates resources, meticulous planning, and robust organization (Azer, 2011). Aiming to provide practical guidance, it emphasizes pivotal challenges in creating such programs and suggests viable solutions to common obstacles encountered (Azer, 2011). Evidence suggests that PBL has several advantages over traditional systems, serving as the driving force for this shift in most instances (Amoako-Sakyi & Amonoo-Kuofi, 2015; Azer, 2011). Apart from encouraging students to actively participate in their own education, PBL enhances critical thinking and promotes collaboration among students (Amoako-Sakyi & Amonoo-Kuofi, 2015). Problem-based learning inherently allows the integration and organization of learned information for easy recall and application, making PBL graduates lifelong learners with the cognitive flexibility to use varied knowledge sources in solving different problems (Amoako-Sakyi & Amonoo-Kuofi, 2015; Azer, 2011). Converting to or developing a PBL program at a health professions program will come with great rewards for the institution, faculty, students, and the healthcare profession. The rewards are directly proportional to the amount of work that will be needed to establish a good PBL program.

References

Abraham, R. R., & Ramnarayan, K. (2016). Heutagogic approach to developing capable learners. *Medical Teacher, 39*(3), 295.
Albanese, M., & Mitchell, S. (1993). Problem-based learning: A review of literature on its outcomes and implementation issues [Review of Problem-based learning: A review of literature on its outcomes and implementation issues]. *Academic Medicine, 68*(1), 52.
Amoako-Sakyi, D., & Amonoo-Kuofi, H. S. (2015). Problem-based learning in resource-poor settings: Lessons from a medical school in Ghana. *BMC Medical Education, 15*(1), 221.
Azer, S. A. (2005). The qualities of a good teacher: How can they be acquired and sustained? *Journal of the Royal Society of Medicine, 98*(2), 67.
Azer, S. A. (2011). Introducing a problem-based learning program: 12 tips for success. *Medical Teacher, 33*(10), 808.
Bahri, A., & Idris, I. S. (2018). Development and validation of learning strategy for metacognitive skills empowerment: PBLRQA (PBL integrated with reading, questioning, and answering). *Journal of Physics Conference Series, 1028*, 12028.
Bashith, A., & Amin, S. (2017). The effect of problem based learning on EFL students' critical thinking skill and learning outcome. *AL-TA'LIM Journal, 24*(2), 93.
Bell, S. (2010). Project-based learning for the 21st century: Skills for the future. *The Clearing House: A Journal of Educational Strategies Issues and Ideas, 83*(2), 39.
Chang, B. (2016). Problem-based learning in medical school: A student's perspective. *Annals of Medicine and Surgery, 12*, 88.
Dolmans, D., de Grave, W., Wolfhagen, I. H. A. P., & van der Vleuten, C. (2005). Problem-based learning: Future challenges for educational practice and research [Review of Problem-based learning: Future challenges for educational practice and research]. *Medical Education, 39*(7), 732.
Finucane, P., Shannon, W., & McGrath, D. (2009). The financial costs of delivering problem-based learning in a new, graduate-entry medical programme. *Medical Education, 43*(6), 594.
Ge, W., Zhu, X., Lin, J., Jiang, J., Li, T., Lu, Y., & Tung, T. (2025). Critical thinking and clinical skills by problem-based learning educational methods: An umbrella systematic review. *BMC Medical Education, 25*, 455. Retrieved from https://bmcmededuc.biomedcentral.com/articles/10.1186/s12909-025-06951-z
Glew, R. H. (2003). The problem with problem-based medical education: Promises not kept. *Biochemistry and Molecular Biology Education, 31*(1), 52.
Hamdy, H., & Agamy, E. (2011). Is running a problem-based learning curriculum more expensive than a traditional subject-based curriculum? *Medical Teacher, 33*(9), e509-14.
Khoo, H. E. (2003). Implementation of problem-based learning in Asian medical schools and students' perceptions of their experience. *Medical Education, 37*(5), 401.
Kober, N. (2015). *Reaching students: What research says about effective instruction in undergraduate science and engineering*. The National Academies Press.
Kokotsaki, D., Menzies, V., & Wiggins, A. (2016). Project-based learning: A review of the literature [Review of Project-based learning: A review of the literature]. *Improving Schools, 19*(3), 267.
Li, T., Wang, W., Li, Z., Wang, H., & Liu, X. (2022). Problem-based or lecture-based learning, old topic in the new field: A meta-analysis on the effects of PBL teaching method in Chinese standardized residency training [Review of Problem-based or lecture-based learning, old topic in the new field: A meta-analysis on the effects of PBL teaching method in Chinese standardized residency training]. *BMC Medical Education, 22*(1), 221.
Lim, W. K. (2012). Dysfunctional problem-based learning curricula: Resolving the problem. *BMC Medical Education, 12*(1), 89.
Maloney, S., Nicklen, P., Rivers, G., Foo, J., Ooi, Y. Y., Reeves, S., Walsh, K., & Ilić, D. (2015). A cost-effectiveness analysis of blended versus face-to-face delivery of evidence-based medicine to medical students. *Journal of Medical Internet Research, 17*(7), e182.

Nendaz, M., & Tekian, A. (1999). Assessment in problem-based learning medical schools: A literature review [Review of Assessment in problem-based learning medical schools: A literature review]. *Teaching and Learning in Medicine, 11*(4), 232.

Pinthong, P., & Chaisongmuang, P. (2019). *Development of problem-based learning model at the faculty of nursing*. Ubon Ratchathani University.

Rehman, N., Huang, X., Mahmood, A., Al-Gerafi, M. A., & Javed, S. (2024). Project-based learning as a catalyst for 21st-century skills and student engagement in the math classroom. *Heliyon, 10*(23), e39988.

Savery, J. (2015). *Overview of problem-based learning* (p. 5). Purdue University Press.

Shrivastava, S., & Shrivastava, P. S. (2023). From tradition to transformation: Revolutionizing medical education for the digital age through virtual problem-based learning. *Indian Journal of Medical Specialities, 14*(3), 121.

Ungaretti, T., Thompson, K. R., Miller, A., & Peterson, T. O. (2014). Problem-based learning: Lessons from medical education and challenges for management education. *Academy of Management Learning and Education, 14*(2), 173.

Walsh, K. (2013). Tutor-less problem-based learning in a large classroom setting—Could it also save costs? *CBE—Life Sciences Education, 12*(3), 315.

Wang, J., Xu, Y., Liu, X., Xiong, W., Xie, J., & Zhao, J. (2016). Assessing the effectiveness of problem-based learning in physical diagnostics education in China: A meta-analysis. *Scientific Reports, 6*, 36279. Retrieved from https://www.nature.com/articles/srep36279

Zeng, H., Zhu, Z., Hu, J., & Cui, Y. (2025). Application of ChatGPT-assisted problem-based learning teaching method in clinical medical education. *BMC Medical Education, 25*(1), 50.

Zhan, H.-Q., Zhang, X., Qin, R., Fei, J., Dong, G.-Y., & Hao, J. (2023). Application of integrated problem-based learning combined with lecture-based classroom teaching in undergraduate medical education: An effective teaching model in a Medical School in China. *Medicine, 102*(34), e34792.

MIX
Papier aus verantwortungsvollen Quellen
Paper from responsible sources
FSC® C105338

If you have any concerns about our products,
you can contact us on
ProductSafety@springernature.com

In case Publisher is established outside the EU,
the EU authorized representative is:
Springer Nature Customer Service Center GmbH
Europaplatz 3, 69115 Heidelberg, Germany

Printed by Libri Plureos GmbH
in Hamburg, Germany